P9-DYZ-664

Managing Health Care Business Strategy

George B. Moseley III

JONES AND BARTLETT PUBLISHERS
Sudbury, Massachusetts
BOSTON TORONTO LONDON SINGAPORE

World Headquarters
Jones and Bartlett Publishers
40 Tall Pine Drive
Sudbury, MA 01776
978-443-5000
info@jbpub.com
www.jbpub.com

Jones and Bartlett Publishers
Canada
6339 Ormindale Way
Mississauga, Ontario L5V 1J2
Canada

Jones and Bartlett Publishers
International
Barb House, Barb Mews
London W6 7PA
United Kingdom

Jones and Bartlett's books and products are available through most bookstores and online booksellers. To contact Jones and Bartlett Publishers directly, call 800-832-0034, fax 978-443-8000, or visit our website www.jbpub.com.

Substantial discounts on bulk quantities of Jones and Bartlett's publications are available to corporations, professional associations, and other qualified organizations. For details and specific discount information, contact the special sales department at Jones and Bartlett via the above contact information or send an email to specialsales@jbpub.com.

Production Credits
Publisher: Michael Brown
Production Director: Amy Rose
Associate Editor: Katey Birtcher
Production Editor: Tracey Chapman
Production Assistant: Roya Millard
Marketing Manager: Sophie Fleck
Manufacturing Buyer: Amy Bacus
Composition: Paw Print Media
Cover Design: Anne Spencer
Cover Image: © Handy Widiyanto/ShutterStock, Inc.
Printing and Binding: Malloy, Inc.
Cover Printing: Malloy, Inc.

Library of Congress Cataloging-in-Publication Data
Moseley, George B.
Managing health care business strategy / George Moseley.
p. ; cm.
Includes bibliographical references and index.
ISBN-13: 978-0-7637-3416-9 (casebound)
ISBN-10: 0-7637-3416-0 (casebound)
1. Health facilities—Business management. 2. Health facilities—Finance. 3. Strategic planning. I. Title.
[DNLM: 1. Financial Management—methods. 2. Health Facilities—economics. 3. Health Services Administration—economics. W 80 M898m 2008]
RA971.3.M65 2008
362.11068'1—dc22

2007045896

6048

Printed in the United States of America
12 11 10 09 08   10 9 8 7 6 5 4 3 2 1

DEDICATION

Dedicated to my good friend and one of the most competent attorneys in Palestine, Tawfik Abu-Ghazaleh.

CONTENTS

ABOUT THE AUTHOR

George B. Moseley III holds the position of Lecturer in Health Law and Management on the faculty of the Harvard School of Public Health. He currently teaches the courses Introduction to the New American Health Care System: Law, Policy, and Management; and Leading and Managing People in Health Care Organizations. He is the author of *Managed Care Strategies: A Physician Practice Desk Reference*. He is a consultant on strategic management for new biotechnology ventures, physician group practices, and hospitals, and he conducts research on the adoption of new technologies by healthcare organizations. He received his MBA from the Harvard Business School and his JD from the University of Michigan Law School.

PREFACE

Both the healthcare and biotech industries are sorely in need of the application of modern and innovative professional management principles, as well as a new generation of managers skilled in using those principles. The purpose of this book is to teach knowledge and skills of strategic management to the students who will become the healthcare and biotech executives of the future.

Healthcare organizations began two decades ago the transition from entities that were passively administered to ones that are actively managed. Many of the larger hospitals, physician group practices, integrated delivery systems, and managed care organizations have completed the transformation to run efficient business operations. Those that have been acquired by for-profit corporations or have converted to for-profit status were compelled to adopt modern management practices very quickly. There still are a great many healthcare businesses that are lagging in making this transition. Many of them are smaller and medium-sized, or of nonprofit status.

The pharmaceutical and biotechnology industries are also at turning points. The development of new drugs has become much more expensive, it takes years longer to complete the research and development process, and the probabilities of creating blockbuster products that are worth the investment are declining. The hope that was placed in new small, highly innovative research-oriented ventures and startups has not been borne out. The existing research and financing models for development of new healthcare technology no longer seem to be effective. New models are being tested and tried.

In particular, these industries need to practice strategic planning and management. The environments in which they operate are in constant ferment. The national healthcare "system" is undergoing persistent, radical changes and adjustments. There is an accelerating flow of proposals for revolutionary reform of the system at both the state and national levels. The market for healthcare services has become increasingly competitive. Some might argue that strategic planning does not make sense in such a fluid environment. Quite the contrary. An organization needs a thoughtful long-range perspective if it is to chart an optimal course through this turbulent sea of threats and opportunities.

Health care and biotechnology do not need to invent new management practices. There is a wealth of proven management models and techniques from other industries. However, there are features and characteristics of healthcare delivery and payment, and of biotechnology research, that distinguish them from all other industries, and that make it inappropriate to apply blindly the strategic management principles that are practiced in most other industries. Those principles do provide a solid foundation of knowledge and practice, which must then be interpreted and tailored to the healthcare and biotechnology settings.

These trends have created a demand for skilled managers who are both trained in modern management principles and familiar with the conditions of the healthcare market and industry. Healthcare management has become a viable and promising career path. A number of business and other schools, both graduate and undergraduate, are now offering degrees, concentrations, and courses in healthcare management.

Because the demand for professional managers in health care has emerged only recently, it has taken some time for related books and other materials to be developed. Although there is a fairly substantial booklist dealing with healthcare operations, relatively few books attempt to discuss strategic issues in the healthcare context. Most of these are not designed as textbooks. They do not include material to facilitate the learning process. Some are idiosyncratic in their explanations of basic strategy concepts. Some do not offer comprehensive coverage of the full range of established principles of strategic planning and management. There is a need for textbooks and other learning materials for people at the beginning of their careers, studying modern business management for the first time, seeking a foundation in professional management concepts, particularly relating to strategic thinking and acting, but as applied to the healthcare and biotechnology industries. That is the idea behind this book.

The book has been conceived from the beginning with an audience in mind of students who are excited by the prospect of a career that takes them to high-level executive positions in healthcare or biotechnology organizations. Its purpose is to help them, with the aid of their instructors, to comprehend the basic principles of managing strategy in those organizations. Throughout the book, the emphasis is on the practical application of those principles. The goal is to give students knowledge and skills that they can employ directly in the jobs that they will hold. It is assumed that most of them will have no or very little previous exposure to management, strategy, or the healthcare industry. The intention is that students who complete a course using this book will be well positioned to assume strategic management responsibilities with any organization they join.

The book incorporates numerous features designed to provide optimal learning value to the students. The foundation of the book lies in the fundamental strategic management principles and practices that are well established in professionally run organizations throughout the world. These principles are interpreted and applied in the healthcare and biotechnology contexts. There are frequent references to specific applications in those fields. At the end of each chapter, there are study questions that do more than ask students to repeat information found in the text; rather, they encourage students to do creative thinking about the issues they have just studied. Even more stimulating are the learning exercises that call for interviews with strategic decision-makers, research on strategic challenges facing real-world organizations, and the preparation of consultant-like recommendations on strategic issues.

The chapters are arranged in a natural progression that follows the traditional strategic planning and implementation process. After establishing and explaining basic strategy concepts in Chapter 1, the next four chapters are devoted to the ground-laying assessments that must precede serious strategic planning. These include an internal audit of the organization's strategic assets, assessment of general factors in the organization's external environment, assessment of the markets and customers that it is serving, and assessment of the industry in which it operates and competitors that it faces there. The separate chapter examining market and customers, so important in the healthcare field, is unique among strategic management textbooks. On the basis of those assessments, the organization defines its future direction in the ways described in the following chapter. Actual formulation of strategies is explained in the next two chapters. One concentrates on strategy at the level of the large multi-unit corporation, while the other explores strategy within individual business units and functional areas. The next chapter addresses another topic often given inadequate attention in strategic management textbooks—the implementation of the strategies selected. The final step in a superior strategic and management process is for monitoring and fine-tuning of the strategies, and is examined in the following chapter. A separate chapter is dedicated to the critical topic of strategic financial management. The final chapter in the book covers alternative organizational types that are so prevalent in the healthcare field—not-for-profit organizations, public/government agencies, and new ventures/startups.

The book content is based on my own training and experience in general business management, strategic management, and the U.S. healthcare system. It reflects case studies I have researched and written about healthcare organizations, my professional contacts with healthcare industry leaders and biotech entrepreneurs, and consulting work that I have done on strategic matters for physician groups, hospitals, and new technology ventures.

I wish the students who read this book, with the coaching of their instructors, great success in their careers as healthcare and biotechnology executives.

CHAPTER 1

Basic Strategy Concepts

Learning Objectives

After reading and studying this chapter, you should be able to:

- Explain the difference between the strategic initiatives and operating activities of a health care organization.
- List the numerous benefits that an organization receives from the practice of strategic planning and management.
- Understand the different types of competition that make strategic planning necessary.
- Distinguish the several different organizational levels at which strategic planning and management can take place.
- Recognize the ability of a person to engage in "strategic thinking."
- Differentiate between "incremental" and "revolutionary" strategies, as well as "intended" and "actual" strategies.
- Describe in a basic way the fundamental steps in a good strategic planning and management process.
- Explain the concept of "strategic direction" and the critical role that it plays in the strategic planning process.
- Understand how strategic management often goes wrong, due to both management failures and inherent organizational barriers.
- Identify the powerful environmental forces that affect organizational efforts at strategic planning and management.

Alice, in conversation with the Cheshire Cat:
"Would you tell me, please, which way I ought to go from here?"
"That depends a good deal on where you want to get to," said the Cat.
"I don't much care where—" said Alice.
"Then it doesn't matter which way you go," said the Cat.
"—so long as I get SOMEWHERE," Alice added as an explanation.
"Oh, you're sure to do that," said the Cat, "if you only walk long enough."
—Lewis Carroll, *Alice's Adventures in Wonderland*

It might not seem to make much sense to do a lot of long-range strategic planning and management in an industry like health care where the ground rules are changing constantly and so many of the options depend ultimately on reimbursement rates set by the Centers for Medicare and Medicaid Services (CMS) in Washington, D.C., or on federal and state health care laws and regulations. Or in the biotechnology industry, which depends so much for its funding on the whims of venture capitalists or congressional appropriations for the National Institutes of Health. Yet, even in these fluid, often chaotic environments, meaningful strategic planning and management is not only possible, it is essential for an organization to survive and, then, thrive.

■ DEFINITION OF THE CONCEPT OF "STRATEGY"

It is best to begin a conversation about strategic management by coming to an understanding of what "strategy" is and what it is not.

> THINK ABOUT THIS: Have you ever used the term "strategy" in conversation? Exactly what did you mean by it? Some people claim to have a strategy for mowing the lawn or shopping for a new car. Are those really strategies or are they some kind of "plan"? What is the difference between a strategy and a plan, and does it really matter?

In the true business management sense, strategy is distinguished by several key dimensions.

- A strategy aims to steer the direction of the overall organization. It affects the long-term well-being of the organization.
- A strategy has a long time horizon, usually measured in years rather than months or weeks. A typical strategic plan may set goals to be achieved five or more years in the future.
- A strategy has an impact that is more likely to be felt throughout the entire organization rather than within a single component of the organization.

- A strategy builds on and exploits to the fullest extent the organization's resources and abilities.
- A strategy aims to create the best possible fit between the organization and its mission, on one hand, and the organization's external environment, on the other hand.
- Strategic decisions require major resource commitments and are difficult to reverse.
- A strategy is distinguished by the strength of the organization's commitment to it and reluctance with which it considers changing it.
- For those organizations in a competitive environment, a strategy is frequently aimed at gaining an advantage over competitors.
- In order to focus its resources and energies, an organization or business unit normally will pursue only a few distinct strategies at one time, perhaps no more than six or seven.
- A strategy is future oriented and marked by uncertainty and risk.
- A strategy calls upon the organization to do something that it is not doing now. This inevitably requires change, sometimes profound, in many aspects of its operations.
- A successful strategy is the result of an integrated/collaborative effort by many parts of the organization.

What is regarded as long term will depend on the organization and the industry or market in which it operates. It may mean five years or longer for a small community hospital located in a modest-sized city in rural Kansas, where it faces no competition. In contrast, a large teaching hospital surrounded by several other teaching hospitals in a vibrant, highly competitive market for hospital care in Boston or Los Angeles may find it hard to think much further than two years into the future.

> THINK ABOUT THIS: Is there any reason that a component of the overall organization cannot have a strategy or a strategic plan? Is it possible for both a teaching hospital and its department of orthopedic surgery to have strategic plans? What advantages might this offer? What problems could it present? Might a surgeon working in that department have a personal strategic plan?

It may be easier to understand the concept of "strategic" planning by contrasting it with two other forms of planning—"operational" and "tactical." A *strategic plan* is concerned with the widest scope of organizational activities, frequently encompasses the broadest geographic area, affects and involves the largest number of employees (often everyone in the organization), costs the largest amount of money (usually millions of dollars), and takes the longest period of time (several years) to implement. An *operational plan* deals with activities of narrower dimensions, impacts subgroups of the workforce (a single department or professional category), involves the expenditure of more modest sums (tens or hundreds of thousands of dollars), and typically takes no more than a year to carry out. A *tactical plan* is at the lower end of the planning continuum: it embraces activities affecting smaller segments of the organization, may require the participation of very few people (one or two, or a small ad hoc task force), entail quite modest expenditure (sometimes no additional outlay at all, perhaps hundreds or thousands of dollars at most), and stretches over a few days or weeks.

A health maintenance organization (HMO) based in Ohio may adopt a strategic plan that sets an objective of expanding from its present market base in the northern part of the state around Cleveland and Akron further south into Columbus and eventually Cincinnati over the next two years. Its synchronous operating plan may be to enroll at least 25,000 new members in Columbus over the next year. As a tactical step toward achieving that goal, the HMO's marketing department may carry out a direct mail and television advertising campaign during the month of October.

When the planning and implementation process is executed expertly, the efforts at the strategic, operational, and tactical levels merge into a seamless continuum of forward-looking activity intended to ensure the survival and growth of the organization. Fulfillment of the tactical plans contributes to meeting the objectives of the operational plans, which in turn advance the end purposes of the strategic plans.

THINK ABOUT THIS: Does an organization that does not face competition need to have a strategic plan? Examples are NFP organizations and government agencies. What benefits would a strategic plan bring to them? Do they in fact have competitors?

Perhaps more than any other industry, health care delivery and financing is performed by a diverse collection of for-profit (FP), not-for-profit (NFP), governmental, and quasi-governmental organizations. 60 percent of the hospitals are organized as NFP corporations, in addition to which the federal government agency Veterans Administration operates well over 1,200 hospitals, clinics, and other facilities. Many states and cities own and run public hospitals and clinics. Some of the oldest, largest, and best-known HMOs are NFP: Kaiser Foundation Health Plans, Harvard Pilgrim, and Group Health Cooperative of Puget Sound, among others. All the Blue Cross/Blue Shield health insurance companies are NFP entities. The largest health care payer in the country is the Medicare program administered by the federal Centers for Medicare and Medicaid Services (CMS). In many states, the state-level Medicaid financing program accounts for the largest portion of the state budget. The health care industry can also be considered to include the large number of federal, state, county, and municipal agencies concerned with regulation of and reporting on the activities of hospitals, insurers, managed care organizations (MCOs), physician practices, and health care professionals. Do not forget the NFP organizations that accredit provider entities (Joint Commission on Accreditation of Healthcare Organizations or JCAHO, National Committee for Quality Assurance or NCQA). There are numerous associations representing the various health care professions, and others seeking cures for the most common diseases.

The professional management of all these organizations demands a strategic mindset and the preparation and execution of a strategic plan. Many of them face a form of competition that must be confronted in a systematic fashion. Government agencies compete with each other for a share of the overall budget and for the attention and support of taxpayers. NFP organizations fight constantly to win the hearts and minds of potential donors, either individual or institutional.

However, strategic action is about more than responding to the competition. It is necessary to constantly adapt the organization to the changes taking place in its external environment. Imagine how unsuccessful a hospital built in 1955 would be if it had made no adjustments during the wave of managed care that swept the industry in the 1980s and 1990s. In fact, many hospitals did not see the need for change quickly enough or lacked the resources to carry it out, and subsequently closed down or were acquired. Internal organizational changes also may drive strategic action. For instance, a medium-sized physician group practice may have depended for much of its past growth and reputation on a highly accomplished, well-known oncologist who has announced that he will be retiring within two years. Immediate steps will be necessary to either replace him (a daunting task) or strategically refocus the group.

■ PURPOSE OF STRATEGIC MANAGEMENT

Every organization in existence is engaged in some current activities designed to create products or services for sale, delivery, or distribution to its customers, clients, patients, or beneficiaries. This is true for a pharmaceutical company selling its drugs to retail drug chains, a durable medical equipment (DME) manufacturer selling its parenteral nutrition pumps to managed care organizations, electronic medical record (EMR) system vendors selling their software and hardware solutions to physician group practices, an NFP hospital selling its clinical services to patients, a small biomedical research firm licensing its drug discovery patent to a large pharmaceutical company, an NFP health care advocacy group lobbying legislators on universal coverage for uninsured people, a municipal public health agency offering newborn immunizations to residents of low-income neighborhoods, or a state Medicaid agency providing health care coverage to medically needy disabled adults. The willingness of the customers to accept, demand, receive, or pay for the goods and services can shift over time—as a result of changes in their desires and preferences or the availability of superior product and services from competing organizations.

An organization employs strategic management to continually adapt itself to these changing circumstances. The adaptation may involve altering virtually any aspect of the organization's operations—the products and services it creates, the way in which it creates them, and the customers to whom it offers them.

The organization generally makes these adjustments for any of three reasons:

- to satisfy and reward its stakeholders,
- to pursue and fulfill its mission, and
- to survive.

In the case of a profit-driven corporation, the primary stakeholders are the equity shareholders, the legal owners of the corporation, and the lenders and bondholders, sources of debt capital. If corporate performance does not deliver the performance expected by these groups, they will be reluctant to provide the capital the organization relies on to fund its operations and strategies.

In the case of an NFP corporation, the stakeholders receiving the greatest attention are charitable contributors and the debt capital providers. The performance results sought by the two groups are different. The lenders and bondholders want to feel secure in the principal and interest payments on their loans, just as debtors for FP corporations do. The donors give money in support of a defined cause or mission, and they wish to see it carried out as fully as possible. If either group is dissatisfied with the organization's performance, it can withhold its funds.

The key stakeholders of public entities like government agencies are the general population of the jurisdiction in which they operate. The citizens' wishes and expectations for agency performance are interpreted by the legislative and executive branches of government, which provide funding and direction. Citizens' unhappiness with that performance can lead to reductions in funding and, in extreme cases, dissolution of the agency.

All of these organizations must keep their primary stakeholders uppermost in their minds as they constantly manage and adjust their operations.

In order to satisfy its stakeholders, an organization must engage itself in some focused undertaking, rather than a set of random, aimless activities. This enterprise is defined as the organization's "mission"—its reason for existing and operating. The mission provides the contextual basis for the organization's strategies. The operational adjustments that they entail are designed to keep the organization's resources, activities, and efforts focused on the mission. Many equity shareholders and debtors of for-profit corporations are not particularly concerned with what the mission is as long as it is pursued competently enough to provide them with the rewards they are seeking.

Beyond the rational strategy motives of pleasing stakeholders and carrying out a mission, most organizations are also driven by an almost primal impulse simply to survive. Even when stakeholders have given up and the mission has become untenable, some organizations struggle to keep going. An example is a community hospital in a small city, most of whose patients have been redirected to a larger teaching hospital in a city twenty miles away. The local residents prefer the convenience of a nearby hospital, but the revenues are insufficient to support it. In a strictly rational health care system, this hospital would not continue to operate. Yet, almost everyone associated with it—board of directors, managers, and employees—will go to great lengths over a number of years to try to keep it alive.

Even if an organization faced no competition at all, it could count on the world around it changing—both the internal and external environments. New laws are enacted (Health Insurance Portability and Accountability Act, or HIPAA), consumer demographics shift (aging, ethnicity), a key employee retires (researcher, physician, executive). It would be necessary to implement strategies to make appropriate operational adjustments to accommodate these changes (new compliance policies and procedures, additions to and deletions from product and service lines, new hires and redefining job assignments). It would be imperative that these adjustments be made with all due haste, but the pressure to do so would not be extreme.

Virtually every organization also must deal with some kind of competitors. Competition is an accepted feature of corporate life for profit-driven organizations. A good example is pharmaceutical companies vying with each other to sell their individual variations of a drug to treat particular diseases. NFP corporations also engage in competition. It is not uncommon for FP and NFP hospitals to coexist and compete in the same markets; the same is true of managed care organizations. Competition occurs even when all the providers of a product or service line in a given area are NFP. In Boston, three major teaching hospitals, Brigham and Women's Hospital/Massachusetts General Hospital, Beth Israel Deaconess Medical Center, and Tufts–New England Medical Center compete vigorously with each other and with several smaller NFP hospitals. Even public government agencies may engage in a form of competition—not so much for customers, but for the attention of legislators and political leaders.

In addition to their competition in the marketplace for customers, organizations also engage in a different form of competition in the marketplace for financial capital. Equity investors buy shares of stock in companies whose financial performance meets their return on investment (ROI) criteria. Money lenders make loans to, or buy the bonds of, FP and NFP entities with high credit ratings that ensure their ability to make interest and principal payments. Wealthy citizens and charitable organizations make donations to NFP organizations that are doing the best job of supporting a cause that they value. Legislators appropriate tax revenues for the budgets of government agencies whose work meets the needs of their constituents.

The way that an organization succeeds in the competition with its rivals is by doing something that gives it an advantage in the eyes of the consumers of its products and services, and the sources of its capital—a "competitive advantage." An advantage is not worth much if it lasts only a few weeks. Ideally, an organization wants to create a "sustainable competitive advantage" that will persist for as long as possible, at least months if not years.

If an organization is going to achieve an advantage over its rivals, it will come through things that it does—the activities performed by its employees. The organization will gain no advantage if it does exactly what its rivals do—creating the same products and services by the same methods, distributing them through the same channels, and selling them at the same prices. Instead, an organization must distinguish its activities from those of its competition. It has three generic choices:

- It can perform activities that are different from its competitors' activities.
- It can perform the same activities as its competitors do but in different ways.
- It can perform the same activities at lower cost than its competitors.

The purpose of formulating and implementing a new strategy is to engage the organization in performing activities that are different from those of its competitors in at least one of these three ways.

■ LEVELS OF STRATEGY

Good managers observe their competition all the time and speculate on what particular strategy those organizations are following. In fact, strategic planning and management may be occurring at three or more different levels in an organization. It will look like a cascading hierarchy of strategic initiatives that build and depend upon each other. Ideally, each level fits into and is guided by the one above it.

Corporate or Organization-Wide Strategy

The highest-level strategy work encompasses the entire organization. The scope and nature of that work is a reflection of what the organization does and how it is structured to do it. Consider the Hospital Corporation of America (HCA). At the end of 2006, HCA was composed of 179 hospitals and 104 freestanding surgery centers in 21 states. During 2006, HCA reorganized those nearly 300 facilities into East, West, and Central groups.

Strategic activity at this level is concerned primarily with managing the portfolio of businesses and groups of businesses that compose the corporation and securing financial capital for allocation to them. It may also define the values that will be practiced throughout the organization, provide varying degrees of direction to the specific strategies adopted by the groups and facilities, facilitate the sharing of resources and capabilities among the groups and facilities, and offer strategic support services to them. Corporate-level strategy is explained in greater detail in Chapter 7.

Strategic Business Unit or Product/Service Line Strategy

Most companies start out—or start up—by offering a single product or service within a single market. If the product or service is well received in the marketplace, the company will thrive and grow. Many businesses continue operating in this fashion, at this scale (one or a few products in a single market), for many years. As long as their stakeholders are satisfied and they are not overwhelmed by competing businesses, there is nothing wrong with this approach.

At a certain point, however, in order to maintain the growth, increase returns to stakeholders, and resist competitive threats, the company will take steps to diversify and expand into other products or services and other markets. Eventually, the company will conclude that it cannot direct the operations and strategies for multiple products competing in multiple markets with a single management team. It will reorganize itself (or actually organize itself for the first time), at first perhaps into several distinct, though not autonomously governed, product or service lines managed by separate sets of managers. The product/service lines often then evolve into strategic business units (SBUs) with significant degrees of autonomy. Each is run by a strong management team that reports to a relatively small corporate headquarters office. Together, the SBUs make up the parent corporation's "portfolio."

These original SBUs are the results of internal development within the corporation. Further along the corporation's strategic path, it may choose to add SBUs to its portfolio through acquisition or merger.

An SBU is distinguished by several features.

1. It serves a discrete external market or market niche different from that of any other SBU.
2. It offers unique product or service lines that are different from those of any other SBU.
3. It is usually a separate structural component of the parent company—a division, group, subsidiary, or department.
4. It is operated as a profit center by the parent company, meaning that the SBU has its own mission, objectives, and strategies and its management is responsible for bottom-line performance.

Strategy at the SBU level is explained in greater detail in Chapter 8.

> **Word Usage Note:** Throughout this book, the term "corporation" will always refer to a for-profit entity composed of multiple SBUs. The terms "business," "company," "firm," "entity," and "organization" will be applied, depending on the context, to individual SBUs, independent freestanding units, and any other type of strategy-making legal structure, either for-profit, not-for-profit, or public. Where the text discussion is relevant only to one type of organization (say, for-profit rather than not-for-profit), that will be made clear.

Functional Area Strategy

Each SBU is further subdivided into functional areas, which make their individual specialized contributions to the unit's operations and strategic initiatives. Traditional functional areas include marketing, manufacturing or production, research and development, human resources, and finances. The functional areas found in a hospital are more likely to be something like medical staff departments (specialties like medicine, surgery, and obstetrics and gynecology), nursing, ancillary services (radiology, clinical laboratory, and pharmacy), support services (medical records, housekeeping, and food service), financial (admitting, billing, and claims filing), and legal (compliance, payer contracting). Sometimes, every SBU will contain all the necessary functional areas for it to carry on its operations. It may have all the characteristics of an independent, freestanding business, except that it is not a separate legal entity and relies for investment capital on its parent. Alternatively, certain of the functions may be provided by the parent for all the SBUs in its portfolio. For example, a hospital that is offering and marketing a unique package of women's health services will rely on the food service, claims processing, radiology or pathology service, and pharmacy service functions used by other clinical areas of the hospital.

These functional areas frequently will prepare and execute their own strategic plans that support the strategies of their respective SBUs. These plans are the responsibility of the departments and workgroups that make up the functional area.

STRATEGIC THINKING OR STRATEGIC MINDSET

Do you have a "strategic mindset"? Can you think "strategically"? It is not surprising that these qualities are common, virtually mandatory expectations of executives as they rise higher and higher in an organization.

Strategic thinking is an ability constantly to view an organization's operations, issues, and problems in a very broad situational and environmental context and with a very long time perspective. A department manager with a strategic mindset will, while thinking about the challenges in the department, keep in mind their impact on other departments and the overall health of the organization. In determining the causes of problems, the manager also will look outside the department and even outside the organization, to customers, competitors, and the entire external environment. This attitude, this mental outlook, is a form of "systems thinking" that recognizes the interconnections between a project or problem in a single department and many other people, departments, organizations, and environmental forces.

A strategic thinker also constantly projects his understanding and analysis of issues well into the future. She may be measuring the effects of actions occurring now on events three or four or more years from now.

It is not an easy task to contemplate simultaneously an almost infinite number of influences and dependencies on the problem at hand, as they transform and evolve over years. Furthermore, this ability does not occur naturally in most people and frequently requires rigorous development.

In the explanations about why managers, with their MBA degrees, and physicians, with their MD degrees, clash so often when they must work together in hospitals and managed care organizations, the point is often made about their very different professional mindsets. The physician is trained to concentrate his attention on the patient in front of him and to mobilize all available resources to resolve the patient's medical problems in the shortest time possible. The ultimate measure of success is clinical outcomes. The value of this training is particularly obvious in the emergency department or the operating room. The manager is trained to think about markets composed of thousands of customers, the coordination of numerous functional areas and departments, the threats posed by competitors, and the long-term future of the organization. The ultimate measure of his success is fiscal outcomes. This perspective reaps its greatest

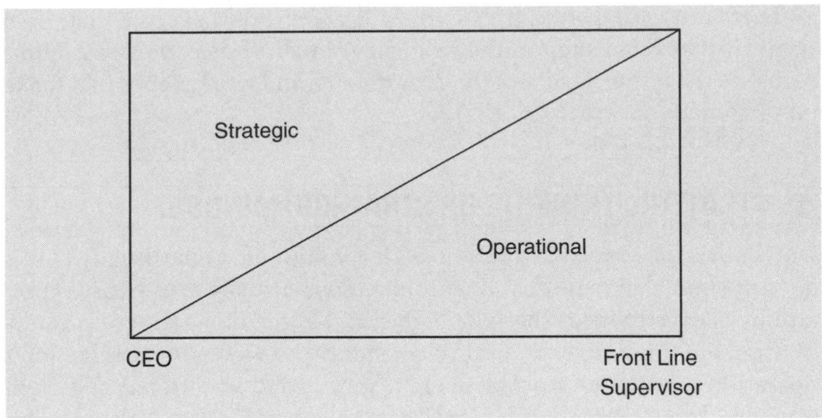

Figure 1.1 Work Focus Shift from Operational to Strategic

rewards when preparing annual financial statements, meeting with Wall Street analysts, or trying to impress shareholders.

It is not surprising that people with such different work culture backgrounds would be in conflict. However, it is also true that many managers never truly develop a strategic mindset. In the lower echelons of the organization, supervisors and junior managers must focus almost exclusively on the current operations within their organizational scope of authority—a department, an office, a task force, or a unit. Their sole responsibility is to keep that component operating as smoothly and efficiently as possible on a day-to-day basis. They are not expected to think strategically and normally do not have the time to do so.

As managers are promoted through the organization, their duties take on an increasingly strategic nature. They become less concerned with the short-range, routine operations of a particular department and look further into the future, to other units within the organization, and outside the organization to forces in the external environment. By the time a manager reaches the position of CEO, she spends her entire working day on strategic issues. The shift in work focus from operational to strategic could be pictured as shown in Figure 1.1.

It is a challenge not only for individual mid-level managers but also for the organization as a whole to find an appropriate balance between current operations and long-term strategy. The actual work of a health care organization is carried out in the present: treating patients, filling prescriptions, performing diagnostic tests, researching new drugs, and processing claims—the multitude of activities that fulfill its mission. The purpose of strategic thinking is to prepare the organization for the actual work that it will carry out in the future and move it toward realization of its vision. The work activities that provide value to stakeholders (like customers and shareholders) today may not be the activities that do so two or three years from now.

■ INCREMENTAL VERSUS REVOLUTIONARY STRATEGY

Formulation and implementation of a new strategy is a statement that an organization intends to make some sort of change in its operations. The change can vary greatly in the extent to which it is a departure from the current state of operations. The degree of change can range along a continuum from incremental to revolutionary. For instance, a physician practice may decide to begin introducing its patients to alternative medicine options. A modest, incremental first step would be to place literature in the waiting room describing acupuncture, yoga, and herbal medicine. At the more revolutionary extreme, the practice could hire an acupuncturist and a yoga teacher, and start promoting itself as a holistic healing center. Strategy planners must be conscious of how much they are asking of the organization and its people; it has implications throughout the strategic management process.

- An incremental change is more likely to be carried out satisfactorily; revolutionary change may stir greater resistance that slows or prevents success.
- A revolutionary strategy may be necessary to give the organization a breakthrough in gaining a sustainable competitive advantage over its competitors. To be incremental when a revolution is called for could be a mistake.
- In contrast, a well-conceived incremental strategy that leverages a unique resource, competence, or value activity may be more effective than a dramatic, high-risk, mistargeted revolutionary strategy.
- The type of strategy must be consistent with an organization's culture. A firm with a tradition of risk avoidance probably should not attempt a revolutionary strategy.
- The chosen strategy type must be backed by sufficient resources, particularly financial. A revolutionary strategy may require more working capital to sustain it until the strategy succeeds and finances reach the break-even point.

■ INTENDED VERSUS ACTUAL STRATEGY

Books on strategic management sometimes make it seem like a pretty cut-and-dry process. An organization does a nice, thorough job of examining itself, its markets, and its competitors and uses its best judgment in formulating a few good strategies. If it can implement them properly, most of them will be successful and produce something close to the intended results. In practice, it rarely works that way.

What happens is that even with a deliberate, structured, and forceful strategy-making process, other factors come into play that can produce different outcomes.

- Assumptions about the external environment, including competitor actions and customer preferences, cease to be valid due to unanticipated changes. Management decides that it no longer makes sense to proceed with the strategy, or it chooses to make significant modifications in the strategy.
- Strategic support that was expected from important stakeholders, such as suppliers, investors, or legislators, is not forthcoming. The strategy must be cancelled or overhauled.
- If strategies are implemented at all, it is through many small routine actions, decisions, and behaviors on the part of individuals and subunits within the organization. Most of the time, these activities are carried out without the close oversight of a strategist and without close attention to the strategic plan. Nonetheless, they can have the cumulative effect of subtly moving the organization in a definite strategic direction. That direction may be a little bit or a lot different from the intended direction.
- One of the most influential lower-level decisions in shaping an organization's strategic movement has to do with the allocation of resources. There is always competition among individuals, projects, programs, and departments for the limited amounts of money, space, time, equipment, personnel, and influence available. The way those resources are distributed may not follow the strategic plan closely or at all. However, they do contribute unintentionally to a strategic momentum.
- All organizations are characterized by a unique collective personality or "culture," often described as "the way things are done around here," an undocumented set of values, customs, beliefs, and habits. When employees need to act and make decisions under the conditions of uncertainty and ambiguity that prevail in rapidly changing environments, they often instinctively fall back on traditional patterns and practices that they know best. Unconsciously, that can create its own strategic direction.
- Strategies are carried out by people and, wherever people come together to work toward a common end, internecine politics come into play. Rather than the result of a dispassionate, objective dialogue, strategy often is determined by biased, passionate bargaining. The participants bring different educational backgrounds, professional cultures, experience bases, and values and mindsets to the

negotiations. Their hidden agendas may be to protect a personal power base, enhance a department's status, increase a budget, or simply protect and maintain traditional practices. The strategic welfare of the organization may be a secondary consideration.

The net result of these forces is that several different kinds of strategy development paths can occur within an organization. First, there is the strategy intended by the planners and executives. It is based on careful analysis of prior history, current circumstances, and projected future developments. It is a description of how the managers would like things to turn out in an ideal world. Then there is the implemented strategy, the one that the firm puts into operation. Because the implementation is not well conceived, does not receive the necessary resources or attention, or is not competently executed, the resulting strategy can be significantly different from what was intended. In the end, the actual strategy that is pursued and impacts the marketplace can be even more at variance with the original intention. This may be due to changed environmental conditions, customer preferences, or competitor behaviors. There is also a category of strategies that simply "emerge" or develop without much prior planning in the course of the firm's operations. These *emergent* strategies may be conscious, spontaneous responses to new opportunities or threats that show up in the normal course of events, after the formal strategic plan has been prepared. Sometimes, they arise almost unconsciously as managers and employees make instinctive, often small adjustments to subtle shifts in the world around them. Finally, there are the planned and intended strategies that never actualized. Changed circumstances or failed assumptions may render the strategy irrelevant, or the organization may fail to implement the strategy competently or at all.

■ STRATEGIC PLANNING AND MANAGEMENT PROCESS

Traditionally, the process of making business strategy was described as strategic planning and management (SPM), or even simply "strategic planning." Those phrases are significant. One of the most daunting parts of the process is the preparation of the strategic plan. It often receives such a disproportionate share of corporate attention and energy that the management step is overlooked or never really carried out. In fact, it might be better to use the term "management" to describe the entire ongoing process of directing an organization's available resources and competencies in the preparation and execution of strategic plans that move the organization closer to achievement of its chosen vision. It is important to be clear about the full range of tasks that go into making successful strategy for an organization.

These are the fundamental steps in the process. They may be referred to by different names. They are rarely performed sequentially, one after the other, fully completing one step before moving on to the other. Some steps may be carried out simultaneously or jointly with other steps. Some organizations may prefer to reorder the steps slightly, putting one later or earlier in the process. Each organization tends to develop its own unique way of making strategy. What is important is that certain strategic management activities are p'erformed; how they are structured or designated is less important. These steps are explored more fully in the remaining chapters of this book.

Mission—what the organization is doing right now.

Vision—what the organization wants to be doing five or ten years from now.

Values—behavioral principles which employees will follow in performing their duties.

Grand strategic objectives—a few, broad organization-wide thrusts that will move it toward its vision.

Specific organization-wide strategic plans (at corporate and SBU levels)—complex, systematic, expensive, long-term programs for achieving the strategic objectives.

Benchmarks, metrics, targets, goals within those plans—standards by which strategic plans and performance are judged.

Functional area strategic plans—coordinated plans in support of the organization-wide strategic plans.

Action plans—more detailed, shorter-term sets of activities designed to carry out the organization-wide and functional area strategic plans.

Implementation of strategic (corporate, SBU, and functional area) and action plans—actual performance of the steps and activities described in the plans.

Monitoring and adjustment of plan implementation—constant measurement of plan progress coupled with appropriate fine-tuning.

STRATEGIC DIRECTION

If strategic planning and management is about moving an organization in a rational "strategic" direction, how does the organization decide what that direction is? Can it go in two or more strategic directions at once? How many possible strategic directions are available to a particular organization? When an organization decides on a strategic direction, how does it describe it? Where is it found in the organization's documents? Do you

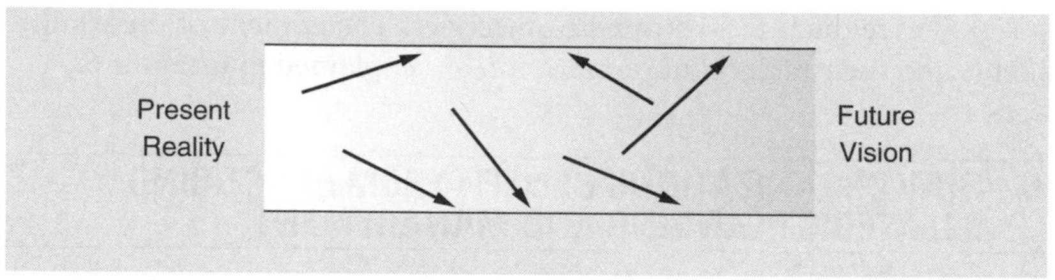

Figure 1.2 Misdirected Strategies

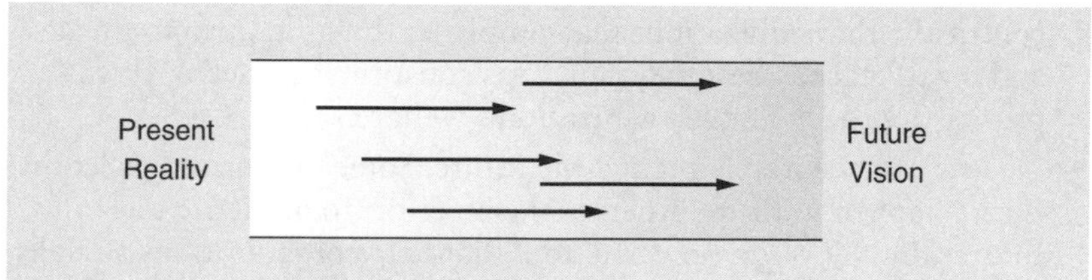

Figure 1.3 Multiple Strategies Moving Toward the Same Goal

know what the strategic direction is of organizations for which you have worked?

It is possible for a business to implement very successfully a strategy that does not move it one bit closer to realization of its vision. In fact, the strategy may move it farther away from that vision. The business may be better off with no strategy than one that is misdirected (Figure 1.2).

Quite often, a business will be in the process of implementing five or six distinct strategies at one time. Ideally, they should all work in unison to move the business along a desired path. Without careful thought, it is easy for strategies to conflict with one another and reduce their respective chances of success (Figure 1.3).

The penalties for pursuing strategies that are not aligned with some vision for a future state are that the business never arrives at a place that it truly wants to be. It never accomplishes goals that have been chosen deliberately by its executives and managers. For all its efforts, the business does not deliver optimal value to its stakeholders. In the process, it wastes financial resources, human energy and focus, and the most valuable commodity of all—time. Ultimately, for all these reasons, it may fail as a competitive entity.

Every forward-looking organization must define a strategic direction for itself. That is traditionally accomplished through the preparation of four documents or statements: a mission, a vision, a code of values, and a set of a few long-term strategic objectives. The content of these statements and their method of preparation are explained in Chapter 6.

HOW ORGANIZATIONS BENEFIT FROM PRACTICING STRATEGIC PLANNING AND MANAGEMENT

A great many benefits accrue to organizations that practice SPM. Most would not be as successful as they are without it. Some examples include:

- By engaging in SPM, an organization is taking an aggressive, proactive approach to maintaining and growing its operations. This is in contrast with organizations that simply let things happen to them and try to react as best they can. This constitutes an active versus a passive approach to an organization's welfare.
- No one can accurately predict the future. Some organizations let the future happen to them, others make an effort to influence their futures, but SPM is a powerful tool that helps organizations actually create the future that they most desire.
- The plan and its execution increase the likelihood that the organization will actually arrive at that desired future, the place where it wants to be.
- The process of preparing a strategic plan forces the organization to develop a clearer sense of its strategic vision. In fact, when organizations begin doing strategic planning, they frequently realize for the first time that they can and should have a strategic vision.
- The motivating effects of a well-founded strategic initiative with carefully gauged "stretch" goals result in higher levels of organizational and individual achievement than would be possible under "status quo" operations.
- The preparation of a strategic plan and the management of its implementation require that an organization focus on what is strategically important. It is easy to become so immersed in the tactical and operational details of running an organization that one loses sight of broader, longer-range concerns like strategic direction.
- To prepare a meaningful strategic plan and keep it relevant, an organization is compelled to acquire a better, more comprehensive understanding of its environment. This is particularly critical when that environment is evolving rapidly—as it is in health care and the biotechnology field.
- Every organization—for-profit, non-profit, or government—is limited in the resources that it has to carry out its current operations and plans for the future. The resources include money, people, space, skills, time, and commitment. Common sense says that the

organization that employs its resources more efficiently will do better than the organization that is sloppy and wasteful in its resource utilization. The discipline of SPM allocates resources to the activities that contribute most to the organization's mission, ensuring the most efficient use of those scarce resources.

- The existence of a strategic plan coupled with organizational commitment to its implementation stimulates and energizes the people carrying out the strategy. A strategic plan provides a greater sense of purpose to their work that goes beyond their routine operational duties. It often shows the way that employees can satisfy their personal goals through achievement of the organization's goals. A plan can be a powerful motivating force.
- The strategic planning and implementation process encourages imagination, innovation, and forward thinking in response to an ever-changing external environment.
- A well-conceived strategic plan establishes metrics for success that can be used to plot and evaluate the progress and performance of the organization and its people. The objective, time-limited goals in a strategic plan may be incorporated into pay-for-performance compensation schemes.
- The effect of a well-executed strategic plan is to orchestrate and synchronize the efforts of disparate people and units scattered throughout the organization. This results in higher levels of achievement than would be possible without a coordinated, inspired focus on the future.
- The future is an unpredictable, sometimes scary place. Strategic planning and management secures a desirable future for the organization and its stakeholders.

■ HOW STRATEGIC MANAGEMENT GOES WRONG

Strategic thinking and the practice of strategic management do not come naturally to many senior managers. It is not surprising, therefore, that their efforts to make strategy sometimes run into problems that limit their effectiveness. When that happens, both they and the entire organization can become disaffected from the process. It is worth anticipating and preempting problems.

The firm takes a passive reactive approach to external events, rather than an aggressive proactive one. Organizations with a passive, almost submissive attitude about the world in which they operate frequently do no strategic planning at all. When they do embark upon strategic initiatives, they are often reacting impulsively to a development in the general environment or a threatening move by a competitor. In the latter case, the firm is allowing a competitor to dictate its strategies. An essential element of strategic management is the desire of an organization to take charge of its future, to do all that it can with its resources and capabilities to carry out its mission.

The strategic plan is created at the top of the organization and handed down without further input from other parts of the organization. Sometimes, a special strategic planning unit handles most of the preparation before handing the plan off to senior management for approval. This approach misses out on two opportunities. First, many people throughout the organization can provide valuable inputs to the planning process based on their contacts with customers, suppliers, competitors, and other stakeholders in the course of their day-to-day work. Their knowledge and opinions help ensure a plan that is responsive to its environment. Second, it is the masses of employees below the level of senior management (and the strategic planning unit) that will be responsible for carrying out the plan. Experience shows that they will implement the plan more effectively and enthusiastically if they have been involved in its creation. The importance of their participation cannot be overestimated.

Management fails to build a consensus around the plan before trying to implement it. Even if senior management insists upon creating the strategic plan entirely within the executive suite, optimally effective implementation depends on some degree of buy-in from other employees and other stakeholders who may have a role to play. If these people were not involved in the formulation of the plan, an aggressive effort should be made to "sell" it to them and solicit their support. This usually requires numerous small-group meetings throughout the organization, including extensive Q&A, as well as a willingness to make some adjustments to the plan in response to feedback received.

The strategic initiative begins and ends with the plan; little attention is given to actual implementation. This sometimes happens because the managers involved exhaust themselves in the planning activity and have no energy left to do the things necessary to put it into effect. They also may not understand the additional steps required—breaking down broad goals into narrower actionable tasks, setting time deadlines for completion, delegating primary authority to specific individuals, allocating appropriate resources, constantly measuring progress, and making small and large adjustments. The plan may be broadcast to the organization and its execution left to employees who are more concerned with their immediate operational tasks. The strategic plan is forgotten.

The planning process gets stuck in "analysis paralysis." There is an infinity of information that can be gathered about an organization, its customers, its competitors, and the general environment. It is easy to get so lost in data collection and analysis, always seeking just one more report or making just one more calculation, that the plan is never completed, let alone implemented. Experienced strategists know when to halt the quest for greater knowledge and precision and move on to translating the information at hand into actionable plans.

The organization follows the plan unquestioningly throughout its term, which may be as long as five years, despite substantial changes in the organization's external and internal environments. By the second or third year, the assumptions on which the plan is based may be invalid and its objectives no longer relevant to the organizational mission. Instead of moving the organization closer to its desired future, the plan may have moved it further away and wasted resources in the process.

Because of low risk tolerance and a fear of failure, the strategic planners set modest, unambitious goals. A good strategic plan stretches the firm and its people. How far depends on the industry in which the firm competes. When the competition is particularly intense, when the external environment is changing rapidly, bold, even audacious strategy is called for. These are the conditions that currently prevail throughout the health care industry. Undemanding strategic goals are less likely to capture the imagination of employees; they will be less motivated to work toward achievement of the goals. As a result, the firm may fall behind the competition and fall behind in pursuit of its vision.

There is a lack of top management support for the strategic planning and management effort. In most organizations, initiatives with far-reaching agendas like strategic management do not go very far without the explicit support of managers at the highest level. Their apparent disinterest sends an implicit message to employees and other stakeholders that the organization does not intend to engage systematically with the competition or its own future. If senior managers responsible for the long-term future of the firm are not enthusiastic about strategic thinking, employees responsible for carrying out any plans that emerge will be no more motivated.

Strategic planning is conducted separately from or totally without functional area planning. The practical details of implementing a strategic plan are laid out within the functional areas of an organization (e.g., marketing, production, clinical services, finance). The area managers should be consulted during the planning process to be sure of their ability to carry out the plan's directives. It is most critical to involve those managers familiar with the firm's access to the financial resources called for by the plan. It is not uncommon for each functional area to back up the overall strategic plan with a strategic plan of its own.

The plan fails to address crucial strategic issues because they seem too difficult or too numerous. As a firm analyzes itself, its markets, competitors, and the general environment, a few especially critical issues will emerge. They may be based on a competitor's announced new strategic initiative (e.g., local teaching hospital will build a new women's health center), changing demographics in the market area (e.g., population aged

25–34 is declining), or proposed new state legislation (e.g., state governor backs a plan for statewide universal health coverage). A responsible strategic plan will acknowledge such issues and offer some response. Management may choose not to because either it does not fully comprehend the issues or there seem to be too many to cope with. It is better to make a mediocre attempt to answer the challenge than to ignore it. If the number of critical issues is overwhelming, some probably are not as critical as others and the list should be prioritized.

The strategy implementation phase lacks flexibility and responsiveness to subsequent changes in the environment. A well-researched strategic plan is based upon the best possible projections of how competitor and customer behavior are likely to evolve in the future, and of events and trends likely to occur in the general environment. Many of the plan assumptions will turn out differently, sometimes so much so that the strategies, as originally conceived, are no longer relevant. In some cases, they may be rendered counterproductive. An essential piece of strategy implementation is the ongoing monitoring of conditions that might impact the strategy, coupled with a willingness to make minor or major compensating adjustments in the strategy itself. It would be a rare strategic plan that, two or three years into its implementation, did not have to be radically altered. This is particularly true in the tumultuous health care and biotechnology industries.

The plan does not address or focus on the most critical issues. The plan is a thoughtful, well-structured document that is implemented with great effect. The problem is that it does not tackle some of the core strategic issues facing the organization. Some of them may be too difficult or too painful to even think about, so they are bypassed in favor of less-stressful, less-perplexing issues. In contrast, in an attempt to be thorough, the plan may attempt to cope with far too many issues. They cannot all be critical. The result is that none of them, including those most important to the business's future, get the attention and the resources they deserve.

BARRIERS TO STRATEGIC MANAGEMENT

If SPM is such a good idea, why do so many organizations fail to practice it? These are some of the reasons.

- Organizations have poor reward structures, no positive reinforcement. Businesses do not formally recognize success in performing strategic planning and management. Some might not even be able to define "success" at the strategic level. If a firm is aware of when it has succeeded strategically, managers do not notice the people who contributed to the success. And, if managers can see that some

The Changing Pace of Modern Strategic Management

One way to picture the frequency and intensity of strategic activity within an organization is through the metaphor of a boat traveling down a long river. Through most of its length, the river current moves slowly and calmly; the boat captain does not have to work too hard. He must make sure that the craft stays more or less in the middle of the river without running into either of the banks or aground on a sand bar. Occasionally he puts a line over the side and brings some fish up from the river. It is not particularly challenging or stressful work. The crew have relatively little to do.

Every once in a while, however, there are rapids in the river, caused by the presence of a jumble of rocks or a narrowing in the river course. The water turns white with foam, moves more swiftly, twists and crashes against the rocks. If the boat is to negotiate the rapids safely, the captain's attention and alertness must increase, and he must look further down the river to plot a course through the rocks and standing waves. It may be necessary for all crew members to pick up a paddle or oar to help steer the boat along the path chosen by the captain. With experience, skill, and some luck, the boat and all the people on board will get safely through to the calmer water on the other side. Everyone then can relax for several miles until the next rapids appear.

In the current environment within the health care industry of hyper-competition, relentless pressure for lower costs and higher quality, a steady flow of new laws and public policies, and expanding demands from consumer-patients, it could be said that strategic decision-makers are now operating in conditions of "constant white water." Events move faster, are more fluid, and are ever-changing. A health care business must face rapids every day of its life. There are no calm, restful periods.

The more frenetic pace of life and activity in a twenty-first-century health care organization requires a different model of strategic planning and management. Strategy-making as a series of sporadic, discontinuous events, a sort of "punctuated equilibrium," no longer works. It cannot keep pace. Instead the formulation and evolution of strategy must become a persistent, continuous process, carried out by every member of the organization almost without thinking.

people are making a difference in moving the firm into the future, they simply do not reward them, monetarily or otherwise for their efforts. There are no incentives for spending time on strategic matters or doing well at them.

- Organizations are focused on operational or tactical activities or, even worse, on crisis management. Historically, the management of health care organizations, most of them not-for-profit in noncompetitive environments, was concerned exclusively with relatively routine operational matters. Some managers have never made the transition from that more benign milieu to the current industry situation that demands constant attention to markets, competitors, and the future. Health care management, in general, has become more complex, more intense, and more demanding. It is easy to get so caught up in trying to keep a hospital or a physician practice running on a day-to-day basis that there seems little time left to indulge in the luxury of long-term thinking and planning.

- Organizations fail to appreciate the delayed link between strategic planning and management efforts now and concrete operating results in the future. In a culture constantly seeking immediate, certain gratification, and in businesses with predominantly short-term horizons, strategic management has two unpopular aspects. It is concerned with creating effects in the future and, because it is impossible truly to predict the future, those effects are uncertain. The subjects of strategic decision-making are dealt with on a timescale measured in years. Decisions made today will produce changes so far in the future that some people lose patience and interest. Under such conditions, engaging in strategic management seems pointless.
- If an organization has no prior experience with strategic management, at least some of its members will have to acquire new skills and comprehend new concepts. A few people must develop the ability to think strategically. For those nearly overwhelmed by their current responsibilities, there is no desire to make the effort to learn.
- When an organization feels that it is doing quite well currently, and perhaps has been successful for a number of years, there may be a tendency to believe that it is doing all the right things. Strategic management then seems superfluous. The firm's leaders are content with the way things are and assume that they will never change. Or, they become overconfident in their ability to adapt and improvise in response to any challenges that may appear.
- At the other extreme, some executives believe that their organizations are operating in environments that are changing so rapidly that any attempt to look and plan ahead will be made irrelevant by unanticipated circumstances and conditions. An attitude like this would not be surprising in the turbulent climate of today's health care industry.
- Managers have had unhappy prior experiences with strategic management. It is possible that managers in health care have worked previously for organizations that did practice some form of strategic

planning. However, the experience may have been so dysfunctional, unpleasant, or nonproductive that they assume that all strategic management initiatives are similar and avoid repeating them.
- Some managers without prior experience or education in strategic planning and management believe that it can or should offer a 100 percent probability of success and, when they learn that the outcome cannot be ensured, refuse to engage in the process at all.
- By definition, strategic management sets out to create fundamental changes in an organization structure or operations. A few managers with a vested interest in the status quo may fear the loss of money, status, or power, and will purposely avoid strategic management and even attempt to sabotage the process.

For all these reasons, organizations choose not to invest the time, the money, or the personnel that even a modest strategic planning effort would require.

FOCUS ON THE HEALTHCARE AND BIOTECHNOLOGY INDUSTRIES

The scope of this book is the planning and management of strategy in particular industries—those associated with the delivery and financing of health care in the United States. The term "health care" is interpreted in its broadest sense to include the following, among others:

Managed care organizations
Health maintenance organizations
Preferred provider organizations
Independent practice associations
Solo physician practices
Small group practices
Large group practices
Academic physician practices
Multi-specialty group practices
Teaching hospitals
Community hospitals
Specialty hospitals
Integrated delivery systems
Health plans
Health insurance companies
Community health centers

Pharmaceutical companies
Biotechnology and biomedical companies
DME manufacturers
Public health regulatory agencies
Public health financing agencies (CMS)
Public health delivery agencies (Veterans Health Administration, or VHA)
State departments of public health

Taken together, these industries account for expenditures approaching one-fifth of the gross domestic product of the United States.

There are several reasons for devoting a book to an explanation of the practice of strategic planning and management by organizations in these particular industries. The strategic challenges that they face and the competitive milieu in which they operate are strikingly different from those in other economic sectors. In few other industries do federal, state, and local government agencies play so significant a role through regulation, financing, and direct service delivery. In few other industries are the choices of which products and services to buy, the payment for those products and services, and the consumption of those products and services carried out by different people. More than in any other industry, the structures, products and services, practices, and costs of health care and biotechnology are the subject of close scrutiny and constant debate by the media, politicians, scholars, executives, professionals, and members of the public. Even though many of the strategy concepts and principles are generic, it is more useful to explain them in terms and contexts familiar to the health care and biotechnology executives who must employ them.

ENVIRONMENTAL FORCES THAT AFFECT STRATEGY-MAKING IN THE HEALTHCARE AND BIOTECHNOLOGY INDUSTRIES

It is worth acknowledging some of the significant forces in the external environment that influence the strategies that health care organizations choose to adopt—or are virtually compelled to adopt if they wish to survive. These forces are present in every area of the organizations' external environment. Because of the constant ferment in the health care industry, some of these forces may weaken or disappear completely within a few years while others will become stronger and more influential. New environmental forces with impacts on health care strategies will emerge. The process of assessing and monitoring a firm's general external environment is discussed in Chapter 3.

Legislative/Political. At both the federal and state levels, legislators are introducing bills designed to provide various forms of universal health care coverage. It is particularly noteworthy that a number of states have seized the initiative to create individual statewide universal plans. Some have been enacted and are being implemented. Many of the candidates in the 2008 presidential election, primarily on the Democratic side, are speaking openly about the need for sweeping national health care reform. Regardless of who is elected, proposals for significant changes in the financing and structure of the health care system are likely to be on the legislative agenda of the next administration. There will continue to be more regulation of health plan activity—concerning abusive treatment of patients or providers, disclosure of policies (denial of coverage, provider financial incentives), publication of prices for common services and procedures, mandated coverage of specific services, and protection of patient privacy interests. Ongoing legislative efforts can be expected to try to slow the steadily rising national health care budget.

Economic. Though the rate of growth waxes and wanes, the national health care budget continues its inexorable climb. Although more money available for spending on health care might seem like a good thing for health care organizations, the trend also increases the likelihood of more limitations on reimbursements under Medicare and Medicaid because of their budget constraints.

Social/Demographic. The baby boomer cohort continues to work its way through the population, increasing the numbers of elderly requiring the expensive health care services that come with aging. Contributing to this trend is the slow, steady improvement in life expectancy of Americans. The ethnicity of the overall population and, therefore, prospective patients is becoming more diverse. The education level of the population also is increasing; this has special implications for the changing role of patients under "consumer-driven health care." The income disparities within the population are growing, affecting the ability and willingness of patients to pay for their care. That trend is leading to a three-tiered system of access to care: privately insured patients, publicly insured patients (Medicare, Medicaid), and uninsured patients. Patients often experience forced mobility from one health plan to another, and from one provider to another, as employers change their mix of health plans and patients change their jobs. The proportion of the population that is either underinsured or completely uninsured increases steadily. There are critical shortages of nurses and primary care physicians, coupled with physician surpluses in certain geographic areas and in certain specialties.

Technological. The introduction of new clinical technologies that has typified the health care industry for at least two decades continues apace in areas like drug design, imaging, minimally invasive surgical procedures, genetic mapping and testing, gene therapy, and vaccines. The momentum is even greater for medical information technologies such as electronic medical record (EMR) systems, computerized physician order entry (CPOE) systems, automated practice guideline prompts, integrated clinical/cost analyses to demonstrate cost effectiveness, electronic claims filing and processing, and telemedicine. For provider organizations, the availability of these new technologies offers strategic opportunities to gain competitive advantage although often at substantial costs. For the developers and vendors of these technologies, the markets for their products seem to have promising futures.

Industry (competitive). New models of drug discovery and development have created a major new industry composed of small and startup biomedical and biotechnology companies that research products (often no more than one per firm) that are licensed or sold to major pharmaceutical companies for the ultimate market introduction. The trend of consolidation among health plans, among hospitals, and among group practices into networks and systems continues in response to unrelenting cost pressures and heightened competition. The principles of professional business management that are applied in most other industries are steadily working their way into the day-to-day running of health care organizations. Those businesses that embrace these concepts rather than resist them will reap the benefits sooner and gain at least temporary competitive advantage over their rivals. The principles are often first introduced by entities organized as for-profit corporations and their executives with prior experience in predominantly for-profit industries. The for-profit ethos is transforming managerial decision-making and organizational cultures in the health care industry.

Study Questions

1. If a health care organization, such as a hospital, carefully formulates and implements a strategic plan, exactly what differences can it expect to see in four or five years?
2. Try to describe the type of organization that would have no good reason for carrying out strategic management.
3. Under what circumstances should an organization attempt to execute a "revolutionary" strategy, and when should it be satisfied with "incremental" strategy?
4. Draw a diagram of the strategic planning and management process described in this chapter. Elaborate upon the process, inserting additional steps and sub-steps, and drawing lines to show the connections between the steps.
5. Do some Internet research on health care/biotechnology companies that have had substantial, public business problems in the last few years, and try to identify the possible strategic causes of those problems.

What apparent mistakes in either the planning or implementation of strategy led to the problems?

6. Choose a very large corporation in any part of the health care or biotechnology industries, and identify the individual SBUs that make up the corporation. What are the features that distinguish those SBUs from a department or division?

Learning Exercise 1

There is an organization that does research and development in the area of new drug discovery. It was founded four years ago and recently licensed the patent for its initial research output to a large pharmaceutical company. It is now in the very earliest stages of work on two additional research projects in related areas. Up until now, the decisions about the scientific focus of the firm's research efforts have been made by the researchers involved. The patent licensing decision seemed like an obvious way to bring in the significant new financial resources that the firm now enjoys. However, there remains within the firm some general uncertainty about the future.

You have been hired as a consultant by the organization's board of directors to persuade top executives that strategic planning and management is a worthwhile pursuit. The executives have expressed some of the reasons described in this chapter for avoiding any strategic activities up until now. Think of a rational, constructive response to each of those barriers.

Learning Exercise 2

The purpose of this exercise is to design a simple instrument to help you determine whether another person is able to "think strategically." Prepare a series of about ten questions that explore the various dimensions of strategic thinking as explained by this chapter. The answers to the questions may be brief open-ended essays, multiple-choice, assignment of scores or ratings, or anything else that seems appropriate. You may want to test it on a few classmates. When you have it in a final form, administer the instrument to people (friends, relatives, colleagues, coworkers) whose attitudes about strategy are unknown to you. On the basis of their answers, make a judgment about their ability to practice "strategic thinking." How do you feel about the results that you have achieved? Does this exercise give you a better understanding of strategic thinking, either in yourself or in others?

References

Aaker DA. *Developing Business Strategies*. 6th ed. Hoboken, NJ: John Wiley & Sons; 2001.

Coulter M. *Strategic Management in Action*. 3rd ed. Upper Saddle River, NJ: Pearson/Prentice Hall; 2005.

David FR. *Strategic Management, Concepts and Cases*. 10th ed. Upper Saddle River, NJ: Pearson/Prentice Hall; 2005.

Dixit AK and Nalebuff BJ. *Thinking Strategically*. New York NY: W. W. Norton; 1991.

Fitzroy P and Hulbert J. *Strategic Management, Creating Value in Turbulent Times*. Hoboken, NJ: John Wiley & Sons; 2005.

Gavetti G and Rivkin JW. How strategists really think. *Harvard Business Review*. 2005; 83(4):54–63.

Grant RM. *Contemporary Strategy Analysis*. 5th ed. Oxford: Blackwell; 2005.

Harrison JS. *Strategic Management of Resources and Relationships, Concepts*. Hoboken, NJ: John Wiley & Sons; 2003.

Harrison JS and St. John CH. *Foundations in Strategic Management*. 3rd ed. Mason, OH: Thomson/South-Western; 2004.

Hax AC and Majluf NS. *The Strategy Concept and Process: A Pragmatic Approach*. 2nd ed. Upper Saddle River, NJ: Prentice Hall; 1996.

Hitt MA, Ireland RD, and Hoskisson RE. *Strategic Management, Competitiveness and Globalization: Concepts*. 7th ed. Mason, OH: Thomson/South-Western; 2007.

Johnson G, Scholes K, and Whittington R. *Exploring Corporate Strategy*. 7th ed. Upper Saddle River, NJ: Prentice Hall; 2005.

Pitts RA and Lei D. *Strategic Management, Building and Sustaining Competitive Advantage*. 4th ed. Mason, OH: Thomson/South-Western; 2006.

Porter ME. *Competitive Strategy, Techniques for Analyzing Industries and Competitors*. New York NY: The Free Press; 1980.

Porter ME. *Competitive Advantage, Creating and Sustaining Superior Performance*. New York NY: The Free Press; 1985.

Rothschild WE. How to ensure the continuous growth of strategic planning. *Journal of Business Strategy*. 1980;1(1):11–18.

Wheelen TL and Hunger JD. *Strategic Management and Business Policy*. 9th ed. Upper Saddle River, NJ: Pearson/Prentice Hall; 2004.

CHAPTER

2

Internal Audit of Strategic Assets: Resources and Competencies

Learning Objectives

After reading and studying this chapter, you should be able to:

- Explain the concept of an internal audit of a firm's strategic assets and the role that it plays in preparing a strategic plan.
- Describe the three different approaches to an internal asset audit—financial performance analysis, resources and competencies review, and value chain evaluation.
- List and define the key metrics in an analysis of an organization's financial performance and condition.
- Understand the correlation between a business's financial performance and its ability to execute strategic plans.
- Define "resources" and "competencies," the differences between them, and the ways that they depend upon each other.
- List the different generic types of organizational resources, and provide examples of typical organizational competencies.
- Explain how resources and competencies may be "strengths" or "weaknesses" for an organization.
- Describe the ways that an organization can manage and use its resources and competencies.
- Define and describe graphically the internal value chain of a business.
- Show how to employ the value chain concept to reduce costs or add value.
- Understand the difference between performing activities differently and better.

The very first step in a strategic planning and management process is an organizational self-examination, an internal audit of what the organization has to work with. Such an internal audit is conducted at the corporate and SBU levels of an organization. The purpose is to identify the assets (both strong and weak) that the organization possesses for exploiting opportunities and resisting threats in its external environment. In doing this, the organization will leverage its strong points and offset or improve its weak points.

Several different approaches can be taken to examining and understanding the internal functioning of an organization and its ability to implement strategies. They are analysis of its historical and current financial performance, review of its strategic assets as resources and competencies, and breakdown and evaluation of its value chain. There is some overlap among these methodologies, but each provides a unique picture of the organization's strategy-making potential.

■ ANALYSIS OF HISTORICAL FINANCIAL PERFORMANCE AND CURRENT FINANCIAL CONDITION

The common denominator of current operations and future strategies in most organizations is money. The availability of strategic alternatives and their successful implementation depends to a large degree on the capital funds accessible to the firm. The very success of the strategies often is measured in financial terms. Strategic management employs several types of financial metrics and for several different reasons. (These issues are addressed in greater depth in Chapter 11.)

Sales, market share, and profits. The current levels of sales and profits are a measure of the success of past strategies and the need for new strategies. If they are steadily growing, they indicate that customers value the firm's products and services so much that they will buy them in larger and larger volumes and pay a premium (over the cost of production) for them. This would be a positive indication of the firm's ability to survive and prosper. In such circumstances, there is not as great an urgency to create new strategies. In contrast, declining sales or steady sales with declining profits may indicate that certain products or services, market segments, distribution channels, or other operating parameters are no longer competitive. These data can help in deciding whether strategic changes are needed and where they should be focused.

Growth trends in these numbers may show that the firm is reaching the point on the company growth curve when economies of scale, economies of scope, and learning curve advantages will begin to kick in. Rapid growth also implies that the business will be consuming more cash than it generates. When sales growth begins to slow and level off, it may be the sign of a maturing business that can be counted on as a source of cash.

It is important to measure sales and profits over time to demonstrate the trends, and relative to other companies in the industry and to the industry as a whole. A sales growth rate that looks impressive on its own may be lower than what has been achieved by competitors. For this reason, many businesses also pay attention to their share of the market in which they are competing.

Free cash flow. Because of the different delays in its payments and receipts, as well as expenditures on capital investments, a firm's "net profits" are not usually indicative of the funds available for spending on new projects. The "free cash flow" shows how much money is left after the firm meets its existing operating and strategic cash commitments. Where the firm is in its life cycle often determines whether it has negative (during growth) or positive (during maturity or decline) cash flow. The free cash flow must be compared with the cost of the strategic initiatives that the firm is contemplating. If the firm is growing rapidly or has great strategic ambitions, internal cash flow may not be enough to finance the strategies.

External capital sources. When a business finds that it cannot finance its new strategic initiatives through internally generated capital, it will have to turn to external sources. The two general categories of external capital are debt and equity. Debt is secured by either borrowing money or issuing corporate bonds. Equity capital is raised through the sale of stock. All external capital has a cost that must be taken into account when planning new strategies. For strategic planning persons, a firm needs to know how much it can borrow and at what interest rate, how large a bond issue it could float and at what interest rate, and the size of a stock offering it could make and the per-share price it could expect.

Capital project hurdle rate. The hurdle rate is the minimum return a company expects on any new strategic investments. It is composed of its cost of capital plus the profit margin that it aims to earn on everything it does. The cost of capital is weighted for the amounts of different types of debt and equity that the firm has outstanding. If a proposed strategic initiative cannot earn a return that meets or exceeds the hurdle rate, it should be disapproved.

Other capital demands. Every business has a finite amount of capital available from internal and external sources, and demands on that capital that inevitably exceed the amount available. There will be other strategic proposals. During a given fiscal year, some projects may already have been approved for funding. There may be required expenditures on plant and equipment that are substantial but not truly strategic in nature. Prudent financial management may suggest that the firm pay a dividend to its shareholders or buy back some of their stock. Strategy planners must be aware of all these capital demands that compete with their own.

Shareholder value. If the firm is a publicly traded for-profit entity, the value that it delivers to its shareholders is a primary factor in their continuing willingness to invest their money in the firm. That value also affects the firm's ability to raise additional equity capital in the future. Because it incorporates the cost of equity capital, use of the hurdle rate mentioned above is one tool for addressing shareholder value. It leads to several generic rules for maintaining or increasing that value.

- Achieve the existing level of profits with less invested capital.
- Increase the profit level without investing additional capital.
- Decrease the cost of equity capital—by raising the debt-to-equity ratio or buying back existing stock.
- Invest more capital in new strategic projects that earn a rate of return higher than the average for the firm's current operations.

The challenge for business strategists is to satisfy the often ill-advised desire of shareholders for short-term returns on their investment while focusing the firm's strategic momentum and capital investment on long-term initiatives.

Current financial strength and performance. Knowledge of a firm's current financial performance has two important applications. It is an indicator of the viability of the current operations and the success of strategies implemented in the recent past. If the metrics show signs of fiscal weakness, it may be necessary to make changes in operational methods and tactics or launch bold new strategies that take the firm in new operational directions. Financial analysts and credit rating firms also rely heavily on these data in making their decisions about whether a business is creditworthy and deserving of additional injections of capital—debt or equity.

Well-established metrics exist for measuring financial strength and performance. Calculation of the metrics starts with the current financial facts of the organization, as reflected in a few traditional financial statements.

The **balance sheet** is a snapshot of the organization's financial position at a particular point in time. The data contained in a balance sheet can be analyzed in a variety of ways to provide a rather sophisticated understanding of the financial infrastructure and integrity of the organization.

The **operating or income statement** describes the financial currents within the organization over a period of time, typically a month, a quarter, or a year. It is a measure in financial terms of operating activity as the organization carries out its mission and strategies.

The **statement of cash flows** records the actual flows of money in and out of the organization. This is different from the income statement, which shows revenues that have been earned, though not necessarily received, and costs that have been incurred, though not necessarily paid. The information is an indicator of the organization's ability to continue meeting its operating expenses and invest in new strategies. By some reckonings, cash is the most important financial variable. Eventually, all the other fiscal measures are reduced to cold, hard cash.

The **statement of changes in owners' equity (for-profit) or net assets (non-profit)** indicates the increase or decrease in the amount by which an organization's assets exceed its outstanding liabilities. The greater the excess, the greater the value of a stockholder's interest in a company and the greater its financial strength.

The information contained in those financial statements are stark, absolute dollar figures that have no meaning by themselves. The figures must be interpreted and related to one another and to industry standards. The primary tool for this interpretation is a set of ratios that are relied on by anyone seeking a practical understanding of an organization's financial condition. Investors and creditors apply ratio analysis to financial data in order to predict future earnings and the ability to service debt. Managers use the ratios to predict the future and plan strategies that will influence the future. There are four categories of analysis ratios:

1. **Liquidity ratios** define the organization's ability to meet its short-term obligations. "Liquidity" measures state how readily corporate assets can be turned into cash for paying debts like loans or bonds that have come due; bills for materials, supplies, and equipment; and wages and salaries.

   Current Ratio $\dfrac{\text{total current assets}}{\text{total current liabilities}}$

   This is a basic indicator of financial liquidity. Higher values mean better debt-paying capacity. If the ratio is too high, it may indicate that too much cash is being held in the form of more liquid bank accounts or short-term securities rather than being invested wisely in longer-term strategic projects.

   Average Collection Period $\dfrac{\text{net receivables}}{\text{net patient service revenue/365}}$

   This is the number of days' worth of average daily revenue that has been earned but not yet received, showing up on the balance sheet as "accounts receivable." It is an indicator of how long the average patient/customer takes to pay the bill after being discharged or receiving the product/service. Lower values mean that the organization is collecting on those bills more quickly and therefore has the cash available for paying its own debts or investing for strategic purposes.

Days Cash-on-Hand, ST Sources $\dfrac{\text{cash + marketable securities}}{\text{(total expenses – depreciation expenses)/365}}$

This is the number of days' worth of average daily cash payouts that the organization has on hand in the form of liquid assets. It is an indicator of how long the organization could go on paying its outstanding debts if its cash receipts stopped completely.

Average Payment Period $\dfrac{\text{total current liabilities/}}{\text{(total expenses – depreciation expenses)/365}}$

This is the number of days' worth of average daily incurred expenses represented by the organization's total liabilities (e.g., accounts payable, short- and long-term debt). The larger this number, the longer it is taking the organization to pay those expenses, presumably because it does not have sufficient cash. A larger number will be more worrisome to creditors.

2. **Profitability** defines the ability to maintain and grow operations by measuring the relationship of revenues to expenses. In FP health care corporations, investors always seek the highest possible level of profitability. In NFP health care organizations, too much profit may bring criticism from the community, the IRS, and state tax authorities; too little profit may lead to criticism from the board of directors.

Operating Margin $\dfrac{\text{operating income}}{\text{total operating revenue}}$

Measures how much a firm's operating revenues are left over after paying the expenses incurred in generating those revenues. This represents the traditional, popular view of a firm's profits. A higher margin is better.

Total Margin $\dfrac{\text{excess of revenues over expenses}}{\text{total revenue}}$

This measure is similar to the operating margin except that it includes investment income in the revenues figure. It represents profits from all sources—both operational and nonoperational activities. A higher total margin is always preferred.

Return on Net Assets $\dfrac{\text{excess of revenues over expenses}}{\text{net assets}}$

This ratio shows how well the firm is using its assets (debt and equity) to generate profits. The more profit "bang" that it can get from every "buck" borrowed or invested, the better.

3. **Operating efficiency** ratios measure how efficiently a company is using its assets to create products and services in its operations. The higher that level of operating efficiency, the more likely that the business can meet its debt obligations and increase the value of its shareholders' investments.

Total Asset Turnover $\dfrac{\text{total operating revenue + other income}}{\text{total assets}}$

This is a calculation of revenue from all sources as a multiple of the total assets employed to generate the revenue. The higher the multiplier, the more efficiently the organization is utilizing its assets.

Non-Financial Operating Indicators

While money is the lifeblood of an organization, and the owners of for-profit businesses tend to focus primarily on financial measures of performance, numerous nonfinancial indicators are used to measure the success of operations and strategies. They tend to be specific to the industry in which the industry operates. These are some of the most popular metrics for hospital operating performance.

Average Length of Stay (ALOS)

$$\frac{\text{patient days}}{\text{discharges}}$$

This number measures how long the average patient spends in the hospital between a particular admission and discharge. Care must be taken in using this figure to compare hospitals. It can vary dramatically depending on the types of patients admitted, the specific diseases/ailments for which they are treated, and the severity of their conditions. The acceptability of the actual number depends on how the hospital is reimbursed. A lower ALOS is desirable in the case of DRG or capitated reimbursements, while a higher figure is preferred if payment is on a per diem or fee-for-service basis.

Occupancy Rate

$$\frac{\text{patient days}}{365 \times \text{licensed beds}}$$

This metric shows how full the hospital is—what percentage of its beds are occupied by patients. It is in the firm's interest to keep the occupancy rate as close to 100 percent as possible, in order to spread the fixed costs of operating the hospital facility across a larger number of patients.

Outpatient Revenue as % of Total Revenues

$$\frac{\text{outpatient revenue}}{\text{total revenue}}$$

This metric reveals the percentage of total hospital revenues that are accounted for by patients served on an outpatient basis. A higher percentage is desirable because of the preference throughout the health care system to treat patient conditions in the lowest-intensity setting possible. This means that outpatient revenues are almost always preferable to inpatient revenues.

Full-Time Equivalents (FTEs) per Occupied Bed

This is a measure of the number of employees in all categories that it takes to support each bed with a patient in it. A lower ratio suggests that the hospital has found a more efficient way to provide services to its patients. However, maintaining staffing levels too low may detrimentally affect the quality of those services. A facility's optimal FTE-to-bed ratio will depend on the mix of patient cases that it typically sees.

Fixed Asset Turnover $\dfrac{\text{total operating revenue + other income}}{\text{net fixed assets}}$

This calculates the operating efficiency ratio for fixed assets only. It shows how productively the firm is employing its plant and equipment.

Inventory Turnover $\dfrac{\text{total operating revenue + other income}}{\text{current assets/inventory}}$

Certain businesses must maintain inventories of raw materials, work-in-progress, and finished goods to carry out their operations. Examples are pharmaceutical companies, DME producers, and most other manufacturers of products. Inventory management is of somewhat less concern to service-oriented entities, like hospitals and physician practices. The items held in inventory have a cash value that the firm would like to keep to the minimum necessary to support operations. This ratio shows total revenues as a multiple of the inventories used to generate them. A higher number suggests greater operating efficiency, but may also result in lost production and sales because required stock was not available. In contrast, low inventory turnover may mean that too much cash was tied up in inventories.

4. **Capital structure ratios** describe the composition of the package of capital that an organization has available to fund its endeavors. The capital may come from a variety of sources (the basic broad categories being debt and equity), and the mix of those sources is a major factor in determining the organization's long-term liquidity and ability to raise additional capital. Creditors and bond rating firms look at capital structure in evaluating creditworthiness.

Net Asset/Equity to Total Assets $\dfrac{\text{net assets (or equity)}}{\text{total assets}}$

This is a ratio between a firm's equity capital and its total capital. Creditors like to see a higher ratio here; the higher proportion of equity capital means more funds are available to meet debt obligations. In an NFP corporation, net assets are increased through retained earnings or charitable donations. In an FP corporation, it is through retained earnings and sales of additional stock shares that equity is increased.

Long-Term Debt to Net Assets/Equity $\dfrac{\text{long-term debt}}{\text{net assets (or equity)}}$

This ratio shows the proportion between long-term debt and owners' equity or net assets. Debt is a desirable source of capital, particularly when a business is profitable and growing. At a certain point, however, the burden of paying the interest on a large body of debt may make creditors reluctant to lend additional funds to or buy more bonds from the organization. In the interest of raising additional debt capital in the future, a lower ratio is better.

Debt Service Coverage

$$\dfrac{\text{excess of revenue over expenses (or net income) + depreciation + interest}}{\text{principal payment + interest)}}$$

This ratio is simply a measure of a business's capacity for making the interest and principal payments on its long-term debt. It is watched closely by investment bankers and bond rating firms.

All these data are gathered and the metrics calculated continuously, then compared, both with the organization's historic performance, to reveal trends, and with industry averages and numbers for individual competitors. The metrics measure only what they were designed to measure, which may or may not be relevant to the organization's chosen strategies. In practice, it usually is necessary to devise unique criteria to measure the progress toward achievement of the objectives set for particular strategies. Some examples are patient satisfaction for physician practices and hospitals, Healthcare Effectiveness and Data Information Set (HEDIS) ratings for health plans, and National Committee for Quality Assurance (NCQA) accreditation ratings for managed care organizations.

On the basis of ongoing analysis of its performance, the business will reach conclusions about areas in which improvement seems necessary. It may even get clues about the exact changes in strategy or strategy implementation that are called for. However, final decisions on adjustments to existing strategies or adoption of new strategies depend on a review of the business's resources and competencies available to support strategic initiatives, as well as further assessment of its industry and competitors, its markets and competitors, and a variety of external environmental factors among which the strategies will be played out.

■ RESOURCES AND COMPETENCIES

Every organization can be viewed as simply a bundle of resources and competencies. The "resources" are either tangible or intangible. The resources have "competencies"—latent abilities to perform "activities." It is through activities that current operations are conducted and future strategies pursued. Depending on how well they contribute to the performance of an organization's operations and the implementation of its strategies, resources and competencies may be considered "strengths" or "weaknesses."

What an organization is able to accomplish depends upon the resources that it possesses, the competencies of those resources, and how the organization combines them to carry out activities. Some organizations have more resources with better competencies than other organizations. Some organizations do a better job of combining and mobilizing the resources and competencies that they do possess in order to achieve their operational and strategic goals. This ability is at the core of most successful organizations.

It is not enough for a firm to possess an outstanding collection of resources and competencies. The firm must be capable of translating the resources and competencies into the activities required by the strategies that it intends to implement. If that is not the case, the firm must either modify its strategies or acquire the necessary resources and competencies. In the first case, the firm would reexamine what it is capable of doing and look for strategies that are possible within those constraints. Alternatively, it would choose the most optimal strategies with the understanding that it would have to hire new employees, retrain existing ones, or outsource some functions, purchase new equipment, develop new systems and processes, and combine them in ways that allow execution of the strategies.

Resources are things that are owned by a business; they may be either tangible or intangible. By themselves, they accomplish nothing. A sophisticated piece of medical imaging or laboratory research equipment, sitting idle, produces no value for the organization. A highly skilled radiologist or research scientist, employed but unoccupied, performs no strategic function. What makes a difference is what they are capable of accomplishing when they are in action or operation. This latent potential of resources constitutes a firm's competencies. A competence that is triggered is an activity. The performance of activities serve as the building blocks of an organization's operations and strategies.

Resources can be grouped in the following categories.

Tangible—visible, touchable, measurable

Financial—free cash flow, credit rating

Organizational—control and reporting systems, integrated clinical-cost management systems, service-line organizational structure

Physical—real estate, buildings, equipment, geographic location

Technological—proprietary technologies (patents, copyrights, trademarks, trade secrets)

Intangible—unseen, amorphous

Human—staff skills and experience, managerial judgment and insight, workforce morale, congenial labor-management relations, individual and organizational knowledge

Creative—innovation, problem-solving, clinical research capabilities

Perceptual—reputation with customers, suppliers, strategic partners, media, politicians, and competitors, public perceptions of specific product qualities and organizational integrity

Competencies are usually the product of combinations of resources, the most important being human resources. Examples are a person operating a piece of equipment, a person sending a report through a management control system, a person performing a patented research procedure, or several people working together to accomplish a task. Any competence with strategic potential is worth noting, preserving, building, and utilizing. An organization needs a wide variety of competencies just to conduct its day-to-day operating activities, even if they result in no more than competitive parity with its rivals. These are some examples of health care–related competencies.

- Ability to maintain low in-hospital infection rates (hospital)
- System for minimum-error dispensing of medications (hospital)
- Ability to move a drug through the Federal Drug Administration (FDA) approval process with a minimum of cost and delay (pharmaceutical company)
- High proportion of research discoveries translated into commercial products (small biomedical research firm)
- High submission rate of accurate medical claims not returned by payers (physician practice)
- Efficient scheduling of operating room procedures (hospital)
- First-mover in adopting new patient-friendly technologies like e-mail scheduling and prescription renewals (physician practice)

Synergy in the OR

A good health care example of the synergistic combining of resources and competencies is a multidisciplinary operating room (OR) team composed of physicians, nurses, and technicians. The lead physician may be a Harvard Medical School graduate and board certified, with twenty years of experience during which she has performed a particular surgical procedure hundreds of times. She is a valuable *resource* of the hospital. Her training and numerous repetitions of this and other procedures have made her highly *competent* in their performance. The benefit to the organization occurs every time that she actually performs the procedures.

Of course, the surgeon cannot carry out the procedures without the support of the other members of the OR team. Each one of them is a resource with specific competencies. They act together in carefully orchestrated unison. If the team was assembled carefully and subsequently nurtured, it may function with unique proficiency that completes procedures more quickly with clinical outcomes of higher quality. It may be hard to identify exactly what the team members do that permits them to function together so smoothly. The well-designed and equipped operating rooms help; so do the policies and procedures that are trained and enforced. This OR team is a resource with competencies that may contribute to a hard-to-duplicate competitive advantage over other hospitals.

- Effective at maintaining good relations with contracted providers (managed care organization)
- Adept at assimilating newly acquired/merged small biotech research firms (large biotech firm)

When an organization is able to develop a competence that gives it a real "competitive advantage," it is said to be a "core competence," critical to the organization's strategic success. Such competencies have two vital characteristics: (1) because they are major contributors to product costs or features that customers are willing to pay for, and because they can be used to exploit opportunities or defend threats in the external environment, they are *valuable* to the organization, and (2) because they allow the organization to perform activities that its competitors cannot, and create customer value that the competitors cannot offer, and because competitors do not possess them, the competencies are considered *unique*. Even better is the competitive advantage that can be sustained for an extended period of time. To serve as the basis of such a "sustainable competitive advantage," a competence must be difficult, expensive, or impossible for a competitor to *imitate*, and there must be no *substitutes* for it—that is, other competencies that could serve the same strategic purpose.

It would be too time consuming to compile an exhaustive list of all the resources and competencies possessed by an organization and then determine their specific competencies. They would number in the thousands or tens of thousands. There are two more selective approaches for identifying the most significant resources. A focused approach that yields useful results is to identify those resources and competencies that are strengths and weaknesses of the organization. This knowledge can inform three important categories of decisions.

1. New strategies must have their foundation in resources and competencies where the organization is strong. If a strategy depends, even inadvertently, upon areas in which the organization is weak, it is much more likely to fail.
2. A business may decide that it wishes to implement a highly advantageous strategy for which it lacks some of the appropriate resources and competencies. To permit this, it can take steps to develop or acquire them. It may accomplish this by buying specific resources, hiring new personnel with necessary skills, retraining current staff in the needed competencies, contracting with outside firms to provide the competencies, or merging with/acquiring entire businesses that already possess the desired resources and competencies.
3. If a business faces strategically aggressive competitors, it can expect that they may target its points of weakness. It can anticipate such

attacks and take steps to correct the weaknesses or minimize the damaging effects of the attacks.

This approach begins by asking key managers with knowledge of major areas of the firm's operations to identify the strongest and weakest resources and competencies within their areas of authority. It often makes sense to work with the heads of the various functional areas of the organization to come up with this information. Top management also needs to have input to this list for those resource and competence items that are organization-wide or cut across several functional areas.

Another approach is to rate the selected competencies by their degree of strength or weakness. Then, compare them with the same resources and competencies possessed by competitors. The contrasts can be highlighted through presentation in graphic formats.

Strategic Uses to Which Resources and Competencies Can Be Put

Resources and competencies are the tools that strategists have to use in carrying out their plans. It is not the number or the sophistication of a firm's resources and competencies that determines what it can accomplish, but how well the firm is able to leverage those resources to perform strategically appropriate activities. There is a variety of generic ways that a firm can manipulate and deploy its resources and competencies to maximum advantage.

Discovery. It may sound strange, but some businesses have resources and competencies that they are unaware of. Tangible resources are not likely to go unnoticed, but a firm may more easily forget about certain credentials that employees possess or intellectual property that it owns. Even more likely to be missed are unique competencies of employees, machines, or computer software. Think of a billing clerk who learned several useful nursing procedures before dropping out of nursing school, the PET scanner that has always been operated at its default medium-resolution setting, or the un-utilized coding accuracy review feature of a medical claims filing program. An organization limits its strategic possibilities by not learning about all the resources and competencies it already owns.

Creation. A business need not feel constrained by the strategy options allowed by the bundle of resources and competencies that it currently possesses. It can and must be willing to create additional assets if they will enable the implementation of strategies deemed essential to its mission and objectives. It is possible to acquire these assets by a variety of means. (See the sidebar on active management of firm resources and competencies.)

Combination. Resources and competencies have certain strategic potentials when deployed individually; they allow the performance of a great many more activities when they are used together in various combinations. Possible combinations include machines working in synchronization, human

Active Management of Firm Resources and Competencies

A firm's strategies must be matched to the strategic assets—the resources and competencies—that it has available if the strategies are to be successful. However, the firm is not restricted to the bundle of resources and competencies that it currently possesses. The firm should manage its strategic assets portfolio actively and dynamically, constantly assessing its operational and strategic requirements and taking steps to make sure that the required resources and competencies are in place when and where needed. There are several ways to accomplish this.

- Purchase the resources, which may be equipment, systems, technology, intellectual property, buildings/facilities, or real estate.
- Hire new employees with the required experience, credentials, or skill sets to interact with other resources, both nonhuman and human.
- Train and develop existing employees to have the required competencies and to perform the required activities.
- Contract with outside businesses ("outsource") to provide whatever resources and competencies are required, but that the firm cannot readily acquire or develop.
- Merge with or acquire entire organizations that already possess the desired resources or competencies.
- Enter into strategic partnerships with other organizations to share resources and competencies that each requires for its strategic purposes.

resources employing equipment and tools in different ways, people with different skill sets working in unison toward common goals, and systems being integrated with other systems and with the people who interface with them. Artful blending and balancing of a firm's assets can produce powerful new synergies that open up new strategic opportunities.

Preservation. Resources and competencies with strategic or operational value must not be allowed to degrade or disappear. It may take greater recognition or more regular use of an asset to keep it alive. A good example is a complex surgical procedure that a surgeon must perform a minimum number of times in a year if he is to remain competent in it. In addition, the value of some resources and competencies can actually be multiplied by reusing them when they may otherwise seem to be used up, by sharing them with other units in the organization, or by finding new uses for them beyond their original design.

Concentration. A very important guideline for strategic asset deployment is to use just the right resource or competence for just the right purpose at just the right point in the implementation of a strategy. This also implies using the full volume of resources or competencies necessary in a concerted effort. The value of assets can be wasted if they are dissipated or committed in inadequate amounts.

■ BREAKDOWN AND EVALUATION OF THE INTERNAL VALUE CHAIN

Because an organization ultimately aims to create and deliver value to its customers, a second useful way to describe its inner workings is as a sequential series of activities that cumulatively build value in a product or service until it is turned over to the customer. Michael Porter captured this entire process in a concept he called the "value chain." It is composed of primary activities (directly associated with the manufacture and distribution of a product) and support activities (assist in accomplishing the primary activities). His generic value chain is shown in Figure 2.1.

The value chain is based on the traditional manufacturing company model, which brings in raw materials as inputs at one end and outputs finished goods at the other end. Value chains in the health care and biotechnology fields have their own unique features. See Figures 2.2 and 2.3 for examples of value chains for a hospital and a pharmaceutical company.

Within each of the categories in these chains (inbound logistics, production, outbound logistics, sales and marketing, and service) are performed hundreds, if not thousands, of activities. Every one of them does, or should, create some small increment of value for the customer. Each activity can be performed well or poorly. In many cases, the same value could be created through the performance of a different activity. It also is possible frequently to create an entirely new form of value through the

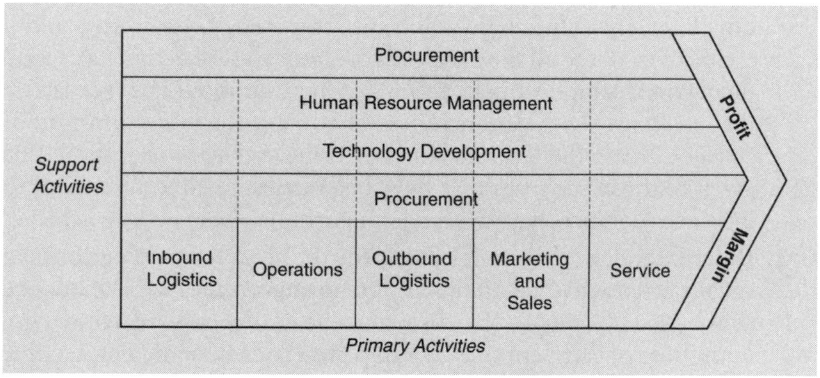

Figure 2.1 Porter's Generic Value Chain

Source: Adapted with the permission of The Free Press, a division of Simon & Schuster, Inc. © 1985, 1988 Michael E. Porter

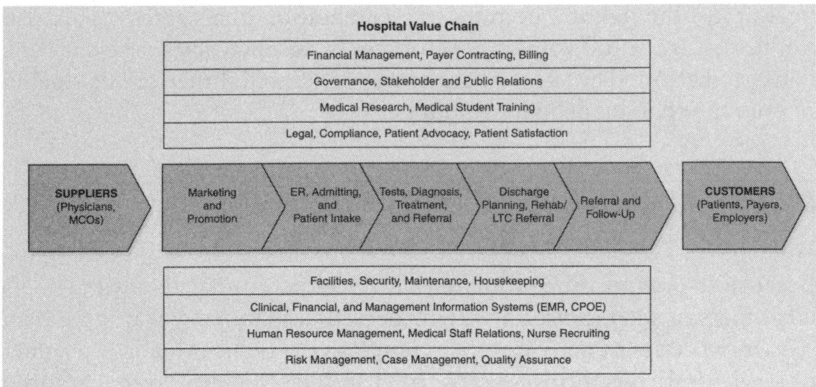

Figure 2.2 Hospital Value Chain

performance of new activities. Competitors are using their own variations of the value chain to manufacture goods and services. When a firm studies its competitors, it compares its own value chain with theirs, activity by activity. (This is discussed in more detail in Chapter 5.)

In analyzing its own value chain, a firm is looking for the points at which the most cost is incurred and the most value added. Every activity does both to some degree. No activities are free and, if they are not contributing (directly or indirectly) to product or service values, they should not be part of the value chain. The purpose of the analysis is to find opportunities for reducing costs or adding more value—in ways that the competition cannot easily copy. It is possible to describe a methodology for accomplishing this.

1. Starting with Porter's value chain model, break down the firm's operations into its component activities. A decision must be made about how finely the value chain will be decomposed. There is no point in trying to evaluate all the hundreds or thousands of activities carried on in large, complex organizations. Attention should be focused on the few, most significant activities that incur the largest portion of costs or create the largest shares of value. Special focus should be given to those activities that have been determined to be critical to whatever competitive advantage the firm has been able to achieve.
2. Describe and, where possible, quantify the actual costs of performing each selected activity. Additionally, try to identify the factors that drive those costs. Compare the costs and their drivers for each activity with those of competitors. This step presumes a competent, flexible cost accounting system. Even then, it may be difficult to isolate the cost elements associated with individual activities. Good approximations based on reasonable assumptions are still better than no

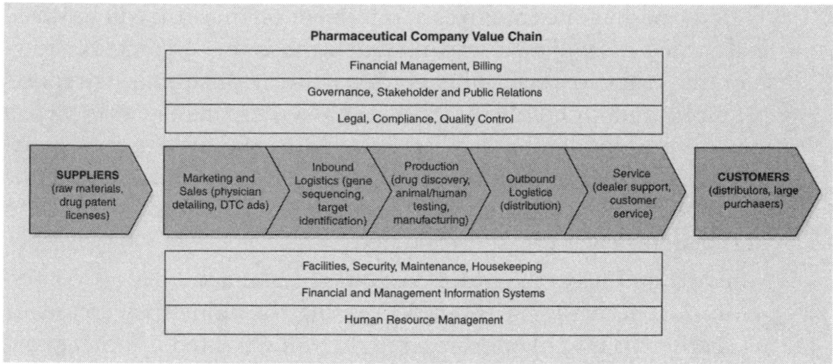

Figure 2.3 Pharmaceutical Company Value Chain

understanding at all of where and how costs are accumulating in the value chain.

3. Describe and, where possible, quantify the amount of value created by each selected activity. More daunting than measuring activity-related costs is defining the incremental value that each activity adds to the firm's services and products. To begin with, this assessment can rarely be quantitative. The value added by a claims filing clerk when she enters the Current Procedural Terminology (CPT) code for a surgical procedure in a claim to be submitted for payment is hard to quantify and is significantly different in type from the value added by the surgeon who performs the procedure. In most cases, what is needed is a clear, practical, qualitative description of the value increment. If it resists description or does not appear to be "valuable" in nature, perhaps no value is really being added.
4. In making these determinations of cost incurred and value created, be sensitive to inter-activity linkages and synergies that might be disrupted by changes in individual activities. This complicates even further the process of assigning the costs incurred and defining the value created by each activity. By failing to note the relationships and synergies among activities, the firm risks making a decision to alter or delete an activity in order to reduce costs or add more value that actually results in a disruption in the value chain, causing the costs of other activities to increase and the amount of value they add to decline.

   For instance, an employee may perform the task of gathering weekly payroll reports from several departments in an organization, doing little more than punching holes in them so they can be collected in a loose-leaf binder, and then sending the binder to top management for review. A suggestion is made to eliminate this task and have each department send its reports directly to top management.

The cost of that one employee's time spent on this task will be saved and the reports will reach top management sooner. In practice, however, the employee nagged each department to submit its reports promptly and, by combining them, enabled top managers to view a single report binder that facilitated comparisons among the departments. After the change, top management received the reports one at a time, sporadically, many of them late. The cost-control function of the reports was greatly weakened.

5. Study to find ways to reduce costs of specific activities (or combinations of activities) without decreasing the value they create, or increasing the cost of or decreasing the value created by other activities. These next two steps (5 and 6) are the primary purposes of this exercise. Assuming that no value otherwise is lost, the cost of an activity can be reduced by performing it more efficiently, performing it differently (by reengineering or redesigning the activity processes), reducing the costs of performance (reap economies of scale by increasing volume, lowering labor costs, improving productivity), replacing it with another equivalent activity, outsourcing the activity to an external contractor, or eliminating it entirely. The study and

Performing Activities Differently or Better?

There is a critical difference between performing an activity in a different way and performing it better in the existing way.

It is important to perform existing activities as best as possible, but the most that this will gain the firm is competitive parity. Competitors are often performing the activity in the same way and they will quickly imitate any efforts to do it better.

Many initiatives in health care, as in other industries, are designed to improve "operational effectiveness." Some examples are:

- Continuous quality improvement
- Pay-for-performance
- Balanced scorecard
- Benchmarking
- Practice guidelines
- Patient-centricity

None of these should be mistaken for strategies.[1] A genuine "strategy" is composed either of different activities or the same activities performed differently. Only with these types of activities is it possible (not certain, but possible) for a firm to gain an advantage over its competitors that can be sustained for an extended period of time.

reduction of activity-based costs is critical to the execution of a "low-cost leadership" strategy, as explained in Chapter 8.

6. Study to find ways to create greater value in the value chain, without disproportionately increasing costs, by either performing the same activities differently—not just better—or by performing entirely new activities, either in place of or in addition to existing activities. Because the concept of value is so amorphous, discovering ways to increase value can be especially challenging. The ability to accomplish this is particularly important for a firm pursuing a "differentiation" strategy. To maximize the cost-saving or value-adding synergy of the value chain, check to make sure that the activities are tied to each other and to activities outside the organization in an optimal configuration.

In the course of analyzing the value chain, it is useful to identify the specific resources and competencies associated with the performance of individual activities. This information tells the firm which existing resources and competencies it must work especially to protect and which new resources and competencies it needs to develop or acquire. A graphical diagram of these elements (resources, competencies, activities) and their interconnections would be a powerful display of how much organizations, especially those in health care, are complex, self-sustaining "systems." It also makes it much easier to identify points in the system that might be manipulated for strategic advantage and the effects that might have throughout the system.

The sequence in Figure 2.4 summarizes the connection between a company's resources and competencies, and its pursuit of strategic competitive advantage.

Cost reduction and value enhancement do not have to be pursued as sporadic, intermittent actions. Much of the success of Japanese manufacturers has been attributed to their practice of "kaizen"—a commitment to constant, continuous improvement of all aspects of business operations. In this case, it means regularly looking for opportunities to lower costs or create greater value. It means never being satisfied with the current level of efficiency or achievement. It is a practice that can become embedded in the organizational culture. In the dynamic health care and biotechnology industries, the rules of the game are constantly changing, creating new opportunities for improvement.

Study Questions

1. Sit down with a friend or classmate who is not studying strategic management and explain to that person the concept of "competitive advantage" until it appears that he or she understands. Do the same thing for "sustainable" competitive advantage.

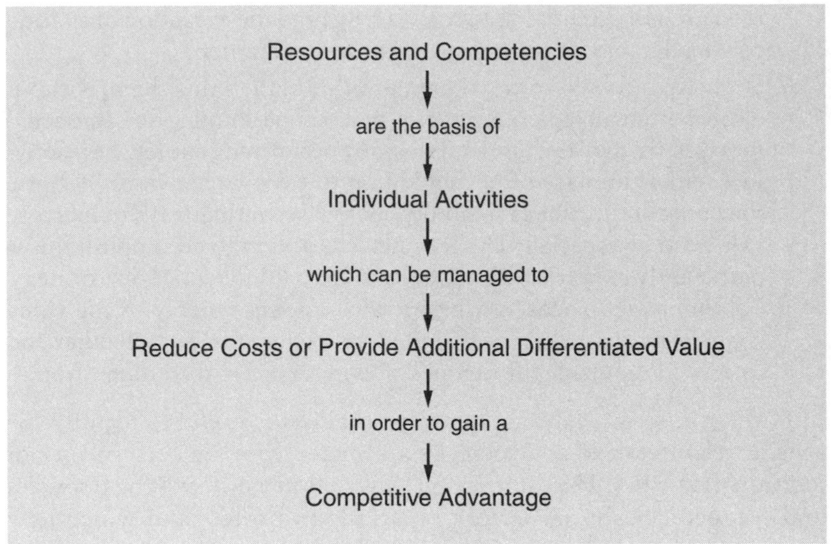

Figure 2.4 How Resources and Competencies Are Transformed into Competitive Advantage

2. What is the difference between a "resource" and a "competency"? Prepare a list of ten competencies that you possess.
3. Lay out the steps that an organization would follow in acquiring or developing a strategically important competence that it lacks. This is probably easier to do if you select a competence that a health care organization is likely to have.
4. Of what strategic value is knowledge of a firm's historic financial performance? After all, it is a record of what was accomplished in the past, which may or may not indicate what is possible in the future.
5. Every organization is a complex bundle of many competencies. How do the managers make sure that those competencies integrate well with each other, so that the result is a smoothly functioning organizational machine rather than a collection of autonomous individuals who perform their individual jobs extremely well but without much concern for the overall mission of the organization?

Learning Exercise

Identify a health care organization for which a significant amount of information is available, in books, journals, reports, or on the Internet. Conduct an audit of the organization's strategic assets. This will not be as thorough and detailed an audit as the organization itself might conduct. You will not have access to the same inside information that its managers do. Do your best to gather and report the following information.

The first part of your audit should concern the organization's historical financial performance and its current financial condition, as described in the first part of this chapter. A lot of the necessary data can be found in the organization's annual report and its filings with the Securities and Exchange Commission (SEC) and state-level government regulatory agencies. Look also at sources like business journals, magazines, and other media that report on these organizations.

The second part of the audit should describe in as much detail as possible what you consider to be the major resources and competencies of the organization. This may be more narrative than quantitatively analytical. Try to identify assets that appear to be unique to the organization and that give it some competitive advantage over its rivals. Also make a note of areas in which the organization is weak, which might be the target of strategic attacks by those rivals.

In the third part of the audit, draw a diagram of the internal value chain of the organization. You might start with one of the templates provided in this chapter and adapt it according to specific information you discover about the organization. As you are constructing the value chain, try to imagine ways in which it could be reengineered (either within its individual links or at the interface between links) to lower cost, improve quality, or otherwise differentiate the product or service that the organization is offering.

When you have completed this audit, you should be in a position to think about the types of strategies that the organization is capable of pursuing. In contrast, if you were a competitor preparing this audit, you could now use this knowledge in planning how to compete with the organization.

Notes

[1] Michael Porter does a good job of explaining this important distinction in Porter, ME. What Is Strategy? *Harvard Business Review*. Nov–Dec 1996;61–78.

References

Barney JB. Firm resources and sustained competitive advantage. *Journal of Management*. 1991(17):99–120.

Barney JB. The resource-based theory of the firm. *Organizational Science*.1996;7:469.

Barney JB. Is the resource-based view a useful perspective for strategic management research? Yes. *Academy of Management Review*. 2001;26(1):41–56.

Collis DJ. Research note: How valuable are organizational capabilities? *Strategic Management Journal*. Winter 1994;143–152.

De Carolis DM. Competencies and imitability in the pharmaceutical industry: An analysis of their relationship with firm performance. *Journal of Management.* 2003;29:27–50.

Dees DL, De Carolis DM, and Coombs J. Dynamic capabilities and new product development in high-technology ventures: An empirical analysis of new biotechnology firms. *Journal of Business Venturing*. 2000;15:211–229.

Douglas TJ and Ryman JA. Understanding competitive advantage in the general hospital industry: Evaluating strategic competencies. *Strategic Management Journal*. 2003(24):333–347.

Goes JB and Park SH. Inter-organizational links and innovation: The case of hospital services. *Academy of Management Journal*. 1997;40:673–696.

Govindarajan V. Implementing competitive strategies at the business unit level: Implications of matching managers to strategies. *Strategic Management Journal*. 1989;10:251–269.

Grant RM. The resource-based theory of competitive advantage: Implications for strategy formulation. *California Management Review*. Spring 1991;114–135.

Hamel G and Prahalad CK. Strategic intent. *Harvard Business Review*. 1989;67(3):63–76.

Hamel G and Prahalad CK. The core competence of the corporation. *Harvard Business Review*. 1990;68(3):79–91.

Hawawini G, Subramanian V, and Verdin P. Is performance driven by industry or firm specific factors? A new look at the evidence. *Strategic Management Journal*. 2003;24(1):1–16.

Helfat CE and Peteraf MA. The dynamic resource-based view: Capability lifecycles. *Strategic Management Journal*. October 2003;997–1010.

Hitt MA and Ireland RD. Relationships among corporate level distinctive competencies, diversification strategy, corporate structure, and performance. *Journal of Management Studies*. 1986(23):401–416.

McGahan A and Porter ME. How much does industry matter, really? *Strategic Management Journal*. 1997;18(special issue):15–30.

Peteraf MA. The cornerstones of competitive advantage: A resource-based view. *Strategic Management Journal*. 1993;14(3):179–192.

Porter ME. The value chain and competitive advantage. Chapter 2. *Competitive Advantage: Creating and Sustaining Superior Performance*. New York, NY: The Free Press; 1985:33–61.

Prahalad CK and Hamel G. The core competence of the corporation. *Harvard Business Review*. May–June 1990;79–91.

Rumelt RP. How much does industry matter? *Strategic Management Journal*. 1991;12(3):167–186.

Senge PM. The leader's new work: Building learning organizations. *Sloan Management Review*. Fall 1990;32(1):7–24.

Wernerfelt B. A resource-based view of the firm. *Strategic Management Journal*. 1984;5(2):171–180.

West GP and DeCastro J. The Achilles heel of firm strategy: Resource weaknesses and distinctive inadequacies. *Journal of Management Studies*. 2001;38:417–442.

CHAPTER

3

External Environmental Assessment: Law, Economics, Demographics, Technology

Learning Objectives

After reading and studying this chapter, you should be able to:

- Appreciate that an organization is both a system unto itself and a component in a much larger system of its external environment.
- Understand that the external environment is composed of a firm's market and customers, its industry and competitors, and general environmental factors like demographics, economics, politics, and technology.
- List the benefits that an organization enjoys by conducting an assessment of its general environmental factors.
- Explain why some organizations have difficulty carrying out such assessments.
- Describe in detail the steps in the process for conducting an external environmental assessment.
- List the basic categories of external environmental factors in the health care and biotechnology industries.
- Identify examples of the factors in each of those categories.
- Understand how those factors are not isolated, but rather interact with and upon each other.

- List the wide variety of sources of information on external environmental factors.
- Describe some strategic uses to which external environmental information might be put.

Most people have no trouble understanding that a business organization is a "system" made up of parts that interact with each other to create the goods and services that it offers to the outside world. But it is more than that. The organization does not exist and function in isolation. It is an "open system" that is linked unconditionally to virtually every aspect and element of that outside world. Events occur in the organization's external environment that affect the organization's plans and actions. Simultaneously, the organization's activities can impact the external environment. The interplay is constant, pervasive, and usually unnoticed. Furthermore, events in one part of the system, whether internal or external, may be separated by time and distance from other parts, with the result that a small catalytic event can produce a much delayed and greatly magnified effect at distant points in the system.

To recognize all this is to engage in "systems thinking." This type of thinking is essential to effective strategic management.

The external environment is the arena where a business's strategies are played out. In that environment, there are forces that enhance the chances of strategic success, other forces that may hinder them, and still others directly opposed to an organization's strategies. It also is in that external environment that opportunities can be found to be explored as well as threats that must be countered. Finally, those conditions external to the corporation are constantly evolving. For all these reasons, strategies cannot be formulated and implemented without a deep, sophisticated understanding of the external environment.

For strategic planning purposes, a firm's external environment can be considered to be made up of three components. One component is the industry (or industries) in which the firm is active and the competing firms that it must deal with there. The industry and competitors are examined in Chapter 5. Another component is the market (or markets) to which the firm is trying to sell its products and services and the customers who make purchases there. The market and customers are examined in Chapter 4. The third component consists of all the other general environmental forces that may influence the firm's choice of strategies and how successfully it is able to implement them. Some examples are demographics, legal developments, new technologies, and sociocultural trends. These forces are the subject of this chapter.

The process by which a firm examines its environment for strategic purposes goes under different names. It may be called assessment, analysis, monitoring, or scanning. The last two terms suggest the importance of paying continuous attention to the environment, monitoring or scanning it on an ongoing basis rather than conducting occasional one-time examinations.

STRATEGIC BENEFITS OF A GENERAL EXTERNAL ENVIRONMENTAL ASSESSMENT

It is possible to point to specific strategic benefits that come from a firm's assessment of its general external environment. The most obvious reason for devoting the resources to gathering and assessing all this information about the external environment is that it enables strategic plans that are more responsive to that environment and likely to be implemented successfully. Through the assessment, the firm acquires knowledge that informs the decisions that managers make about strategy planning and implementation, knowledge pertaining to the setting in which their strategies will succeed or fail. It has the potential to provide "early warning" of positive and negative environmental changes, enabling managers to exploit the positives and resist or avoid the negatives. The assessment may identify resources in the general environment that the firm may be able to employ in carrying out its strategies. If the organization has the mind and the resources to do it, it can use the information to plot ways to actively influence specific components of the external environment. One way of looking at it is that the assessment process allows an organization to align itself with its environment. The net result is likely to be superior firm performance.[1]

DIFFICULTIES IN CONDUCTING A GENERAL EXTERNAL ENVIRONMENTAL ASSESSMENT

There are some challenges in creating a system for regularly assessing the general external environment. The volume of potentially relevant information can be overwhelming, particularly if an expansive "open system" view is taken of the firm. Tracking all the organizations, people, trends, and forces that might impact the firm could consume immense amounts of time, money, and energy. The business must be selective in carrying out this important function. The first time that an organization performs an assessment, it should be broad in scope, covering as much ground as possible. After digesting the mass of data acquired and discussing their strategic implications with key managers, specific topics and sectors of the environment can be selected for continual, intensive monitoring. Less-relevant environmental factors can be assessed less frequently or not at all.

The value of an environmental assessment process depends greatly on how quickly that environment is evolving. If a firm's monitoring system produces a review for top management twice a year, it may be reporting on new legislation that was enacted five months ago. It is necessary to strike a balance between the investment that the firm is willing to make in an ongoing assessment process and the usefulness of its results to the formulation and management of strategy.

In attempting to determine what the general environment is doing and where it is headed, a firm is likely to make forecasts and project trends. Although the science of prognostication has become quite sophisticated, it still is impossible to know the future with certainty. This should be kept in mind when interpreting the output of an environmental assessment.

These are some specific reasons or problems why a business might not be able to perform the kind of environmental assessment that it should have.

Problem: The business lacks the expertise to conduct a good environmental assessment.

Solution: It should do the best it can now and take steps to gradually acquire higher level expertise.

Problem: The business does not have sufficient resources (people, money) to dedicate to environmental assessment.

Solution: Even a minimal effort—one person spending a couple hours a week finding and reviewing a few key data—could contribute to a better understanding of the external environment. As the data are used to plan strategies that grow the company, more resources will become available for an expanded assessment effort.

Problem: Conditions in the environment are changing too rapidly for the business to keep up.

Solution: It is better to learn about events and trends a little bit late than to never hear about them at all.

■ STEP-BY-STEP PROCESS FOR ASSESSING THE GENERAL EXTERNAL ENVIRONMENT

Keeping a steady eye on the external environment is so important to the strategic management process that a firm needs to dedicate resources permanently to the process. A formal environment assessment system should be instituted. The responsibility for the information-gathering tasks, the analysis of the raw data received, and communicating the conclusions to the appropriate managers should be assigned to specific individuals. Depending on the size of the organization, this may be the work for just part of a single full-time employee or for two or three people in a dedicated unit. They will be backed up with sufficient funding for the scope of the job.

A good process will follow these steps:

- The process begins by identifying the environmental forces that may have some impact—positive or negative—on the organization or business. The strength of the impact may be weak at the moment, but it may change in the future. Managers throughout the organization can suggest factors that should be watched. The first listing should be as comprehensive as possible; it can be pruned later.
- In addition to basic forces in the general environment, critical issues specific to the organization, its industry, and its customers are identified. These are issues that implicate a variety of different environmental factors. For instance, the movement toward "consumer-driven health care" grows out of the continuing increase in national health care costs, the apparent desire of consumers for a greater role in choosing their health care, the apparent desire of employers to offload some of their responsibility for financing health care, and the notion that consumers will adopt healthier lifestyles if they have to pay for the consequences when they do not.
- A rough analysis is made of the possible impact of the numerous forces and issues identified on the organization's strategic plans. The analysis needs to be only deep enough to enable a selection of those to which the organization will pay attention.
- A manageable number of environmental categories, forces, factors, and issues are selected for close, systematic monitoring. These factors will be the ones that appear to be changing most rapidly or are deemed to pose the greatest threat or offer the greatest opportunity to the organization.
- It is important at this point to determine the information sources that will be consulted on each of the environmental forces and issues. There is little value in trying to monitor an item for which reliable data are not available.
- If the organization has never performed an environmental assessment before, it will conduct an initial appraisal to establish a baseline of knowledge. This step includes creating a description of the current position and status of the forces.
- Using the information gathered, the organization also endeavors to forecast future directions, trends, and changes in the selected factors and issues. It further attempts to gauge the pace at which the change is taking place.

- The next critical step is to estimate the specific impact that those forces—changing in the directions and at the paces projected—are likely to have on the organization at particular points in the future.
- Those estimated effects then must be translated into practical implications for the organization. If events transpire as projected, exactly what new actions will the organization consider taking? What new strategies should be adopted, and what existing strategies should be modified?
- The data-gathering system will also include rules on which managers should receive alerts about new developments in various categories of the general environment. The information must be passed on to persons in a position to take action on it.
- In some cases, the firm may wish to establish "trigger points" in environmental trends at which specified action will be taken. For instance, when the percentage of physician practices in the local market that have installed EMR systems reaches 20 percent, the firm (an HMO) will issue an interoperability standard for all its participating physicians and offer incentives for them also to install such systems. Or, if the federal government removes its moratorium on the establishment of specialty hospitals, the firm (a group practice of cardiac surgeons) will immediately meet with an identified developer to explore establishing such a hospital specializing in cardiac surgery.

BASIC CATEGORIES OF EXTERNAL ENVIRONMENTAL FACTORS AND FORCES IN HEALTH CARE AND BIOTECHNOLOGY

An organization's external environment can be best understood by breaking it down into several basic categories, and then identifying the individual factors within each. The relevant environmental factors depend on the firm's mission, the industries in which it competes, the markets in which it sells, and the types of strategies that it is pursuing. The following environmental factors pertain to organizations in health care and biotechnology.

Political/Government

This sector of the environment encompasses government agencies (both regulatory and financing), career administrative bureaucrats, politicians (in legislative and executive positions), and their policies and decisions, at the federal, state, and local levels. Specific areas of health care–related interest in this sector are:

Specific election results. Before the election, the firm will have studied the candidates' positions on issues of relevance to the firm. It will notice their political platforms, and their prior experience in the legislature and in the industry. The election results will provide a small indication of the likelihood for new legislation that is favorable or unfavorable to the firm's strategies. The firm will pay attention to not only individual candidates but also the general ideological tenor of the legislative body.

Specific politicians elected to or voted out of office. It is important to continue following politicians after they have been elected. Their public pronouncements, the bills they introduce or sponsor, and their policy positions will offer greater insight into their potential to influence, positively or negatively, issues of significance to the firm.

Political ideological mood of the country, or the local area. This information offers subtle signs of the direction of the public's thinking on issues of interest to the firm. It typically will be discovered by reviewing election outcomes (on candidates and referenda), examining public opinion survey results, and reading media and journal articles interpreting both elections and polling surveys. The 1990s brought growing reports of consumer impatience with the constraints of managed care. State legislatures responded with statutory prohibitions against certain practices (e.g., physician gag clauses) and certain mandatory treatment terms (e.g., minimum-length hospital maternity stays). The continuing indications that consumers wanted a greater role in choosing among health plans, providers, and procedures has been a contributing factor in the development of "consumer-driven health care."

Opportunities for lobbying. To help decide whether it wishes to try to directly influence the political process as it applies to the firm's strategic objectives, a firm will want to know which legislators sit on committees addressing issues important to the firm and their openness to conversations with the firm about those issues. The firm may be the member of an industry association that engages in lobbying efforts, in which case it may want to follow and comment upon its specific initiatives.

Chief executives' and agency heads' positions and announcements on key industry-related issues. The statements made by mayors, governors, the president, and the heads of key agencies are strong indications of the programs and policies to which they will lend their support. These pronouncements from the residents of such high offices can also steer public opinion and lead the policy debates on key issues.

Government spending, generally and specifically. Total spending by government, particularly at the federal level, can have a powerful impact on the overall state of the economy. It can drive economic expansion and growth, or stimulate a moderation in economic activity. Specific budget line items can have a more immediate effect on the firm. The level of funding for the CMS or the NIH can create palpable opportunities or threats for health plans and provider organizations, and for biotechnology firms, respectively.

Government policies on health and research-related matters. Apart from actual budget appropriations, administrative decisions by government agencies (coming out of the agencies' policies and practices) will be of concern to health care and biotechnology firms and organizations. The power of the purse wielded by the CMS allows it to dictate many conditions of practice to the providers participating in the Medicare program. These conditions include data collection and reporting requirements, relationships with other providers to whom patients are referred, and procedures for submitting claims, among others. State Medicaid agencies have a similar authority over their providers.

Vigor of government's regulatory role. Several government agencies are responsible for enforcing laws and regulations that apply to the health care industry. The Antitrust Division of the U.S. Department of Justice applies several antitrust acts to the mergers, acquisitions, and general competitive behavior of health care organizations. The Office of the Inspector General in the Department of Health and Human Services enforces several laws on fraud and abuse against the same entities. Depending often on the ideological bent of the current administration, these and other regulatory agencies may vary in the aggressiveness with which they pursue offenders. The Food and Drug Administration is responsible for ensuring the safety and efficacy of pharmaceuticals and medical devices. In the past decade, it has taken steps to streamline and speed up its drug approval process and to loosen the restrictions on "direct-to-consumer" advertising by drug companies.

Government role in addressing critical societal challenges. The general philosophy of government leaders toward the appropriate role of the government in satisfying key societal needs can vary from one political party to another and from one country to another. A good example is the generally acknowledged value of developing a uniform, nationwide electronic health record (EHR) system. Several years ago in the United Kingdom, this need was recognized, agreement was reached on the standards for such a system, and the central government allocated funds to enable every provider to install the necessary hardware and software. Virtually every physician in the United Kingdom now is connected to the national EHR network. In the United States, the federal government began debating the issue several years ago and its primary overt action has been to create a commission that will disseminate interoperability criteria for an EHR system, leaving it up to private sector initiatives to acquire and install the system with its individual provider interfaces. Currently, approximately one-fifth of U.S. physicians have some kind of EHR capability.

Media reports. Reports in the television and print media can be motivators of public opinion and a call to legislative action. In 1987, national media attention focused on the efforts of the parents of Cody Howard, a seven-year-old Oregon boy with leukemia, to raise $100,000 for a bone marrow transplant. The state Medicaid program had previously announced that it would not cover bone marrow and other types of transplants. Howard's parents were $20,000 short of their goal when he died. The controversy over the procedure coverage rules led to the creation in 1991 of the groundbreaking Oregon health care rationing experiment.

Legal

Perhaps no other industry is so closely constrained by the legal system as health care and its related industries (i.e., insurance, pharmaceuticals). For these purposes, the term "legal system" includes laws or statutes, regulations, administrative rulings, and court decisions interpreting and applying all these legal authorities. This category should also include subtle forms of political/moral suasion that politicians at all levels may try to exert on an organization. The general political climate can influence all of these forces.

Events and decisions in these areas can expose businesses to greater or lesser regulation, present them with higher or lower levels of legal risk, increase or decrease public sources of reimbursement (Medicare, Medicaid) or funding (NIH), require substantial new investments in projects (e.g., HIPAA compliance), raise or lower the organization's taxes, or put competitors at an advantage or a disadvantage vis-à-vis the business. Because political and legal issues are fully in the public domain, there is relatively little difficulty for a business to stay informed about them.

Existing laws. Most health care organizations (HCOs) employ or retain attorneys whose responsibilities include understanding the laws that apply to the organizations and the specific situations that they face. These laws encompass a wide range of general coverage laws in the areas of income tax, insurance, and antitrust, as well as a growing body of laws specific to health care, such as fraud and abuse, self-referral, anti-kickback, and medical malpractice. In addition, when HCOs seek reimbursement for their services from payers, both public (Medicare, Medicaid) and private (insurance companies, managed care organizations), they subject themselves to further comprehensive laws, regulations, and contract terms. Legal developments in these areas must be followed at all relevant levels—national, state, county, and municipal.

Numerous strategies are directly affected by these laws. When a corporation attempts to integrate horizontally by acquiring new businesses similar to those it already owns, it must anticipate antitrust limits on its growing market dominance. Strategic plans to collaborate with other businesses in the industry may appear to restrain competition illegally in a variety of ways. Major tax-exempt status considerations come up when a for-profit business seeks to acquire nonprofit entities, as when for-profit Wellpoint began buying and converting several nonprofit Blue Cross/Blue Shield organizations.

Among the most critical laws affecting the operations and strategies of MCOs, hospitals, and physician practices are the budget appropriation laws enacted by the federal congress and the fifty state legislatures to fund the Medicare and Medicaid programs. Reimbursements from these payer programs are the primary source of revenue for many health care providers.

New laws. As the U.S. health care system continues to evolve and transform, the existing legal climate continually adapts. Alert businesses pay attention to proposals for new laws and modifications to existing laws. They follow closely bills that are under consideration by legislative bodies and regulations proposed for adoption by government agencies. It can be just as important to notice when a lawsuit has been filed (not necessarily involving the organization itself) that may conclude with precedents that favor or harm the organization.

Changes in Medicare/Medicaid reimbursement rates can dramatically affect the financial strength and strategic options of health care providers. The amount and disease focus of appropriations for the National Institutes of Health can create opportunities for new ventures in whole new fields of biotechnology or remove the financial underpinnings from existing biomedical research firms. The sudden emergence recently of state-level universal health care coverage bills has the potential to reshape the health care industry. The proposals for national universal coverage coming from candidates for the next presidential election could have even more far-reaching effects.

Profession/Industry

A great many associations represent participants in the health care industry. In general, there are those representing the people, professional and nonprofessional, who work in the industry, and those that represent the organizations, companies, and other entities that operate within the industry.

Professional associations. These include the American Medical Association, numerous physician specialty societies, the American Nursing Association and its local chapters, and the groups that act on behalf of the variety of nonclinical specialists that work in health care. A few examples of the professional groups represented by one type of association or another: Alliance of Claims Assistance Professionals, American Academy of Physician Assistants, American Academy of Procedural Coders, American Association of Medical Billers, American College of Healthcare Information Administrators, Association of Cancer Executives, Association of Operating Room Nurses, and National Association of Health Unit Coordinators. In addition to the nursing associations that frequently engage in collective bargaining, there are also the unions formally representing other job categories in hospitals and other provider organizations.

Industry trade associations. Leading examples of a health care–related trade group are the American Hospital Association (AHA), the Medical Group Management Association (MGMA), and the Pharmaceutical Research and Manufacturers of America (PhRMA). Almost every other definable subset of organizations that operate within health care has created its own association to represent its interests.

One of the primary functions of these associations, acting on behalf of their members, is to formulate and promote an agenda that advances their interests. This may involve gathering data, adopting and publicizing policy positions, making specific proposals for new policies and programs, bringing class action lawsuits, and, perhaps most significantly, lobbying legislators regarding bills before the congress or state legislatures that affect their members.

A firm is interested in the positions and activities of these associations for several reasons.

- These associations represent collectively individuals whom the firm either employs or deals with as independent contractors.
- They represent businesses that are the firm's suppliers or customers.
- They represent businesses that are the firm's direct or indirect competitors. In fact, the firm may itself be a member of the same association—which raises some interesting questions. Membership may allow the firm to acquire useful information about its competitors, which of course can do the same thing about the firm. The firm also may have disagreements with the competitors about which association positions and activities serve its interests best.

The associations themselves do not engage in any activities that help or hinder an organization's strategic ambitions. It is the policy positions they adopt, particularly if they are backed up by aggressive, successful lobbying, that could have a powerful impact on the organization. For that reason, the activities and announcements are watched closely.

Economic (global, national, regional)

The kinds of data covered in an economic assessment include a variety of parameters that can affect a firm's strategic planning in several different ways.

Interest rates. National interest rates are a direct indicator of how much a business will have to pay to obtain the capital it needs to finance its strategic plans. This is especially important information for not-for-profit entities, like hospitals, that rely on bond issues and bank loans for the majority of their capital requirements.

Stock market prices. Publicly traded for-profit companies are also interested in the receptivity of the stock markets to efforts of companies to raise additional capital through the issuance of stock. A critical moment for many young startup companies, such as those in the biotechnology industry, is the timing of their initial public offering (IPO) and the prices at which their shares can be sold.

Venture capital deals. As a major source of seed capital for startups or subsequent early-stage financing, venture capital firms bear watching; the size of the pools of money that they have to reinvest and the risks that they are willing to assume in making those investments wax and wane. These firms tend to follow the general state of the economy as measured by interest rates and stock market prices.

Government budget deficit or surplus. At the national and state levels, budget deficit or surplus is an important indicator of the funding that will likely be available for public reimbursement programs (Medicare, Medicaid) and research programs (NIH).

Inflation rates. The rate at which the purchasing power of money is declining can affect an organization's strategic thinking in several ways. If the prices of the inputs to the firm's value chain increase, it may be necessary to raise the prices for its products or services. The input price rises may include wage and salary increases that must be granted to employees to permit their incomes to keep pace with inflation. The increasing prices for all goods and services may leave consumers with less discretionary income to spend on the firm's products.

Consumer income, disposable income, and debt. Whether affected by inflation or not, absolute income levels of consumers will determine the funds they have available for spending on the firm's products. Personal tax rates and debt levels must be taken into account in establishing how much of that income will be disposable.

Employment/unemployment levels. The ability of people to find compensable work determines their income levels and their anxiety about spending money. The state of the job market also has a bearing on the firm's ability to hire the staff that it needs, particularly for strategic initiatives.

Economic trend impacts. The movements in these various economic metrics do not always affect all parts of the country and population equally. Employers in particular industries, certain demographic groups, and specific geographic areas may bear the effects more than others. The firm will want to know which of those are related to its operations and strategic plans.

Tax rates. Corporate income tax rates have a direct effect on the financial capital available to businesses for their strategic initiatives. They simultaneously have a similar, but opposite effect on the funds available to public agencies. When corporations are taxed at higher rates, more money is subtracted from their bottom lines and added to the general revenues of the government taxing entity. Tax levels are frequent subjects of public debate and legislative manipulation. It is worth paying attention to the possibility of imminent changes, either up or down.

Economic cycle stage (boom versus recession). Many of these economic indicators are connected in different ways with the stage of the overall economy in its up-and-down cycle. It is sometimes possible for skilled economic forecasters to make judgments about whether the economy is expanding or contracting, and prices rising or falling and at what speed.

Global economic metrics. Historically, economic conditions in other countries seemed unrelated to operations and strategies within the U.S. health care industry. That situation is changing rapidly. All large pharmaceutical companies sell their products in every possible national market. Some of them are actually international companies based outside the United States. Physicians, hospitals, health plans, and other care providers must be sensitive to the small but rapidly growing number of patients willing to travel to other countries to obtain health care services. The time is not far away when major U.S. teaching hospitals will have to consider Bumrungrad International Hospital in Bangkok as a significant competitor. When the market for health care services becomes truly international, health care entities everywhere will have to be concerned with economic conditions and currency exchange rates in any countries that might be a source of customers.

A good example of the strategic implications of these economic forces concerns their effects on how much income prospective customers will have to spend on goods and services, which ones they will choose to buy, and how much they are willing to spend. Historically, this has not been a major factor in health care spending. When people suffer trauma or illness, the necessary medical treatment is not optional and, in most cases, the patient does not pay any or most of the cost. Of course, some health care purchases are discretionary—cosmetic surgery and legitimate physical and mental performance-enhancing products, for example. This convention may change with the expansion of "consumer-driven health care" that expects consumers of health care to spend more of their own money in the process. Already there is some evidence that consumers limit their spending when some of the money comes out of their own pockets.

Sociocultural

This environmental category encompasses a broad mix of some softer, more subjective characteristics of important people in an organization's external environment. The characteristics include traditions, lifestyles, values, ideals, aspirations, principles, sense of ethics, attitudes, beliefs, opinions, tastes, political views, and behavioral patterns; the people include immediate customers, prospective customers, influencers of those customers, end users, suppliers, shareholders, bondholders, lenders, government regulators, politicians, media, general public, and other stakeholders.

These qualities affect the way people make decisions about spending their money and the products they desire, the way they live their lives and the effect that may have on their personal health and need for health care services, the features that they require in the products and services they buy, where and how they are willing to make purchases, and the criteria by which they judge the vendors of goods and services. Identifying these characteristics may give indications of the willingness of investors to buy the firm's bonds, or the inclination of legislators to enact new laws either favoring or penalizing the firm. These attributes may also affect the attitude of media in their reporting and government officials in their administrative decisions. The firm's reputation and brand image can turn on factors like these.

Characteristics that can be objectively measured are powerful tools in planning strategies custom-tailored to the world around the firm. Figuring out how to measure them is the challenge. These variables are not subject to easy quantification. They normally require regular attention to very subjective, amorphous information sources and writings. The conduct of periodic and expensive surveys is one method of staying on top of these trends. Increasingly, surveys on topics like these are being conducted by polling services and other entities that often make the results available either for free or for a price.

A major factor to consider is the lifestyle that people follow. People who live more sedentary lives, get less exercise, and eat more fattening, less nutritional diets have poorer health status and are at greater risk of diseases like obesity, diabetes, cancer, and cardiac complications. As people become busier, with more demands on their time, they want their shopping experiences to be speeded up and streamlined, they don't want to travel far to buy products/services, and they don't want to wait once they get there. Customers are increasingly comfortable with technology applications throughout their lives and are willing to shop electronically. As consumers, they are more sophisticated and curious, seeking greater access to information about the products and services they purchase.

Another important cultural element is the attitudes and values that people manifest in their lives, often based on religion and other ideologies. Such values can show up in the health care field around issues like abortion, faith-based healing, consumer activism, and even assertiveness in dealing with authority figures.

In the not-so-distant past, consumers of health care services were relatively passive about the health plans and providers from whom they received those services. However, they generally expected that the costs would be covered by their health plan and that the health plan premiums would be paid for by their employers or a government program like Medicare or Medicaid. Those attitudes about the consumer's role in the health care delivery process are changing dramatically. Many have come to believe that they should be able to make the decisions about plans and providers, and even specific medical procedures and products. They are also coming to accept that they will have a share of the financial responsibility for their health care purchases. This nearly 180-degree turnabout in customer attitudes requires significant changes in the strategic assumptions of the health care industry about those customers.

The market for health care services ebbs and flows with changes in the social and geographic mobility of customers. As people move up and down between social strata, their income levels change, their lifestyles change, and so too do their attitudes about health and fitness. They may be less in need of certain types of health care goods and services and more interested in buying others. Significant numbers of citizens also move regularly to live and work in different parts of the country. Although this may or may not change their preferences for health care goods and services, it certainly increases the size of the market in one area while decreasing it in another. By tracking relocation trends, businesses can detect emerging and declining geographic markets.

The employees that an organization hires to carry out its strategies have unique career expectations and work ethics that have a tendency to change from generation to generation. It is still best to treat employees as unique individuals, but it also is a good idea to notice general trends in the work-related values of different age groups and adjust accordingly.

The United States is rather quickly becoming a multicultural, multilingual society. The language dimension has an impact on an organization's employees and customers that is in some ways complementary. Customers whose first language is other than English frequently feel more comfortable receiving as sensitive a service as health care from providers who can communicate with them in that language. To satisfy that preference, a savvy organization hires employees with the appropriate language skills.

Demographics

Related to the sociocultural factors just discussed, demographics are data describing personal characteristics of the population of consumers to which the firm is selling, either directly—as with a hospital or MCO—or indirectly through a distribution channel—as with a biotechnology or pharmaceutical company. These data include the gender, age, income levels, ethnicity, race, education, family size and composition, geographic place of residence, employment status, birth rates, and life expectancies. Many of these variables define market segments that have unique needs, wants, and preferences, which in turn demand different strategic approaches.

Firms selling goods or services at the retail level (i.e., all varieties of health care providers) will use these data to understand and serve their existing customers better, and to plan strategies for pursuing new customers. The trends in these demographic data may be viewed as opportunities to be exploited or threats to be avoided. They may reveal new market segments opening up that the firm may wish to target. They may show that one of the firm's most significant current customer groups is shrinking, requiring some sort of compensating strategic action. Changes in predominant places of customers' residence may suggest the value of opening new satellite locations for the business.

The bulk of these data are gathered quite effectively by the U.S. Census Bureau, which makes them available for free. More focused sets of demographic data or integrated data analyses, such as education and income levels within particular ethnic groups, are available from private sources or may be prepared by an organization itself.

Technology

Higher-technology solutions have become so pervasive throughout the U.S. economy, and most particularly in the health care sector, that any competitive business must take them into account in planning its strategies. This is a particularly critical time for organizations in the health care industry to think about the role of technology in their operations. New technology shows up in almost every phase of health care service delivery.

- New capabilities, equipment, and systems in clinical treatment and procedure technologies, including biotechnology and biomedicine. Primary examples are pharmaceuticals, medical devices, diagnostic tests, surgical procedures, and treatment regimens. It has been estimated that new clinical technologies account for roughly one-third of the annual increases in the national health care budget.
- New capabilities, equipment, and systems in researching and developing the clinical technologies just mentioned. These include new equipment for carrying out lab work and the new knowledge of human system functioning that underlies much current research. For large drug companies and small biotechnology startups, the research and development of clinical technologies is the essence of what they do.
- New capabilities, equipment, and systems for gathering, recording, and communicating clinical data that inform both current treatments and research of future treatments. Some examples are EMR, EHR, and CPOE systems. There is a growing national consensus that the health care industry must deploy, sooner or later, an electronic medical record system covering all citizens and linking all health care organizations.
- New capabilities, equipment, and systems for gathering and disseminating a range of nonclinical information, such as that dealing with costs, quality, satisfaction, and communication of patient conditions, test results, and physician orders.

Disruptive Technologies/Innovation

Most technological research and development follows a predictable, incremental path that improves the performance of established products along dimensions that mainstream customers in major markets have historically valued and demanded. This phenomenon is referred to as "sustaining" innovation. Clayton Christensen has introduced the concept of "disruptive" innovation that presents to the customer a combination of values and costs that she was not expecting or asking for.[2] Such innovation has the effect of disrupting the competitive equilibrium in that particular market. The innovation can occur not only in the products and services sold but also in the methods by which they are created, promoted, and distributed.

- Other useful technology-related information is the volume of public and private investment in medical research and development (R&D) and the focus of that funding, and the numbers and nature of patent filings that result.

For hospitals, physician practices, and managed care organizations, the clinical and information technologies are items that they must assess and decide whether to adopt. The challenge for them is finding the money to pay for all these sought-after technologies. From the viewpoint of researchers, entrepreneurs, and vendors who discover and sell these technologies, they represent opportunities for creating new businesses or expanding existing ones.

INTERDEPENDENCIES AMONG EXTERNAL ENVIRONMENTAL FACTORS

Once an organization has established a system for regularly gathering data on a variety of external environmental factors, its analysis of the data must include a study of the way that different data items affect each other. Trends in demographics, technology, economics, and sociocultural factors do not proceed in isolation. For instance, as the baby boomer generation enters its retirement years, it leaves behind a relatively smaller group of younger people in their income-producing years, resulting in proportionately lower tax revenues to support growing Medicare expenditures. Technological innovations over the past two decades (computer gaming; Internet surfing; large-screen, high-definition television sets) have led to more sedentary lifestyles for many citizens.

Pinpointing these interdependencies is challenging. One approach is to look at the individual factors themselves and ask the questions, "How is this factor likely to impact specific other factors?" and "How is this factor likely to be impacted by specific other factors?" Eventually, so many different possible links among all the factors are identified that it makes sense to look at them in one large interrelated bundle. A popular way to approach this is through scenario prediction. A "scenario" is an informed speculative description of a business's external environment, encompassing all relevant factors, at some point in the future. Normally, several alternative possible scenarios are described—usually a very optimistic scenario, a more conservative scenario, and a most likely scenario.

As the future unfolds, the firm will notice which assumptions and trends are proving accurate and which are not. In an iterative process, it will constantly rethink and reshape its expectations about the future external environment. Perhaps the greatest value to the business of its effort to assess the external environment lies not in the accuracy of the projections or scenarios but in the enhanced understanding of the external forces and their possible effects on the business's strategies.

INFORMATION SOURCES FOR EXTERNAL ENVIRONMENT ASSESSMENT

There is a great variety of sources of information on the external environment in which a firm operates. Many of them probably overlap with the sources already being consulted in the firm's competitive intelligence and market research programs. In fact, it may make efficiency sense to combine them, in some fashion, in a single, comprehensive, and ongoing data-gathering effort. Although many of the sources are public and free, some organizations charge fees for access to what is often the most useful information. These are some of the most common sources available.

- Newspaper clipping services
- Automated searches of both general-purpose and narrow-focus Web sites on the Internet, which include both traditional news media with Web sites (newspapers, magazines, radio/television) and Web-only news media
- Charitable research foundations
- Think tanks
- Consulting firms
- Government agencies
- Legal research databases (Lexis-Nexis, Westlaw)
- Journals, magazines, periodicals
- Trade and professional associations
- Published survey results

It should be emphasized that data collection by a business in a competitive industry should be a continuous, ongoing activity. The general external environment, the market and its customers, the industry and its competitors, all are changing constantly. A firm cannot plan relevant, effective strategies without staying on top of these changes.

TOOLS AND TECHNIQUES FOR ANALYZING AND MONITORING THE EXTERNAL ENVIRONMENT

An organization can easily become overwhelmed by the volume of undifferentiated information that it will accumulate. Data collection systems must be matched with tools for analyzing and interpreting the output. A few examples are:

- Sorting and classification
- Trend identification and extrapolation (quantitative and qualitative)
- Statistical modeling
- Brainstorming
- Alternative future scenario projections
- Delphi process dialogues
- Role playing
- War gaming

WHAT TO DO WITH THE INFORMATION ON THE EXTERNAL ENVIRONMENT

Applying these tools to the environmental information gathered is meant to provide inputs to the strategic planning process. One way of accomplishing this task is to ask strategists what environmental variables concern them the most and are likely, in their estimation, to have the greatest impact on the strategies they have in mind. Then, in response, provide them with data, conclusions, and projections for those variables. Another approach is to ask and answer a series of generic questions about strategy effects.

- How much more or less money are customers likely to spend on our products?
- What new technologies will we have to acquire in order to maintain competitive parity, and how much will it cost?
- Of the bills presently before the congress/state legislatures affecting our industry, which are most likely to be enacted into law and what would be their effects on our organization?

- What are the likely effects on customer value preferences (product features and price, supporting services, distribution channels) of the projected demographic trends in our marketplace—age, ethnicity, income level, education level?
- How would our strategic planning decisions change if Medicare reimbursement levels over the next five years were 5 percent/10 percent/20 percent higher or lower than our best projections?

The external world is a complex place with an infinity of factors that could affect a business's strategic management efforts. The business will never be able to comprehend fully the interaction among those factors and their possible effects on strategy, but it is most definitely worthwhile to make a good-faith effort to stay informed about what is happening outside the organization.

Study Questions

1. An organization's external environment theoretically includes the entire world and everybody in it. How do the organization's managers decide how much of that environment they will research and follow? They will not have the resources to keep track of everything.
2. Once an organization has a good understanding of its external environment, how does it go about interpreting the possible effects on its operations and strategies? What guidelines could it use for recognizing specific threats and opportunities that deserve attention?
3. Do some library or Internet research on the MIT professor Jay Forrester, who virtually invented the field of "system dynamics." Study what he has to say about the operation of "systems" and apply those principles to be strategic operations of a health care organization.
4. External environmental factors change over time, some at a very rapid pace. Organizations cannot take occasional snapshots of the external environment; they must measure and track it continuously. Review the numerous environmental factors described in this chapter and decide how an organization would follow changes in them over a period of years. The factors subject to quantitative measurement are easy. Try to figure out how you would evaluate the more subjective sociocultural factors from year to year.

Learning Exercise

Select a health care provider organization in the local community, preferably a hospital or a physician group practice. Conduct an external environmental assessment for the organization along the lines described in this chapter. Be sure to cover all the basic categories of environmental factors. Draw a diagram showing the environmental forces you have identified and the interrelationships among them and with the organization.

When you have completed the assessment, make a note of at least five apparent threats that are facing the organization, as well as at least five opportunities. The organization will probably need to respond to the threats to maintain its mission and ensure success. It may take advantage of the opportunities to maximize its accomplishments.

Notes

[1] Subramanian R, Fernandes N, and Harper E. An empirical examination of the relationship between strategy and scanning. *Mid-Atlantic Journal of Business.* December 1993; 315–330; and Daft RL, Sormunen J, and Parks D. Chief executive scanning, environmental characteristics, and company performance. *Strategic Management Journal.* 1988;(9):123–139.

[2] Christensen, CM. *The Innovator's Dilemma.* Cambridge, MA: Harvard Business School Press; 1997.

References

Boyd BK and Fulk J. Executive scanning and perceived uncertainty: A multidimensional model. *Journal of Management.* 1996;22(1):1–21.

Daft RL, Sormunen J, and Parks D. Chief executive scanning, environmental characteristics, and company performance: An empirical study. *Strategic Management Journal.* 1998;(9):123–139.

Garg VK, Walters BA, and Priem RL. Chief executive scanning emphasis, environmental dynamism and manufacturing firm performance close quotes. *Strategic Management Journal.* 2003;24(8):724–744.

Hanke JE, Wichern DW, and Reitsch AG. *Business Forecasting.* Upper Saddle River, NJ: Prentice Hall; 2001.

McConkey D. Planning in a changing environment. *Business Horizons.* 1988;31(5):67.

Ringland G. *Scenario Planning: Managing for the Future.* Hoboken, NJ: John Wiley & Sons; 1998.

Subramanian R, Fernandes N, and Harper E. An empirical examination of the relationship between strategy and scanning. *Mid-Atlantic Journal of Business.* December 1993;315–330.

Thomas JB, Clark SM, and Gioia DA. Strategic sensemaking and organizational performance: Linkages among scanning, interpretation, action, outcomes. *Academy of Management Journal.* April 1993:239–270.

CHAPTER

4

External Environmental Assessment: Market and Customers

Learning Objectives

After reading and studying this chapter, you should be able to:

- Explain the difference between a market and its component segments, and explain why a business must pay attention to the segments.
- Understand why an organization cannot or should not offer its goods or services to all possible customers in the widest possible market.
- Identify the criteria that a health care or biotechnology organization might use to define market segments.
- Describe how a business selects the market segments in which to compete.
- Recognize the importance of accurately defining who an organization's customers are.
- Understand the concept of "value" that a product or service brings to customers.
- List some techniques that a business can use to determine what its customers value.
- Apply the acquired knowledge of customer value preferences to the planning of competitive strategies.

Market and customers make up one of the three major components of the external environment. It is the most congenial of the three; the customers purchase the firm's products and services and generate the flow of revenues and profits that it depends upon for its existence. In contrast, the firm's competitors stand in opposition to its strategic aspirations; they wish to capture the firm's customers and the revenues and profits along with them. The third component, the broad social/political/economic environment, is a generally neutral factor, affecting all industry participants more or less equally.

Interestingly, far more attention in the strategic management literature is given to the analysis of the competition than the study of the customers who are a business's lifeblood. In a fashion similar to the examination of the industry and competitors in Chapter5, this chapter begins with the analysis of the market in which an organization operates and moves on to the characteristics and motivations of individual customers in choosing which products/services to buy and from whom to buy them.

ANALYZING THE MARKET AND ITS SEGMENTS

A good strategy planner wants to know several things about the market in which the strategies will be played out.

The absolute first step is determining the appropriate market. Many businesses that have been in operation for many years take this for granted; they already have a substantial group of customers and simply accept them as their "market." The problem is that they may never have clearly delimited the market; they actually may not have a very good idea of who they are selling to. Furthermore, they may be missing other markets that are more attractive. Defining the market (or markets) as precisely as possible opens up new possibilities for sale of the firm's products and services.

In defining a firm's existing and prospective markets it almost always is necessary to think in terms of "segments" of a larger market. For instance, in the provision of health care services by a hospital located in a major U.S. city, the total conceivable market is about 300 million people, the entire population of the country. (In fact, with the growth of "medical tourism" and Americans traveling overseas for low-cost, good-quality care and foreign citizens coming to the United States for very high quality care, the theoretical maximum market is five billion people.) However, the hospital does not plan strategies to try to sell to this overall market—because it could not plausibly make its services available to all 300 million people. To begin with, the vast majority of them are not within geographic proximity to visit the hospital. Any strategies will be limited to those people within the metropolitan area close enough to travel to the hospital.

There are exceptions to even this general rule. Certain medical centers with national reputations, like the Mayo Clinic, deliberately promote themselves to patients living anywhere in the country. Some hospitals with international reputations, like Massachusetts General Hospital in Boston and Bumrungrad International Hospital in Bangkok, cater to patients coming from outside their countries. Perhaps even the market for clinical health care services is becoming global.

In addition, the hospital's currently available competencies and services may be rather specialized—focusing perhaps on the treatment of children or people with certain diseases (cancer, diabetes). That narrows the scope of the potential market even further. The hospital may have developed a unique competence in delivering care within the constraints of a particular payer's (Medicare, Medicaid) benefit schedule. As a result, it will aim its strategies at that payer's beneficiaries.

Unless a firm is quite large, with substantial resources and competencies, it will have trouble gaining a competitive advantage across the full breadth of a market. The solution is to concentrate the firm's strategic energies on a few pieces of the total market, on selected market segments. The challenge is to find appropriate criteria for defining the segments and, of all the possible segments, select those few in which the firm can have the maximum strategic impact.

What Is a "Market Segment"?

A market segment is a subgroup of actual and potential customers within the larger market whose needs are similar to each other and also significantly different from the needs of customers in other subgroups. A large amorphous mass of consumers in a broad market, like the market for health care services, can be subdivided in an infinite number of ways. The goal is to define segments with unique characteristics that permit an organization to target a meaningful, effective strategy at them.

The task of segmenting a market is made the more challenging by the fact that existing segments can disappear and new segments emerge. The customers do not disappear; the characteristics of a particular grouping become less relevant to strategy planning. At one time, pharmaceutical and medical device companies focused much of their strategic efforts on physicians in solo or very small group practices. Many of those physicians are still in practice, but they have either joined large physician groups or get most of their patients through MCOs that have established drug formularies or must approve use and coverage of new technologies. Solo-practice physicians are no longer a segment that can be exploited profitably by these companies. In contrast, a large number of new segments have developed. Previously, cosmetic surgery procedures were performed primarily to correct physical deformities or reverse the signs of aging in women. It now is a procedure also sought by teenage girls and adult men. Back in the day of solo-practice physicians, the gold standard of outpatient care delivery was the house call. Today, a significant number of consumers prefer to engage with their physicians by e-mail whenever it makes clinical sense.

What this means for firms operating in the market for health care services is that they must follow the constantly shifting mix of market segments in order to become aware promptly of new opportunities and threats with strategic implications.

Bases for Segmentation

Any customer characteristic can be used as the basis for market segmentation, as long as it makes strategic sense to the firm. To be useful, a characteristic should satisfy several criteria. Reliable information on the characteristic should be available with relative ease and economy. The information should be in a form that is objective, preferably quantitative. The segment that the characteristic describes ought to be accessible to the firm's product distribution and marketing efforts. It should be of sufficient size—in terms of number of customers or volume of sales that they are likely to generate—to justify a separate strategy focusing on it. The firm must possess the resources and competencies that will permit it to deliver products and services of value to the segment. The customers making up the segment must desire the kinds of products and services offered by the firm and be able to pay for them.

Following are some of the traits most commonly used to define market segments in the health care and biotechnology industries.

Patient Demographics

When the customer is a patient, a consumer of clinical medical services, basic demographic variables are primary determinants of his or her demand for products and services of firms in the health care industry. The medical problems that a person has are very much a function of age, sex, race, and ethnicity. The elderly have very different clinical needs than children do. Certain health care facilities cater specifically to the needs of these segments: nursing homes and skilled nursing facilities (elderly) and children's hospitals (children). Women deal with unique medical issues not faced by men. Beyond the traditional ob-gyn department, it has become popular among hospitals to establish women's health centers.

Patient Economics

The financial or economic circumstances of a patient will determine his ability to pay for health care products or services, and that patient's suitability as a customer for the firm. Given the current structure of the U.S. health care system, the initial question is whether an individual is covered by some type of health insurance. For many people, health insurance is connected to their employment status. Even when there is insurance, the identity of the payer will make a difference in the services covered, the amount of reimbursement, the requirement for copayments or deductibles from the customer, and the complexity of the process for filing claims for payment by the insurer. Some health care providers attempt to avoid patients covered by Medicare or Medicaid; the strategy of others is to cater actively to those market segments. An individual's discretionary personal income will make a difference in his ability to pay for basic health care services if he is not insured, elective medical procedures like cosmetic surgery, alternative medical procedures not covered by insurance (like acupuncture), and patient-initiated purchases like over-the-counter (OTC) medications and herbal supplements.

Patient Lifestyle

The style in which a person lives her life has a powerful effect on health status and the likelihood that she will require health care services. It also influences her preferences for the ways in which she will receive those services. A frequently criticized feature of current American lifestyles is their increasingly sedentary nature. Many people choose to spend their free time watching television and playing with computers, they ride in cars when they could easily walk to their destinations, and they generally avoid serious forms of exercise. This inactivity is coupled with eating habits that encourage a variety of diseases, including diabetes, cancer, heart problems, and obesity. Ironically, a number of very active people engage in high-risk sports and other activities that increase their exposure to other health hazards, particularly traumas.

Perhaps because of a long history of receiving health care services at little or no personal cost (because the premiums for health plans with generous coverage were paid by employers), many Americans persist in their reckless lifestyles and then, when their health problems inevitably arise, they turn to the health care system and expect to be returned to their original health status. This presents a challenge for health care providers who usually realize that the best way to deal with these problems is to prevent them in the first place. Many of their customers do not want to hear that message, so the providers continue to deliver predominantly curative medicine. American society is slowly coming to grips with this inconsistency by putting greater emphasis on preventive medicine. This shift will present both opportunities and threats for health care organizations.

Another feature of American lifestyles is the accelerated pace at which many people move. They try to accomplish as many tasks as possible in a short period of time and have little tolerance for delay. Americans are famous for their desire for "instant gratification." This trait is reflected in their attitudes toward the health care delivery process. Increasingly, patients are content to interact with health care providers electronically, whether that means making appointments, hearing test results, or renewing prescriptions. When a face-to-face visit with a provider is necessary, they would like to be able to schedule an appointment almost immediately, certainly in no more than a few days, and then on the day of the appointment, spend minimal time in the waiting room. Forward-looking providers are taking these customer preferences into account and making appropriate adjustments in their operating procedures.

Health care organizations can make strategic choices on the basis of these lifestyle characteristics. They can cater to that segment of the overall market that is willing to alter lifestyle behaviors if it is likely to prevent the onset of disease. Some have made a specialty of meeting the health care needs of people who do engage in active, sometimes risky sports.

Patient Sociocultural Factors

This category of market variables includes a variety of factors that can be useful in defining market segments. Families range in size from a single person to much larger extended units comprising parents, children, grandparents, and other relatives. Their health care needs and desires vary considerably. Family size often goes hand in hand with "stage of life," which usually parallels age. It is popular to say that young adults behave as though they were immortal with little thought about possible health care needs. If such needs do arise, their lifestyles and lower levels of income may make it harder for them to pay for the necessary medical services. At the other end of the life continuum, as elderly people approach the ends of their lives, much of their time and thoughts are concerned with health status and obtaining the health care that they increasingly need. Just these two variables present a wide array of market segments that call for very different strategic approaches by health care organizations.

Some very substantial market segments in the United States are defined by the unique cultures and languages of the increasingly diverse population of patients seeking health care. Cultural attitudes and beliefs can affect the ways in which people prefer to interact with the health care system and individual providers. Language differences require health care organizations to develop new communication competencies. Without accommodation of a patient's culture and language, the quality of care that he receives can suffer.

A patient's level of education may affect her ability to describe her health care problems, understand a provider's explanation of their causes and recommended treatments, and comply with the proposed course of treatment. Provider organizations need to make appropriate adjustments in all their patient communications.

The spiritual component in the healing process has received relatively little attention by the formal health care system. However, there is growing awareness of its potentially significant therapeutic role. The "spiritual" includes not only religious prayer or faith healing, but also the ego-defying belief in a source of contentment outside one's self. In addition to practitioners who concentrate on a spiritual basis for their therapies, traditional health care providers are taking it into account in their treatment plans.

Patient Geographic Location

The physical location of prospective patients is a major determinant of whether and how a health care organization will try to market its health care services to them. It may be the location of their residence, their place of work, or where they go for recreation. People may require health care services at any time and, depending on the severity of the need, will seek out the most convenient provider. Related to physical location is a person's willingness to travel for health care services. A good example of a strategy targeting a travel-related market segment is the establishment of retail primary care clinics. One of the first movers on this concept is retail drug chains that are taking advantage of their multiple existing outlets in key locations.

Patient Purchase/Usage Behavior

An absolutely fundamental set of features that define market segments in health care concern consumer habits and preferences surrounding the purchase experience for goods and services. To start with, what is the individual's purchasing style? Emergency room visits aside, does she plan her visits to health care providers well in advance or act spontaneously, perhaps waiting until the discomfort of the illness prods her into action? Does the patient do a lot of personal research on her health condition so that she is well informed and capable of discussing treatment options with her provider? Is she insistent on being involved and consulted on all health care decisions?

The immediacy of a consumer's product or service need can range from elective to necessary to emergency. A health care provider organization must attune itself quite differently to meet these three distinct types of demand for health care services. A related matter is the source of the purchase initiative: Did the patient seek out the provider on his own, was he sent there by the referral of another provider, is he a health plan member being directed to providers by the plan's gatekeeping system, or was he brought to the provider by an ambulance in an emergent condition? Even when a patient appears to be making health care decisions on her own, there may be other people (friends and family) who have strong influence over her.

Two other factors in a consumer's purchase pattern are the purpose for purchasing a product—that is, the particular use to which it will be put—and the intensity of that usage. The product may be purchased for the purpose intended by its manufacturer or for another unintended, unanticipated purpose. The consumer may buy a product for another person. The purchaser's usage of the product may be heavy, moderate, or infrequent. Many health care products are purchased without immediate consumption in mind. They are acquired as a precaution against some possible future health care need.

In selecting health care products and services, a customer will frequently have specific preferences for the brand of the item, the performance and appearance features of the product, the service associated with the sale (before, during, and after), and the price to be paid. Customers will also have different sensitivities to the quality of the products they buy. The many combinations of these variables result in a wide variety of potential market segments. Many traditional health care organizations continue to market themselves, and their products and services, to the entire population of prospective health care patients in their service area. They leave themselves vulnerable to more focused strategic attacks by more creative competitors.

Organization Physical Location

Not all customers in the health care industry are individuals. In fact, there are a great many organizations at every stage of the industrial value chain. On the basis of distinguishing characteristics, they too can be placed in defined market segments. The physical location of organizational customers is quite important for certain products and services, and not at all for others. Certain products can be shipped to an organizational consumer from across the country or around the world. However, a hospital would be unwilling to purchase its laundry services from a firm even fifty miles away. Health care businesses have strategic choices to make about the geographic breadth and distance of the markets they will serve.

Organization Economics

Just as human customers vary in the size of their families and the levels of their income, so too do organizations differ in the volume of their revenues and the rate at which they are growing. These factors, plus their level of profit, are often taken into account by the supplier businesses wishing to serve them. For instance, a distributor of hospital supplies might dedicate itself to meeting the needs of smaller hospitals (less than fifty beds) located in rural areas (more than 100 miles from a major city). This market segment might be unappealing to a distributor that is catering to much larger teaching hospitals and primary metropolitan areas. A customer organization's stage of life might also come into play in strategic planning. A distributor of laboratory supplies and equipment might choose to specialize in selling to biotechnology startups that are relatively small, but rapidly growing by fits and starts.

Organization Purchase Behavior

Significant differences exist in the purchase behaviors of organizations. Some may buy small amounts of a product at more frequent intervals, while others make larger purchases more infrequently. Some purchase large volumes of low dollar value products, in contrast with organizations that buy only a few higher-priced items. A health care business will want to pay attention to the product/service selection criteria that its different customers use. An organization may have strong loyalty to a particular brand, it may be interested in certain product features and not in others, product quality may or may not be a significant concern to it, and it may have constraints on the prices that it is willing or able to pay. Some organizations want and truly need certain levels of service from their suppliers—either before, during, or after the sale. For instance, purchasers of complex equipment may perform their own repair and maintenance, or prefer to rely on the supplier for those services. Different organizations may demand different levels of performance from the same product. Organizational customers often have unique purchase procedures, to which suppliers must adjust. One factor that should not be neglected is the importance of the product or service in the customer's internal value chain. If the customer is absolutely dependent on it or it constitutes a major proportion of the customer's cost of goods sold, the supplier business is in a much stronger position in its dealings with that customer. This multitude of purchase preferences provides a basis for defining numerous market segments on which a health care business might concentrate.

Organization Infrastructure

The very infrastructure of an organization may be a relevant factor in determining the segments that a business will or will not try to serve. This may include the distinction between for-profit and not-for-profit status, as is the case with hospitals. A corporate customer may operate out of a single large facility or through many smaller facilities scattered around a geographic area. The technology that a customer employs can be important: It may affect its ability to integrate certain products into its operations, or to interface with a supplier's electronic purchasing system. The attitude and competence of a company's management may be a consideration in whether and how a business wants to target it as a prospective customer. Even the competitive strategies that a customer organization is following may affect its relationships with suppliers. For instance, the organization may be trying to create greater value for its own customers by refining the way that it deals with suppliers.

It is worth exploring different ways of segmenting the market to see what that reveals about groupings of common customer interests and the firm's ability to cater to them. It is interesting to mix and match various market variables to see what segments pop up. It is sometimes possible to discover reasonably large segments with unique needs that are not being addressed by any other competitor. On the other hand, just because a market segment can be defined and measured does not mean that it is a useful basis for configuring a firm's product/service and marketing strategies. The goal is to identify segments that are well matched to the organization's resources and competencies, ideally allowing it gain a competitive advantage.

The share of each market segment that a firm has been able to capture is important in measuring its performance vis-à-vis its competitors (see Chapter 5). Market share is also an indicator of the firm's experience with its customers. A larger share takes time to build and in that time, the firm learns how to offer its products and services at lower cost. Over a period of years, customers are more likely to develop a loyalty to those products and services.

Choosing the Segments to Target

Once the firm has broken the total market down into meaningful segments, the serious market analysis can begin. Several types of segment data will help it decide which segments to focus on and the strategies to apply to them.

Total Sales from the Segment

The first piece of information about a market segment that the firm will seek is probably its size measured in terms of the total sales of products and services to that segment. If a segment has very small revenue prospects, it may not be worth the firm's efforts to operate within that segment. Generally, larger revenues in a segment will be more appealing. The problem is that what is appealing to the firm is likely also to be appealing to its competitors. The competitive intensity in a large market segment

Is a Market Segment of One Customer Possible?

The theoretical ultimate goal of a business's efforts to differentiate its products is to treat each customer as a separate market segment. The traditional view has been that it is too costly to custom design and deliver products or services to individual customers. Some firms move in this direction by adding features to a basic, mass appeal product and charging a higher price for it. There are good examples in the health care field. The vast majority of patients admitted to a hospital receive the same basic standard of medical care and service. However, some hospitals have created separate sections where patients willing to pay a higher out-of-pocket cost will enjoy more luxurious physical amenities and service, with closer, personalized attention from staff. The quality of clinical care is presumably the same. A recent trend in physician outpatient care delivery is the concierge practice. The patient typically pays a fixed fee per month or year in return for special services like accompanied specialist visits, twenty-four-hour direct physician access, house calls, and same-day appointments. These cases illustrate how creative strategic thinking can overcome established beliefs to give an organization a competitive advantage.

may be so great that a firm concludes that it cannot succeed there and chooses to avoid it.

On the other hand, there may be relatively few rivals active in a smaller segment and the firm may feel that it can more easily garner a large market share there. To put it another way, a 20 percent share of a $20 million market segment is better than a 2 percent piece of a $100 million market.

Average Profits Earned in the Segment

Large sales revenues in a market segment are nice, but the ultimate goal is a high level of profits on those sales. Some segments with substantial sales may be returning very thin profit margins. Because the profit-earning ability of competitors may vary within a single market segment, the metric of interest to a firm will be the average profits earned by all those competitors.

Segment Value Chain Activities and Related Costs

It is important to understand exactly how businesses in the segment serve its customers: how they deliver value to them and how much it costs them to do it. A firm may not want to follow automatically the operating models employed by competitors. In fact, if it seeks true competitive advantage, it will be looking for ways to do things differently. But a competitor's methods are a good starting point.

The process of describing and analyzing an organization's internal value chain is explained in Chapter 5, on industry and competitors. In a market segment analysis, the value chain study is less rigorous. The purpose is to understand the sequence of activities that existing businesses are using to create value for their customers. The firm would like to know what those activities are, the cost of performing those activities, whether it has the resources and competencies to perform those activities as well, whether it is able to perform them at lower cost, and whether it is able to perform the same activities differently or different activities in order to gain a competitive advantage. Certain value chain activities will appear to be more important—because they are most directly related to creating the values most sought by customers.

Segment Distribution Channels

Another question concerns how the products and services are distributed to customers in the market segment. Will the firm sell directly to the end user or will it have to go through an intermediary (distributor, wholesaler, retailer)? If an intermediary is present, how much bargaining power does it have and, as a result, how much of the total profit in the full industry value chain is it able to capture? This information may help a firm decide whether to execute a strategy of either developing alternative distribution channels or integrating forward into the existing channel.

Competitive Intensity

Whether a firm wishes to operate in a specific segment or not will often turn on how many other businesses are already present in the segment and the intensity of their competition with each other. The competitive intensity affects the average profitability possible in the segment. Michael Porter describes the factors driving the level of competition and the resulting profits in terms of "five forces," summarized in greater detail in Chapter 5.

Trends in Market Segment Parameters

The trends in all these market segment parameters are significant. A company's strategies are carried out in the future, so it makes sense to try to understand where the market segment will be several years down the road. Trends can portend strategically relevant changes.

A segment with large revenues may actually be on the decline, while a much smaller segment may be in an early growth stage. Like products and businesses, market segments can have life cycles. They can emerge from nowhere (or with the encouragement of a business), grow to substantial size, remain at that level for several years, and then, slowly or quickly, disappear. Knowledge of where a particular segment is in its life cycle helps a firm decide whether it wishes to compete there and, if so, what strategies to follow. Different strategies are called for in markets that have just materialized, are on a rapid growth curve, have matured and stabilized, or are shrinking.

Trends in profit margins are no less important. They do not necessarily keep step with sales. For instance, profits are often low during rapid growth, become much more substantial when the market matures and sales level off, and may increase even further as revenues decline. In addition to tracking profit trends, a savvy firm will follow the developing changes in the competitive intensity factors. Is the bargaining power of suppliers or customers increasing or decreasing? Are substitute products or services becoming available? Are new competitors entering or existing competitors leaving the market?

One might think that distribution channels would not change very often until the rapidly developing popularity of mini-clinics located in retail malls and larger stores like Target, CVS, and supermarkets is considered.

Close attention to trend data can reveal more attractive sub-segments within less-appealing segments. For instance, although sales may be low and stagnating, with mediocre profits caused by intense competition within an overall segment, deep data analysis may disclose a niche of unserved customers within that segment who could be the source of modest sales at healthy profit margins without immediate threat of competition.

Keys to Competitive Advantage in the Segment

The analysis of a market segment is not complete without an identification of the elements required for a business at least to succeed and eventually to gain a competitive advantage. This includes the resources, competencies, and strategies that have been deployed by the most obviously successful companies in the segment. The methodologies for acquiring this knowledge are described in Chapter 5.

At this stage in the analysis, it is usually possible to begin categorizing the various market segments in terms of size, profitability, growth, price preferences, product feature preferences, competitive intensity, and fit with the firm's resources and competencies. It may be useful to construct four- or nine-cell matrices or charts contrasting key segment variables (e.g., size and profitability, growth and strategic fit) as a prelude to selecting segments in which the firm will actively compete.

Criteria for Selecting Suitable Market Segments

Smart businesses divide large markets into segments and go after those where they are most likely to gain a competitive advantage. However, that wisdom is confounded if a business selects unsuitable segments. Time and resources will be squandered. An ideal market segment for exploitation will satisfy the following criteria.

- The segment can be defined in objective terms, so that it may be studied and customers in the segment can be identified.
- The business can physically distribute its products or services to customers in the segment.
- There are media channels that the business can use to market itself and its products to the customers.
- The customers in the segment are interested in buying the firm's products or services if they are available.
- The customers have the financial resources to buy the products or services.
- The business is able to satisfy the customers' needs and sell products to them at prices that allow it to earn an average or above-average profit.
- The soft characteristics (values, attitudes, behaviors) of the customers in the segment do not conflict with those of existing customers so much that they are alienated.
- There is room in the segment for another competitor. If not, the business will never get its foot in the door.

ANALYZING THE CUSTOMER

To compete successfully in a market segment, a firm needs to know more than just the demographics of the customers who populate the segment.

In order profitably to create value for them, the business must gather considerable detail about how they play out their roles as consumers of the goods and services that are traded in the segment.

Who Is the Customer?

When a pharmaceutical company broadcasts television advertisements promoting one of its prescription medications, it does not expect viewers to recognize their need for the drug and then go looking for one of the company's stores to buy it. Drug companies do not operate retail outlets and, even if they did, a physician's prescription is a prerequisite to purchase by a patient. This highlights the importance of clearly identifying the customer in a particular market segment. In the case of prescription drugs, is it the patient who takes the drugs, the physician who prescribes them, the pharmacy that sells them (on behalf of the drug company), the health plan or insurance company that pays for them, or the employer that pays the monthly premium to the health plan or insurance company?

Identifying the right customer, the person on whom the firm's strategy should be focused, may be more complex in the health care industry than in any other part of the economy. The following people may have a role to play in the purchase of health care services.

- The person who actually receives the services, the person with the illness, trauma, or disease, the patient.
- The person who decides if the patient should receive the services. These are usually one and the same person. However, when the patient is a child, the parents usually make the decision. If the person is incompetent or incapacitated, an appointed guardian may take the responsibility. If the patient is brought in an uncommunicative state to an emergency room, unaccompanied by a legal proxy, the ER staff will make the necessary treatment decisions.
- Any other person who may informally influence the patient's decision-making about receiving health care services, including if, when, where, how, and what. This person may be a friend or family member. In some communities and ethnic groups, it may be the equivalent of a village elder.
- The person who decides from whom the patient will receive the services. This person performs a triage function, initially diagnosing the patient's problem and determining which caregiver she should see first. This is the so-called gatekeeper in a typical MCO. Depending on this person's decision, the patient may immediately receive medication, have an MRI picture taken, be examined by an internist, or be sent to a specialist.

- The person who actually provides the services (or products) to the patient. This person may be a physician, nurse, mid-level provider, technician (operating imaging equipment), or pharmacist.
- The person who will cover and pay for the services. If the patient is covered by insurance, this is the person who decides whether the insurance contract will cover and pay for the services. Whether services are covered is partially determined when the scope of covered benefits is defined in the contract. The insurer (insurance company, health plan, HMO, MCO, Medicare, Medicaid) makes the final determination of coverage after a claim for specific services is filed. If the patient is not insured, she is also the payer.
- The person who pays the monthly premium for the insurance coverage. If the patient is covered by insurance, this may be the patient's employer or the patient herself. Incidentally, when first agreeing to pay the premium, this person (employer or patient) frequently has a choice to make about the scope of benefits that will be covered by the insurance contract.

A firm selling into the health care market, or a segment of it, must be clear about which of these "customers" will be the target of its strategic initiatives. By selecting the wrong individuals, the firm can waste resources and miss opportunities. A strategy can aim at multiple customers, as long as it understands the different roles they play in the purchase process and adjusts the strategy accordingly. For instance, a pharmaceutical company wishing to promote its prescription drugs might deliver television ads to prospective patients, send representatives to talk with physicians who might prescribe the drugs, and negotiate with health plans to have their drugs included in the plans' drug formularies.

When thinking about customers and planning how to increase sales of products or services to them, it is important to keep in mind that they are always specific people, not organizations. It is easy to say that the ABC Health Plan has chosen not to cover a firm's medical devices, but a health plan is an organization and organizations do not make decisions. People do. The task for the firm in plotting its market-focused strategies is to find out who the real decision makers are in each phase of the purchase process.

Sources of Customer Value

After selecting appropriate market segments and identifying accurately the customers within them, a firm needs to discover what those customers value in the kinds of products or services that the firm is selling. There are many attributes of the overall purchase experience that may make a difference to customers. Some examples are the performance features of the product/service (it gets the job done); the appearance features (it looks or feels good); its level of quality (reliable, never breaks, runs smoothly); the setting/milieu in which it is purchased/consumed (pleasant waiting and exam rooms in physician's office); the reputation of the company selling it (big-name teaching hospital); the reputation of the brand name of the product/service (preferred gas chromatograph/mass spectrometers from a particular company); the demeanor of the people selling/delivering it (pleasant "bedside manner" of physician providing care); the service available before (salespeople helpful in explaining and demonstrating research equipment before lab's purchase), during (tasty food during hospital stay), and after the purchase (prompt maintenance and repair of research equipment, phone follow-up by physician's office after visit); and the cost (both initial and ongoing).

Within a given market segment, customers are likely to place importance on different aspects of the purchase experience. The firm will try to learn the most common, popular aspects and concentrate its strategies on them. It is helpful to begin with the *threshold* attributes. These are the bare minimum qualities that customers must have in order to even consider purchasing the product or service. They take them for granted. They will not pay extra for them; they simply will not buy the product if they are missing. In a physician practice, patients might expect a waiting room, a receptionist, office staff wearing uniforms, and a degree of cleanliness. If they don't see them, they will not even walk in the door.

The next level of attributes will determine whether the customer will prefer one competitor over another and whether it will pay a premium for the added-value features. These are referred to as the *critical success factors* (CSF) for that market segment. If a firm has the appropriate resources and competencies and can deploy them to satisfy these factors, it will gain a competitive advantage over other companies in the industry.

Their role in creating competitive advantage points to the strategic importance of a firm's resources and competencies. They need to match up with the critical success factors in the market segments where it has chosen to operate and compete. If they are not in sync, the firm has two choices. It can attempt to develop the necessary resources and competencies, or it can refocus on a market segment to which its existing resources and competencies are better suited.

It takes time and determination to acquire new resources and competencies. It is not always easy to drop out of one market segment and move into another. As a result, many firms continue operating in market segments in which they do not enjoy a competitive advantage, and are not likely to in the foreseeable future. A situation of competitive parity exists among the competitors. In the short run, this situation is not necessarily a bad thing. The firm may be able to perform well financially under such conditions. Eventually, there will be a shift in the general external environment or a competitor will embark on a strategy to create an advantage for itself, and the competitive equilibrium will be disrupted. The firm itself should be the one doing the disrupting.

How to Learn What Customers Value

A firm already has some information about what its current customers value in its product and services. What they buy and do not buy is an indication of their preferences, as reflected in the differences in the characteristics of the products they seek and those they shun. Customers also occasionally volunteer comments during their purchase experience. Firm employees can be trained to notice and record such comments. But that passive information gathering is usually not enough. It certainly does not help with prospective customers or when a move into a new market segment is contemplated.

The firm can use more assertive ways to discover what customers are looking for in a product or service. It might start with the public opinion surveys that are conducted by or for charitable foundations (Kaiser), think tanks (Rand), industry and professional associations (Medical Group Management Association or MGMA, American Hospital Association or AHA), academic researchers, consulting firms, and periodicals (*Health Affairs, U.S. News & World Report*). For results more specific to the entity and its immediate market area, it will have to initiate its own research. It can include appropriate "product value-added" questions on the patient satisfaction survey that it already should be doing. The complaints that customers make, and should be encouraged to make, may be read as signs of what they prefer in their products or services and what the firm is not delivering. Professionally facilitated interviews on product preferences may be carried out with individuals and with groups of customers. Focus groups are another proven method of eliciting candid customer views on product qualities.

The firm also can contract with marketing research businesses to carry out studies of the firm's current customers, potential new customers in its current market segments, or prospective customers in new market segments that the firm might enter. Even more elaborate advice is available from the health care industry practices of most of the major management consulting firms.

This research on customer value preferences must be an ongoing effort, as those preferences change over time. The customers' lifestyles change, they become more sophisticated consumers, or competitors offer products with new features.

Using Knowledge of Customer Value Preferences

When analyzed properly, the knowledge of what customers, current and prospective, value in the firm's products and services can inform several

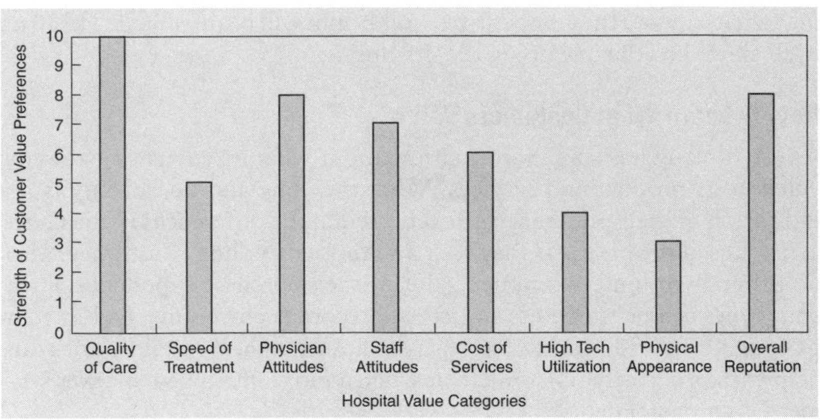

Figure 4.1 Market-Wide Hospital Customer Value Preferences

key strategic decisions. The information may be best understood if presented graphically. Many formats are possible. One example arrays the individual identified value preferences along the X-axis of a graph and a scale showing the strength of the preference for each value along the Y-axis (Figure 4.1). A bar indicates the strength of the average customer preferences for each value category. The resulting bar graph is a profile of what a customer is ideally looking for in the products or services offered by the firm. If average preference ratings are used, the profile can apply to an entire market or market segment.

The next step is to research and prepare variations of the graph that profile customer views of how well their values are met by the firm's products and those of other competitors in the market. By overlaying the profiles on the same graph, it is possible to see how closely the firm's product value profiles match the preferred value profile of its customers (Figure 4.2). Significant gaps between the two profiles may indicate areas where the firm could choose to make product improvements.

By comparing customers' impressions of the firm's products with those of its competitors' products, the firm can recognize points at which it is at competitive advantage or disadvantage. The gaps between the firm's and its competitors' profiles may indicate opportunities for exploitation or threats that must be countered.

The firm may use this customer value graph approach to identify new market segments into which it might wish to move. The graph would reveal opportunities for product enhancements that give the firm an initial competitive advantage.

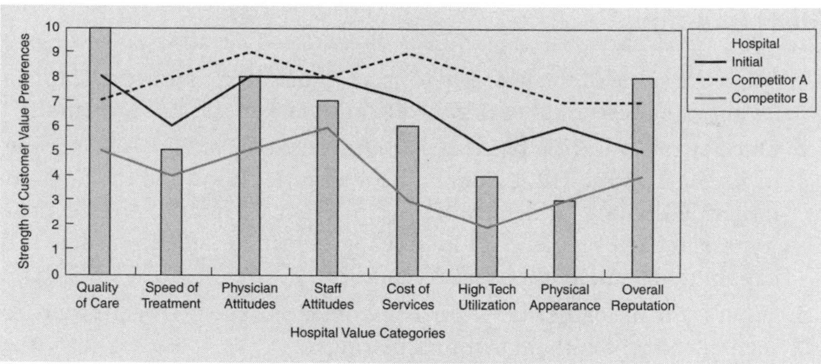

Figure 4.2 Customer Value Preferences Satisfied by Initial Hospital and Two Competitors

PLANNING STRATEGY TO MEET CUSTOMER NEEDS IN A TARGETED SEGMENT

The purpose of gathering and analyzing all these data about markets and customers is to inform a business's strategic decisions. These are some basic steps in the process of translating that information into action.

Start with identifying the threshold product features that customers, either in the firm's existing markets or in segments that it is considering entering, expect and take for granted from any competitor. Remember that product features include appearance, performance, related services, purchase process, location of sales facility, price, and even psychological factors.

Next, identify the additional product features that make a difference to customers, that make them prefer one competitor over another. These are the critical success factors for that market segment. They point to what a business must do effectively if it is to win the interest of customers in the segment.

Assess all competitors in the market segment, including the business itself, for how well they deliver both the threshold and other desired product features.

Compare the business's resources and competencies to the segment's critical success factors to see what it would take to gain a sustainable competitive advantage. Recognize important gaps and determine how easily they could be filled.

Make strategic decisions about whether to dedicate the organization to improving its performance regarding the critical success factors, perhaps by developing or acquiring new resources and competencies, or concentrating on another segment where the firm's abilities better match the critical success factors (CSFs).

Study Questions

1. What are some of the possible sources of data for a strategic planner trying to understand her organization's market and its segments?
2. Once an organization has clearly defined its market, as well as some of its most attractive segments, how does it choose which ones to target? How does it determine the product preferences of the customers in each segment? How does it determine whether it has the capability to satisfy those preferences?
3. What is the difference between a customer and the market or market segment to which that customer belongs?
4. Think about the times that you have needed some kind of health care products or services. These situations could range from an inpatient surgical procedure to remove your appendix to an over-the-counter purchase of a cold remedy. How did you choose which hospital to visit and which surgeon would perform the procedure? How did you choose which drugstore to visit and which brand of cold remedy to buy? How were you influenced in making these choices? In fact, what range of choices did you have? If you were a hospital executive that wanted to persuade a person like you to have their appendectomy performed at his hospital, what would you do to try to reach that person and affect her buying choice? At various points throughout the health care industry, who is the actual customer?
5. Do customers always know what they value in a product? How does an organization sell its products or services to customers who are not aware of their buying preferences?

Learning Exercise

Imagine that you are the head of strategic planning for a 150-bed general hospital located in a medium-sized city with a diverse population representing a cross-section of U.S. society. Compile a list of the segments into which the hospital's overall market could be defined. You might want to start by thinking about the most prominent variables that define a population. It should not be hard to come up with at least twenty or thirty possible segments. Once you have the list in hand, check off those segments that your common sense says are the most likely bases for differentiated product or service offerings. In other words, look for segments that probably want something unique in their hospital services.

References

Aaker DA. *Strategic Marketing Management.* 8th ed. Hoboken, NJ: John Wiley & Sons; 2008.

Berkowitz EN. *Essentials of Health Care Marketing.* 2nd ed. Sudbury, MA: Jones and Bartlett; 2006.

Dickson PR and Ginter JL. Market segmentation, product differentiation, and marketing strategy. *Journal of Marketing.* 1987;51(2):1–10.

Ferrell OC and Hartline MD. Marketing Strategy. 4th ed. Mason, OH: Thomson/South-Western, 2008.

Hillestad SG and Berkowitz EN. *Health Care Market Strategy: From Planning to Action.* 3rd ed. Sudbury, MA: Jones and Bartlett; 2004.

Kotler P and Keller KL. *Marketing Management.* 12th ed. Upper Saddle River, NJ: Prentice Hall; 2005.

Smith WR. Product differentiation and market segmentation as alternative marketing strategies. *Journal of Marketing.* 1956; 21(1):3–8.

CHAPTER

5

External Environmental Assessment: Industry and Competitors

Learning Objectives

After reading and studying this chapter, you should be able to:

- Describe the concept of an industrial value chain, in contrast with a business's internal value chain.
- Understand how businesses in that chain may generate different amounts of the value in the chain and "capture" varying amounts of the reward or payment for that value.
- Explain the Five Forces Model of industry attractiveness and competitive intensity.
- Describe each one of the five forces as they apply to competitors in the health care industry.
- Recommend strategies by which a business might respond to and deal with each of the five forces.
- Decide which of all possible competitors a business should focus its attention on.
- Explain the concept of "strategic groups" and how it applies to the analysis of competitors in an industry.
- Show how to conduct an analysis of individual competitors, particularly which characteristics to evaluate.
- Understand how a business can use the results of competitor analysis to forecast a competitor's likely strategic behavior.
- Discuss the role of "competitive intelligence" in understanding competitors, and the possible sources of such intelligence.

The third major component of a firm's external environment is the industry (or industries) in which it competes and the individual competitors within them. It is in that arena, against those other players, that a firm's strategies will be tested. The primary challenge that the firm will face is the competition from other businesses operating in the same markets and fighting for the same customers. Their goal is to sell as many of their products and services to the customers as they can manufacture. If they succeed, it means that the firm sells fewer of its products and services to those customers. It is a zero-sum game—every customer captured by a competitor is a customer that will not buy products and services from the firm. The harder those competitors fight for the customer's business, the more difficult it is for the firm to function and survive.

A firm is particularly interested in the attractiveness of the industry in which it chooses to operate. An industry's attractiveness is generally measured by the average profitability that can be earned by all the businesses operating there. Profitability, in turn, is determined largely by the intensity of the competition among those businesses. Intense competition tends to drive profits down.

■ INDUSTRY

The word "industry" is a generic term for a group of organizations, usually for-profit (FP) and sometimes not-for-profit (NFP) corporations, engaged in manufacturing and selling similar lines of products and services to similar markets. The word "market" refers to a group of consumers who have demands for similar products and services intended to satisfy similar needs. The two terms are often used interchangeably. One way of distinguishing the terms is to say that an industry is composed of corporations or businesses, and a market is composed of consumers who buy from an industry. From a strategy viewpoint, a firm competes with other industry members for the business of consumers in particular markets. An industry can sell to several different markets.

Opposition to a firm's strategies designed to serve specific markets comes from other competitors in its industry. If the strategies are to succeed, they must be based on a clear understanding of that industry. There are two good methods for comprehending how an industry is structured and operates. They were first explained and popularized by Michael Porter in his seminal book *Competitive Strategy*.

Industry Value Chain

The process by which a product or service is brought to a market for purchase by consumers can be viewed as a long, interconnected chain of sequential activities, each one adding a little bit more value to the product or service until a finished good emerges at the end for sale to a consumer. Porter called this a "value system" or value chain. A classic example of an industry value chain is the Ford Motor Company as originally conceived by Henry Ford in the 1920s. At one time, the company owned mines in Minnesota and northern Michigan from which it extracted iron ore, and mines in Kentucky and West Virginia from which it extracted coal. Both were shipped to mills in Dearborn, Michigan, where they were combined to produce iron and steel. The steel was passed on to rolling mills, forges, and assembly plants to be transformed into springs, axles, and car bodies. Forges converted the iron into engine blocks and cylinder heads. All these were assembled with other components into engines and complete automobiles. If Ford had sold its cars through company-owned dealerships, it could be said to have controlled the entire automobile manufacturing industry value chain.

Firms in most industries operate in only part of their industry's value chain. Typically, they acquire components or raw materials for a product from suppliers, assemble or manufacture them into a partially or fully finished product, and sell it to buyers in the next stage/link of the chain—which may perform additional value-adding operations on the product or simply move it along the distribution channel to the ultimate consumer. Each of those firms can be said to have its own internal value chain that is composed of activities that sequentially add value to raw materials until they become finished products. The internal value chain concept was used to discuss the firm's resources and competencies in Chapter 2.

Different amounts of value are added by different firms in the industry value chain. The pharmaceutical company that researches and develops a new drug and moves it through the FDA approval process would appear to be creating most of the value that goes into the product finally administered to a patient. The shipping company that transports the packaged product from the drug company to a drug wholesaler, the next link in the chain, seems to add relatively little value—simply moving the product a little closer to the end user. Nonetheless, it is an essential link.

Different amounts of customer reward or payment for a product's value are captured by different firms in the industry value chain. If the customer desires the total product value created by the value chain, he will pay a price that is greater than the sum of the costs incurred to create that value. Because of differences in their relative bargaining powers, the firms in the chain may not receive proportionate shares of that profit. For instance, a typical industry value chain for health care delivery in a local market might consist of an employer who pays premiums to an MCO to buy health coverage for its employees. Those employees choose one of the health plans offered by the MCO. The MCO contracts with an integrated delivery system (IDS) to pull together the different providers needed to meet all the health care needs of those employees. The IDS contracts with

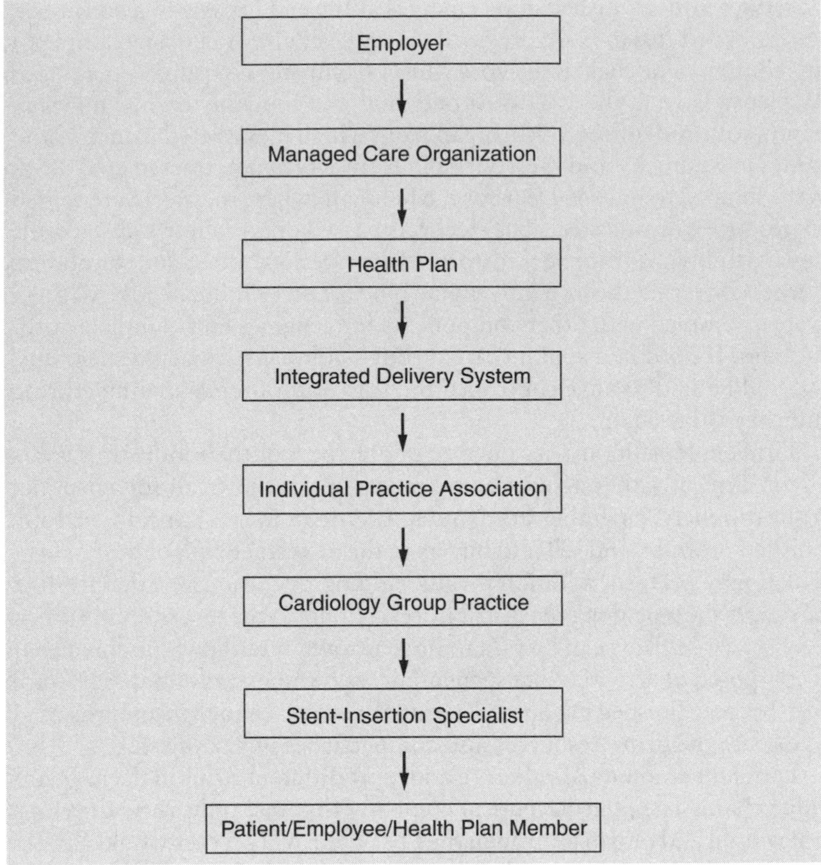

Figure 5.1 Industry Value Chain for Artery Stent Implantation

an individual practice association (IPA) to deliver the physician services required. The IPA contracts with a small group of cardiologist physicians to diagnose and treat heart problems that the employees may have. One of the group's members specializes in the process of inserting stents in arteries. Those stents are inserted in the arteries of a patient who is also an employee of the employer and a member of the health plan. The resulting chain can be depicted as shown in Figure 5.1.

The monthly premiums paid by the employer will cover the costs of providing health care to its employees by all the other parties in the value chain *plus* return a profit. The question is how that profit is distributed among those parties. It does not happen as a result of a centralized joint negotiation among the parties. Instead, the profit each party earns is a result of a combination of the prices that it pays to its suppliers for the inputs to its value chain (e.g., raw materials, personnel), the efficiency with which it performs its value-adding activities, and the price it receives when it sells its products or services to its customers. To a certain degree, the price that a business pays and the prices that it is able to charge are a function of its bargaining power vis-à-vis suppliers and customers.

If the employer is one of several modest-sized companies in the market and the MCO is the primary and dominant source of managed health care, the employer will probably be compelled to accept the MCO's premium demands. If the IDS is relatively large and has contracts with most of the providers in the area, there will be bargaining parity between it and the MCO. The IDS should be able to negotiate reasonable, not extravagant compensation from the MCO. The IPA includes a diverse mix of the best, most highly regarded physicians in the market. Neither the IDS nor the MCO can afford to omit these physicians from their provider panels. The IPA will be able to enforce demands for relatively high levels of compensation. Because there are three equally competent cardiology groups within the IPA, none of them can command unusually high compensation. The physician specializing in stent-insertion procedures is the only one with that expertise in the entire value chain. He can ask for and receive almost any compensation he wants.

Which of the parties in this hypothetical value chain are likely to capture most of the profit flowing from the employer premiums? Because of their stronger bargaining power, the MCO, the IPA, and the stent-insertion specialist will do the best. The profit capture of the IDS will be mediocre. The cardiology group practice will do more poorly.

A significant strategic decision for a firm is where in the industry value chain it will operate. Its choice will depend on its strategic objectives in that industry and on the resources and competencies it can deploy. The ultimate goal is to match so well the firm's resources and competencies with the critical success factors for a stage in the value chain that the firm is able to gain a competitive advantage. An ambitious firm will also aim to capture as much of the profit in the chain as possible. It does not make strategic sense to try to compete anywhere in an industry for which a firm is not qualified and where it cannot achieve superior results.

Once a firm is established at some point in the industry value chain, an available strategic option is to expand forward or backward in that chain. This takes the form of what is called "vertical integration." This concept is discussed in more detail in Chapter 7.

Five Forces Model of Industry Structure

One of the best ways to understand the nature and intensity of the competition in an industry is through the five forces originally defined by

Michael Porter.[1] The interplay of these forces largely determines the profit potential of the industry, and what a firm will be able to accomplish there.

1. Competitive Intensity. When trying to assess the force of competition in an industry, the first thing that often comes to mind is the intensity of the rivalry among the competitors that currently make up the industry. Businesses in adversarial relationships constantly engage in a variety of combative activities designed to gain an edge on competitors or prevent them from gaining an edge on it. Common examples are price increases or decreases, marketing campaigns, new product or feature introductions, and customer service improvements. The frequency, magnitude, and persistence of these activities are measures of the competitive intensity in an industry.

The pace and fervor of competition is increasing in almost every area of the U.S. economy, none more so than in health care, both in specific subsectors (like pharmaceuticals, health plans, hospitals, and physician practices) and throughout the industry as a whole. Some managers may have a gut feeling that they are facing a lot of competitive pressure, but it is still a good idea to examine the several factors that are strong indicators of the level of competitive intensity. Full comprehension of the relevant factors aids the planning of strategies that permit an organization to survive.

Factors Encouraging Intensity of Competition

Large number of competitors. The more competitors in an industry, the smaller their individual market shares, and the hungrier they are to gain market share. Each competitor is smaller, with fewer resources, and may appear vulnerable to aggressive competitive action. The likelihood of such action is increased when the competing firms are relatively balanced in size, resources, and market power.

Slow industry growth. When the total size of an industry is steadily expanding, firms can increase their sales and profits by simply maintaining their market shares. When industry growth has slowed or stopped altogether, the only way that individual competitors can continue to grow is by taking market share from another firm in the industry.

High fixed costs. A firm that has large fixed costs associated with its operations (as a result of long-term contracts with vendors or for plant and equipment maintenance) has a strong need to keep its sales volumes at high levels in order to cover those costs. A classic example is hospitals designed to operate at maximum efficiency when all their beds are filled. They will compete vigorously to keep occupancy rates as high as possible.

Lack of differentiation. If there are few significant differences among the products or services offered by firms in an industry, each will have to work harder to persuade customers to choose its offerings. When a firm's products have unique distinguishing features desired by some customers, the firm may concentrate on selling to specific market segments rather than competing head-to-head with other rivals.

Consider This: Currently there is a strong movement to introduce greater product cost and feature transparency throughout the health care delivery industry. Health care providers are being prodded to calculate and publicize their costs of delivering specific services. Considerable research is being done to find ways to measure nonfinancial aspects of health care, such as the quality of services offered, the competence and performance of individual providers, and patient satisfaction with the services and the providers. This information, too, will be made publicly available. The result may be to make it easier for customers to distinguish among several competitors, in turn requiring those firms to rethink the bases for their competition with each other.

High strategic stakes. Some competitors may have made an especially strong strategic commitment to succeeding in a market or industry. They may be selling only to one market segment or they may have invested substantial financial resources in their strategies targeted at that segment. A firm that is a recent startup will live or die depending on the success of its initial strategies. For any of these reasons, a firm will be a fierce competitor.

An interesting example of this phenomenon might be the emergence in recent years of "specialty hospitals." These are entirely new hospitals, typically for-profit entities created by a group of physicians in a particular specialty, often in league with entrepreneurs. The hospitals focus on treating patients with specific medical conditions or who require surgical procedures. They have tended to concentrate on cardiac, orthopedic, surgical, and women's care. The argument is that through their specialization and economies of scale, they improve quality and reduce costs. One of the main criticisms of these hospitals is that their areas of concentration are the highest-margin procedures that general hospitals in the area use to subsidize lower-margin services.

This trend puts both the specialty hospitals and the general hospitals from which they take patients in strategically precarious positions. The doctors have made large financial and professional commitments to their new specialty hospital ventures, which are at risk if they fail. The financial stability of the general hospitals is threatened by these new competitors. Both parties can be expected to compete strenuously for their survival.

High exit barriers. Competitive intensity will not remain at high levels if an overstressed competitor, unable to keep up, can simply pull out of the industry with relative ease. Factors that make that difficult, if not impossible, force the firm to stay and fight, often with even greater desperation because its survival may be in the balance. Consider a major teaching hospital that is one of several in a large metropolitan area. If the hospital's executives felt that they lacked the resources and competencies to respond to the competitive pressure, several hurdles would stand in the way of their closing the hospital and departing the industry:

- A large capital investment in plant and equipment.
- Facilities that cannot easily be converted for other uses.
- Long-term contracts with suppliers, payers, medical schools, and other providers.
- As a result of the hospital's probable not-for-profit status, difficulty in transferring or disposing of assets.
- Psychological dependencies of many stakeholders of the hospital: patients, the public, uniquely trained employees, and other health care entities (pharmacies, labs, physicians, primary care/outpatient clinics).
- General political resistance from local and state government and legislative officials.
- A strong possibility of lawsuits from any of the affected stakeholders.

High competitor diversity. When there are great variations among competitors in a market segment in terms of values, culture, resources, and strategies, they are more likely to pursue divergent strategies that inadvertently and unpredictably clash with each other. They will not understand each other well and may misread strategic actions. The result can be more intense competition than is actually intended. This kind of diversity is typical of physician group practices, even within specialties. Although physicians do not have a tradition of vigorous competition with each other, this could change in the face of greater demands by consumers for cost and performance data.

The presence or absence in an industry or market of these rivalry factors can change over time and should be watched closely in a firm's strategic environment monitoring program. Competition can heat up quickly if market growth slows, new competitors enter the market with fresh resources and capabilities, or new technologies disrupt the existing competitive equilibrium. For instance, the availability and utility of electronic medical record (EMR) systems provide a new basis for competition among physician groups and hospitals as well as an opportunity for early adopters to get a competitive jump on their rivals.

2. Threat of Entry by Competitors from Outside the Industry. In addition to the competitive energy exerted by the current industry participants, the intensity level can be raised by new firms entering the industry. They may be existing businesses in other industries that see opportunities for expansion and growth in a new industry. Or entirely new businesses may choose to start up in the industry. The likelihood of new competitors emerging depends on the barriers to entry into the industry and the expected reactions from existing competitors.

Barriers to Entry by New Competitors

Economies of scale. At the current level of competition in an industry, competitors have grown to a size that allows them to realize economies of scale that result in lower costs and lower product and service prices. In order to offer comparable prices, a new competitor would have to immediately create a facility that operates at a sufficiently high volume to enjoy the same scale economies. However, it normally takes some time for sales to grow to such volumes. A simple case is the decision of an outside entrant to build a new hospital. It is not possible to start with a ten-bed facility with a commensurate number of doctors and staff, and then steadily expand to accommodate a gradually increasing number of patients. In a major metropolitan area, economies of scale may dictate a minimum 100-bed hospital, even though patient admissions may not fill that capacity for several years.

Product differentiation. A product that has been well designed and managed over a period of years develops a reputation associated with its very name. The reputation may be based on tangible and distinctive product features, the service supporting the product, and clever, aggressive marketing. If the reputation or image thus created fits the preferences of consumers, they can develop powerful loyalties toward that product. It is usually difficult, costly, and time consuming for a competitor to match or exceed this level of loyalty. An example is a solo-practicing physician who, over a period of ten or twenty years, earns the respect, affection, and allegiance of a large number of patients. He practices in the same subspecialty as several other physicians in the market, yet he is preferred over them. His appeal is based on a subtle mix of genuine clinical competence, genial "bedside manner," patient-friendly service, and accumulated trustworthiness.

Capital requirements. Related to the economies of scale barrier is the minimum capital investment required to begin operations. A new competitor trying to enter a market may have to consider a major initial investment in plant and equipment, as well as working capital to cover operating costs until revenues reach the break-even point. The new 100-bed hospital mentioned above is a good illustration. It would require a large physical plant, clinical treatment and test equipment, elaborate data gathering and reporting systems, and a large staff skilled in a multitude of disciplines. The substantial costs of creating such an enterprise would make any business hesitate to build a new hospital.

Switching costs. Whenever a customer switches from an existing vendor to a new one for the purchase of a product or service, there are one-time costs of making the move. If those "switching costs" are low, customers can change vendors easily and quickly, and the vendors must fight harder to hang on to them. If the costs are high, the customers are locked in for at least the near term and the vendors can be a little more relaxed about competing to retain them. The costs do not have to be financial; it may simply be a matter of convenience and possible disruption to the customer's operations. Many physician practices outsource their claims filing, billing, and collections to third-party vendors specializing in such tasks. The practices often must install the vendors' proprietary systems for recording and transmitting claims data, and train their staff in using them. To switch vendors requires new systems, retraining of practice staff, and delays in collections until the practice and the vendor are working together smoothly. A new vendor must offer a lower price, more product features, or better performance to offset those switching costs.

Another example comes from Porter's book: "For example, in intravenous (IV) solutions and kits for use in hospitals, procedures for attaching solutions to patients differ among competitive products and the hardware for hanging the IV bottles are not compatible. Here switching encounters great resistance from nurses responsible for administering the treatment and requires new investments in hardware."[2]

Access to distribution channels. A business that relies on various types of distributors to get its products or services to the ultimate consumer may have a tough time persuading those channels to handle its offerings. For instance, when an MCO decides to enter a new geographic market, its first step is usually to sign contracts with large employers in order to be able to offer the MCO's health plans to employees and enroll them as members. The employers are likely already to offer a selection of health plans; they will be hesitant to add a new plan or replace one of the existing plans unless it has some significant added benefits. Similarly, a physician moving to a new market area normally wants to develop a flow of patients as quickly as possible. The best way of doing this is securing a position on the provider panel of a local MCO. However, if the MCO is selective about the physicians it contracts with and already has several doctors in the new physician's subspecialty, it may need to see something special about her before it adds her to the panel.

Cost disadvantages apart from economies of scale. In addition to the benefits of scale economies accruing to established competitors, they may possess other cost advantages. For example, around the country, there are a number of respected community and teaching hospitals established decades ago in prime urban locations acquired at relatively low cost. It would be financially prohibitive for a new hospital to be built on such sites today. A surgeon in a group practice may develop a pioneering variation of an existing procedure or a novel instrument for use in that procedure. A scientist in a biomedical research firm may invent a new protocol for conducting whole genome scans to identify the genetic roots of common diseases. If these innovations are protected through their patent or trade secret status, they may be a barrier to an outside business attempting to compete with the group practice or research firm. Frequently, a firm or its individual employees become more adept at performing a service or manufacturing a product the more often or the longer they do it. This "learning curve" effect can lead to reduced costs of production or improved product quality. Physicians performing complex procedures tend to have better clinical outcomes when they see large volumes of patients. This phenomenon makes it difficult for a new physician in the market to establish her clinical credentials.

Government policy. In carrying out legitimate public policy mandates, government agencies can create barriers for new firms wishing to break into certain industries. These barriers may take the form of product/facility/personnel licensing requirements, product safety and efficacy regulations, and onerous product-testing hurdles. Satisfying those conditions can be both expensive and time consuming. A classic example is the multistep, multiyear drug-review process of the FDA. Bringing a new drug to market has been estimated to cost pharmaceutical companies an average of about $100 million. These costs of compliance with government regulations are a strong inhibitor to any firm thinking of entering the prescription drug industry.

Likelihood of Strong Resistance to Attempted Entry

If a firm feels confident that it can overcome most of the traditional barriers to entering a new industry, it still needs to think about the reaction its move may provoke among the existing competitors. If one or many of them feel sufficiently threatened, the resistance could be daunting.

A good indicator of likely resistance is a previous history of vigorous retaliation against prior attempts at entry. A firm needs to begin by identifying and analyzing any other businesses that made the effort in the last five to ten years. It is important to know what part of the industry or market they sought to enter, what resources (e.g., financial, managerial expertise, brand name) were behind the move, which existing competitors were most directly attacked, what tactics they used to respond, and what the outcome of the encounter was. With that knowledge, a new entrant might be able to focus, or appear to focus, on a less-sensitive sector of the industry. It might choose to commit greater resources to its entry strategy. It might configure and promote its entry in a way that does not appear to confront the most worrisome competitors head-on. At the very least, the entrant can prepare itself for the reaction it anticipates. A final option is to give up the entry plan.

A prospective entrant will pay particular attention to well-established competitors with substantial resources to hit back. The chances of retaliation also will be heightened in an industry in which previous competition has brought profit margins to very low levels. Under those conditions, the industry participants will not tolerate even a modest increase in competitive intensity.

The barriers to entry and the likelihood of competitor retaliation change over time. The barriers can be raised or lowered; competitors can become more likely or less likely to resist. An entry strategy that seemed doomed at one point could look much more promising just a few years later. Occasionally, the entering firm can take deliberate initiatives that modify barriers. A drug development startup might adopt a new research methodology that significantly reduces capital required for test equipment. A new MCO coming into a market might bring a successful antitrust lawsuit that overturns the exclusive contracts that existing MCOs have with most of the physicians in the area.

3. Availability of Equivalent, Substitute Products. In addition to the competition among firms offering an industry's traditional products, attention must sometimes be paid to very different products that can function as substitutes for the conventional items. The similarities may not be obvious. A true substitute needs only to perform the same function as the mainstream products. In fact, it may be enough that consumers believe that the products are functional equivalents—whether they really are or not.

In the field of health care, "alternative medicine" is a competitive substitute for traditional or conventional medicine. Alternative medicine encompasses a wide variety of medical treatment methodologies like chiropractic, herbal medicine, acupuncture, homeopathy, naturopathy, holistic medicine, aromatherapy, hypnosis, massage therapy, and biofeedback, as well as faith-based healing practices. There is doubt about the efficacy of some of these approaches; research is in progress to determine their usefulness. Already, large numbers of consumers value alternative medicine highly enough to pay out of pocket for it. In response to the demand and the initial research findings, health plans are beginning to offer insurance coverage for alternative medicine treatments.

One of the primary reasons that consumers may be drawn to substitute products is that they seem to offer more performance for the price, or the same performance at a lower price, than the industry's current products. The question for firms in the industry is when to start paying attention to substitute products and how to treat them.

Substitute products deserve notice when they begin to make serious inroads into industry sales or when they otherwise appear to pose a threat. One example is the alternative medicine modalities mentioned above.

Although most of them have been practiced in the Far East for centuries, the U.S. health care industry began to look more closely only within the past two decades when evidence showed that there were more visits to alternative medicine practitioners than to primary care doctors.[3] Since then, industry researchers have been conducting clinical studies that demonstrate the efficacy of some of these treatment methods. Another very different example is chiropractic, the treatment of diseases through manipulation of the spine. This approach was devised in the United States in the late 1800s and has never been shown to have scientific validity. Nonetheless, every state has enacted a chiropractor licensing law that makes such services available.

An industry firm has several strategic choices for responding to the threat of a substitute product. One is to explore it and, if it proves legitimate and inevitable, consider embracing it. This is the position the health care industry has taken on alternative medicine. Hospitals and physicians have begun to provide acupuncture services, and health plans have begun to cover them. Another approach is to meet the threat head-on. The organized profession of medical doctors has vigorously resisted efforts to bring chiropractic into the mainstream of health care delivery. It has done this through lobbying, litigation, public speaking, and scientific research. The chiropractic profession has been very aggressive in advancing its own interests, and a standoff now exists between it and organized medicine. The medical doctors have now adopted a third strategy—to largely ignore the threat of chiropractic in the belief that a certain share of the market will use its services regardless of scientific evidence.

4. Bargaining Power of Buyers or Customers. When a firm's customers have substantial bargaining power in their relationship with the firm, they can exert pressure that increases competitive intensity in the industry. They may be able to force the firm to lower prices, and demand higher quality, additional product features, or better service. In the process, they may try to play industry competitors against each other. A number of factors can give a customer this kind of influence or dispose it to use the influence.

The customer's purchases represent a large chunk of the seller-firm's sales. In such a situation, the seller is highly dependent on the one customer for its financial well-being. There is a threat, implicit or explicit, that the customer will stop buying from the firm if its demands are not satisfied. Imagine a medium-sized market with several competing MCOs and a single large employer that accounts for a third of all potential MCO members in the area. That employer has a contract with one of the MCOs to provide health care coverage to its employees. The contract contributes 40 percent of the MCO's annual revenues. The employer has several other choices of MCOs from which to purchase the health care coverage. The current MCO would have a difficult time replacing the lost revenues if the employer switched. It will accede to many of the employer's demands before it will allow that to happen.

The customer's purchases from the firm represent a large share of customer's costs. As a major item in its operating budget, the buyer will want to obtain the maximum value for its expenditures. This includes reducing that cost element to its lowest possible level. It will wield all the bargaining power it has toward that end. Many employers are in this position with regard to the health care benefit costs for their employees. It is frequently pointed out that health care adds from $1,000 to $1,500 to the sticker price of each automobile produced by the Big Three auto manufacturers. When health benefits represented a relatively small portion of employers' operating budgets, employers were relatively passive about increases in the insurance premiums they paid. As premiums have moved steadily upward, along with budget share devoted to employee benefits, employers have become much more assertive in their dealings with the sellers of health care services and insurance. In the most pointed stimulus to rivalry among health care competitors, many large employers engage in competitive bidding processes with the available health plans. In a few noteworthy cases, employers have moved backward in the industry value chain to contract directly with hospitals and physicians, almost completely removing the health plans and insurers from the chain.

The items purchased are homogenous with few differentiating features. Buyers can count on receiving virtually the same product from any of several sellers. Under these circumstances, they will tend to focus on price and can more easily take their business to another seller. It is an interesting feature of the general health care industry that, until recently, medical care services have appeared to be undifferentiated. A patient assumed that a surgical procedure performed at hospital A was approximately the equivalent of the same procedure at hospital B. This was largely due to the absence of any reliable measures for quality or other distinguishing characteristics of the services. However, as the health care system became concerned about the quality of care that it provided, a great deal of research has been devoted to finding reliable measures of that quality. As competition among health care providers has heated up, the study of patient satisfaction has increased. The growing movement toward consumer-driven health care is spurring the systematic collection, analysis, and publication of data on a wide variety of metrics that consumers might use in making their purchase choices. The differences among health care providers and the services they offer are becoming more transparent.

The costs of switching from one vendor to another are low. When the financial or convenience costs of changing vendors are low, buyers will have no hesitation about switching to get a better deal. This places pressure on competing vendors to work hard to retain the customers they have and gives them an incentive to steal new ones from their rivals.

The buyer's profit margins are low, which compel it to apply pressure to its suppliers. A buyer under some financial strain is likely to be more demanding of its suppliers. This phenomenon occurs in health care when an MCO, under relentless pressure from its employer-customers to restrain the growth in the premiums it charges, turns to its hospital and physician-suppliers for concessions on the reimbursements it pays them.

The buyer has plausible opportunities to integrate backward into the seller's business. If a buyer is unhappy enough with the products or service that it receives from a seller, it may consider going into the seller's business. Not only is the buyer thus assured of getting the products on its preferred terms, it is also able to capture the profit from the value that the seller adds in the industry value chain. This is a serious threat to the seller only if the buyer has the means to carry it out. A backward integration move takes a company into a field of operations in which it may have few competencies. A good example of this is the Buyers Health Care Action Group (BHCAG) founded in 1988 by several large Minnesota employers out of dissatisfaction with their steadily rising health care costs. The BHCAG assumed many of the traditional functions of MCOs to begin contracting directly with health care providers.

The buyer has good knowledge of the sellers' operating costs and negotiated deals with other buyers. With this information, a buyer is aware of the markup over cost represented by the seller's prices and can bargain accordingly. The buyer also can demand the same terms that the seller has given to other buyers. The importance of this factor is likely to increase in the future. It is common knowledge that many providers, particularly hospitals, charge different prices to different buyers, depending on their negotiating power. The highest prices have been levied on the most disempowered buyers—the uninsured. Several of these factors clearly apply only to buyers that are commercial enterprises. It is worth keeping in mind that some of them also pertain to individual retail consumers. Much of this information will become publicly available as a consequence of consumer-driven health care.

It is a fact that a firm can choose which buyers or buyer groups to sell to—selecting those with the least bargaining power. Sometimes, however, there are no other buyers of comparable size in the market. A classic example is the small physician group practice that relies for most of its patients on a single dominant MCO in the market. The MCO's bargaining power allows it to dictate contract terms and reimbursement rates to the doctors. They would prefer to sell their services to a less uncompromising payer, but there are no alternatives available.

5. Bargaining Power of Suppliers or Employees. When a firm's suppliers have disproportionately strong bargaining power, they can threaten to raise prices or reduce quality or product features in order to increase their own profits. Certain circumstances give suppliers more clout in their dealings with customers.

The group of available suppliers is dominated by a few companies and is more concentrated than the industry it sells to. In this situation, each supplier will be larger in size, buyers will have fewer alternatives if they are dissatisfied with one supplier firm, and the few suppliers may function as an oligopoly.

The supplier is not faced by other substitute products to its own for sale to the industry. The availability of substitute products, functional equivalents to the supplier's products, serves as another source of competition. Without them, a supplier feels less pressure to accede to a buyer's demands.

The buying industry is not an important customer of the supplier group. If sales to the buyer industry are not a significant source of revenue to the suppliers, they will not mind foregoing the sales entirely if they do not like the terms.

The supplier's product is an important input to the customer's business. In other words, a buyer cannot conduct its business without the supplier's product. It will make a lot of concessions, in price, product features, and service, to be assured of receiving the product when it needs it.

The supplier's products are differentiated or marked by switching costs. The products are unique and cannot be obtained from any other supplier. If they are available from another source, the financial and convenience costs of switching are prohibitive. The buyer is essentially locked in to the one supplier.

The supplier poses a plausible threat of forward integration. If a supplier has the resources, abilities, and latent desire to integrate forward in the industry value chain, it poses a threat to its buyers. They are unlikely to make demands that might prompt the supplier to become direct competitors of theirs.

When discussing "suppliers," the first thought often is of product and service vendors—of items like computer systems, pharmaceuticals, surgical gloves, cleaning supplies, or food ingredients. In a labor-intensive industry like health care delivery, employees are also a major category of supplier. For the above reasons, many of them can wield substantial bargaining power. This includes scarce, highly skilled personnel (e.g., specialist physicians, clinical equipment operators) and highly unionized staff (e.g., nurses).

Government Policy. Although government policy was listed as a possible barrier to entry by new competitors into a market, it is considered by some to be such an important factor that it should be treated as a sixth force in Porter's model. There are few industries in which government laws, regulations, programs, and policies have so great an influence on competition as they do in the health care and biotechnology industries. Government agencies serve as major payers/customers (Medicare, Medicaid) and direct providers (municipal and Veterans Administration hospitals). Government reimbursement policies have a significant influence on the type and viability of medical education programs. The National Institutes of Health is a major source of funding for research by biomedical and biotechnology firms. A whole range of laws constrain the operational and strategic activities of providers and biomedical product manufacturers (HIPAA, EMTALA, ERISA, Stark I and II, fraud and abuse, nonprofit tax status, antitrust). Companies selling pharmaceuticals and medical devices must submit their products to a lengthy and expensive testing process in order to obtain government (FDA) approval to put them on the market.

Strategic Firm Responses to the Five Forces

The Five Forces analysis and industry understanding provides a solid backdrop for a firm's strategic decision making. The formulation of specific strategies is explored in Chapter 8. It is possible here to describe a few generic responses a firm might make to the forces that it discovers in its industry.

Aggressive-Transformative. The firm can set out to change the forces to its advantage. Through vertical integration—either backward or forward—a firm can defuse the bargaining power of suppliers and buyers. A hospital could purchase and manage the practices of physicians on its medical staff—as many of them did in the 1990s. The hospital could also usurp the power of its health plan payers by developing its own managed care product. When substitute products appear to pose a threat—as some believe that traditional medicine does for conventional medicine—a firm may begin offering the substitute along with the original product. Some health plans do this when they offer coverage for acupuncture and yoga.

Passive-Adaptive. The firm can adapt its strategies to the forces. When a firm clearly understands its resources and competencies, as well as the dynamics of its industry, it can tailor strategies that dovetail the one with the other. When an industry force is particularly strong and the firm lacks the resources to resist, it will do its best to avoid or deflect its impact. It might do this by shifting into a different, related market segment or differentiating its products in a way that deflects competitive pressures. Physicians accomplish this by learning a new procedural skill not available from competing practices or by catering to a narrow subset of patients (e.g., learning Spanish in order to better serve the market's Hispanic community).

Passive-Exploitive. The firm can implement strategies that exploit the forces. One of the forces transforming the health care industry is the growing power of consumerism, reflected in a desire for more convenient ways to obtain health care. Some organizations, like pharmacies and physician group practices, are anticipating this trend by establishing retail walk-in clinics. Physician practices are opening up e-mail channels for distribution of medical advice to their patients.

COMPETITORS

Because all competitors in an industry are not homogenous, it is necessary also to analyze individual competing organizations.

Which Competitors to Analyze?

There are several types of competitors to be concerned with. First are the business's *existing, immediate competitors,* the ones that it has probably been dealing with for many years. Then there are *potential competitors,* companies currently operating in other industries or markets but that show a high likelihood of entering the business's industry or market. Several sources of new entrants to an industry are:

- Firms operating in other geographic regions seeking to expand their markets.
- Firms offering similar and related, but not directly competing, products that wish to expand their product lines.
- Customer firms that decide to integrate backward in the industrial value chain.
- Suppliers attracted by margins may choose to integrate forward in the chain.
- A small, strategically weak firm becomes a serious threat of entry when it is acquired by a company that can reduce or eliminate the weaknesses.
- Firms that feel threatened by a move into their markets might retaliate by moving in the opposite direction.
- Firms that have a possible fit or synergy with the critical success factors in the industry.

Attention must also be paid to *indirect competitors,* those entities offering products or services that may serve as substitutes to the business's products or services in the eyes of its customers. Alternative Eastern medicine has been playing this role for over a decade in the markets for traditional Western medical care. It is best to view as competition any firm that is capable of satisfying the same set of customer wants and needs that the business is now meeting or planning to meet.

Competition With and Among Networks and Systems

There can be a tendency to look for competitors organized as independent freestanding businesses or SBUs within a larger corporation. Within the health care and biotechnology industries, another competitive form has emerged in the last decade or so: the network or system composed of numerous otherwise independent businesses. The best example is the integrated delivery system (IDS), a combination of hospitals, physician practices (primary care and specialists), and other provider entities required to serve all the health care needs of a large regional population. More than one IDS may exist in a market, competing with one another for contracts with payers like HMOs. The HMOs themselves, which are groupings of provider entities with a financing function, compete as systems with each other. To expand their research capability, old-line pharmaceutical companies have been establishing strategic partnerships with smaller, more nimble biotechnology companies, many of them recent startups with promising technologies under development.

This trend has implications for strategic planning. It affects who a business identifies as its competitors and how it assesses their strategic and competitive potential. A hospital whose cross-town rival has just become an integral part of an IDS needs to shift its competitive focus from the individual hospital to the entire system—perhaps by seeking another IDS to join itself. Or, if the hospital just has been acquired by a large multistate hospital network, it now will be backed by considerably greater financial resources. Its parent corporation and its sibling hospitals may have additional resources and competencies that it can share. Management at the corporate center may have specific ideas about the strategies that it wants the hospital to pursue. Anyone attempting to assess the competitive capabilities of a drug company must look at not only its own substantial internal R&D resources, but also the research competencies and potential new products of the strategic partners it may have acquired.

Narrowing the Scope of Competitor Analysis

In some markets, a firm may face a large number of competitors of varying size, competence, and potential threat. Imagine all the other physician practices that a group of doctors in a large metropolitan area must consider to be competitors. Most firms do not have the resources to go after every one of their competitors. There are two solutions to this quandary.

To employ limited resources most efficiently, one approach is to *concentrate* on those competitors that pose the greatest threat, that are most likely to hinder the implementation of its strategic plans. In most instances, primary competitors are quite visible and easily identified. Against whom does the firm usually compete? Which are its most intense competitors? It might make sense, in a rough, informal way, to grade and rank other businesses in the market by their degree of competitive intensity. The firm may then limit its detailed analysis to the most threatening competitors.

Another approach to simplifying competitor analysis for firms with more substantial resources is to divide the industry participants into *strategic groups*. A strategic group is a collection of businesses (such as physician practices) that have similar characteristics, possess similar resources and competencies, and tend to pursue similar competitive strategies. Firms in a strategic group will be affected by and react to industry developments in similar ways.

Knowledge of an industry's strategic groups can be used in several ways. A corporation composed of several SBUs can decide in which strategic groups it will compete, either by moving an SBU from one group to another, developing a new SBU in a new group, or acquiring a firm already competing in the new group. An individual SBU may choose, for strategic reasons, to migrate to a more attractive group or to create an entirely new strategic group. At the very least, a strategic group classification tells a firm which competitors it needs to analyze individually and in greater detail.

There are some basic characteristics that are used in distinguishing the firms that belong to a particular strategic group. These examples apply to physician practices.

- The medical specialties practiced and the degree of concentration on them.
- Any reputation that the practice has earned and the customer loyalty it has engendered.
- The channels through which it delivers its services (hospital-based, office-based, satellite or retail clinics).
- The aggressiveness, extent, and nature of any marketing efforts.
- Market segments served (elderly, women, children, Hispanic, geographic area).
- Contractual relationships with payers (MCOs, Medicare, Medicaid).
- Impressions, and perhaps objective measures, of the quality of services provided.
- How rapidly the practice has embraced new technologies, like EMR and CPOE systems.
- Extent to which it has expanded backward or forward in its industry value chain (specialty hospitals, self-pay patients only).

- How cost efficiently the practice is managed.
- The level of service amenities that it provides to patients.
- Comparison of its fee and charges to those of competing practices.
- How well capitalized the practice is (physician willingness to invest).

Some of these characteristics are better indicators of a competitor's strategic threat potential than others. In defining the strategic groups, it is worth trying different combinations of characteristics to see which produce the most useful, intuitive classifications of firms in the industry. The process for identifying strategic groups is similar to that for categorizing market segments discussed in Chapter 4.

Before it moves on to an analysis of individual competitors, a firm may choose to apply the Five Forces Model to measure the degrees of attractiveness and competitive intensity within strategic groups. One thing that analysis will reveal is mobility barriers that inhibit or prevent businesses from moving out of or into a group. One way to develop a sustainable competitive advantage is to pursue a strategy based on unique resources and competencies that reinforces barriers to competitors.

Whether or not a strategically motivated firm takes the intermediate step of describing the strategic groups in its industry, it will eventually move to an analysis of individual competitors. Solid competitor understanding can suggest opportunities and threats that will merit a response, allow the prediction of emerging threats and opportunities, enable forecast of the likely reaction of competitors to the firm's strategic initiatives, and may identify some strategic uncertainties that will be worth monitoring over time. That understanding comes from an analysis of each competitor that parallels the internal assessment that the firm performs on itself (see Chapter 2). This means gathering competitive intelligence on strategic resources and competencies, company value chains, financial strength and capital-raising capabilities, and strategic intentions.

Individual Competitor Analysis

A firm is interested in two broad areas of a competitor's strategic program. The first is its intentions or desires, the strategies that it is committed to implementing or is considering implementing. The second is the resources and competencies that it possesses actually to carry out those strategies. The firm will be somewhat less concerned with a competitor's strategic intentions that it lacks the means to put into action.

Strategic Aspirations and Commitments

A competitor's strategic thoughts and plans for the future are based on the following types of factors.

Motivations for strategic action. A fundamental question about any competitor is whether it has strategic aspirations at all and, if so, what they are. Even more important is knowledge of commitments that it has made to specific strategic actions. This knowledge permits a firm to determine how unhappy a competitor is with its current operating performance and how inclined it might be to make bold strategic moves. The firm can better assess the threat posed by those moves and the competitor's likely response to the firm's own strategic initiatives.

An indication of a competitor's strategic motivations can be found, first, by observing its financial performance and statements of dissatisfaction with it. Sometimes, managers will publicly announce (to financial analysts, if they are investor-owned) their intentions to improve certain financial parameters. A firm also will pay attention to a competitor's acknowledged shortcomings and plans in other areas like product quality, customer satisfaction, market focus, new technology adoption, and market segments served.

These are some examples of strategic impulses that a medium-sized community hospital might have.

- Revenues have been growing at a rate slightly below the average for its market; profitability fluctuates between 1–2 percent positive (profit) and 1–2 percent negative (loss). Management feels that the hospital's financial and market position is slowly eroding. It believes that corrective action of a strategic nature is called for.
- The hospital has preferred to conduct its affairs in the tradition of nonprofit, charitable provider organizations rather than a tightly managed profit-driven entity. The one member of the hospital's board of directors with substantial high-level business experience has suggested openly that the hospital must move away from this model.
- The rest of the board of directors are either hospital physicians and executives, or various leaders within the community. The outspoken director has advocated that a greater proportion of the board should be composed of accomplished business leaders.
- The hospital recently settled a CMS complaint of Medicare billing errors for $2.3 million that the hospital blamed on seriously outdated financial management and control systems. The hospital CEO said that it needed to upgrade most of its technology-based systems—billing and claims processing, financial reporting and control, clinical outcomes, errors and quality, patient records, and the like.

If the hospital is part of a wider network of hospitals or is a subsidiary to a parent corporation with other SBUs, such as physician practices, primary care clinics, and nursing homes, the strategic aspirations of that parent are also relevant. For instance, how well is the overall corporation performing financially, and how does the hospital's performance compare to the other SBUs? Because the hospital may be the flagship of the corporation's portfolio, it can receive both pressure and support from the parent to be a strategic leader. It may be expected to generate sufficient cash flow to make up for fiscal shortfalls in the other units.

Strategic mindset. All organizations develop a set of attitudes, beliefs, and mental models about themselves and all aspects of their environment. This knowledge can give clues as to what kinds of initiatives they will take, how aggressively they will pursue them, and how they will respond to others' initiatives and to external events. This part of the analysis usually begins by examining a competitor's self-image, how it contrasts that with other competitors in the market and the industry, and its view of its customers. Does it consider itself to be a leader, a follower, or simply a peer among competing firms? Does it have a realistic understanding of how it is viewed by the rest of the industry and by its customers? Is its perception of its customers sympathetic or cynical?

It would be extremely valuable to know what a competitor believes its strengths and weaknesses to be. Even if they are misguided, not grounded in reality, they will certainly be the basis of the business's strategies. The organization may also feel bound by long-standing philosophical or cultural loyalties to certain people, market segments, practices, policies, or products that unduly influence its strategic decision making.

Some organizations evolve strong ethical values that guide their business behaviors. While he served as CEO of Beth Israel Deaconess Hospital in Boston, Mitchell T. Rabkin, M.D., instilled a culture that was recognized for being particularly humane toward both its employees and its patients. Some of the hospital's strategic initiatives bear out that legacy to this day.

Competing firms develop attitudes about their external environments, including industry trends, prevailing moods in public policy, shifts in the political and legal climate, and the threats posed by their rivals—attitudes that influence their strategy making. During the 1970s and early 1980s, some indemnity health insurance companies recognized the trend toward managed care and turned themselves into MCOs; others did not and went out of business. During the late 1980s and early 1990s, many providers adopted constructive attitudes toward managed care and established rewarding relationships with their MCO payers; others struggled in what were more adversarial relationships. Historically, many health care organizations have been focused more on satisfying their providers, usually the physicians, than their customers-patients. Savvy health care businesses now are having to adjust their views in order to compete in a more "consumer-driven" marketplace.

Strategic track record. Knowing how a competitor has made strategy historically can be a strong indicator of how it will act or react in the future. It is useful, therefore, to study several features of a competitor's strategic track record and the infrastructure on which it was based.

The status of a firm's current operations should be viewed as the product of the strategies it implemented three to five years in the past. Notice the ways in which those operations have changed and speculate on the strategies that brought them about. If the firm has been closely monitoring the competitor for some time, it may already be aware of the strategies it has been pursuing. A less competitive, poorly performing rival may have made faulty strategic choices in the past or simply made no choices at all. Perhaps it implemented the choices ineptly. If a competitor has improved its market position, it probably is the result of some recent smart strategic moves. What were they?

It is worth keeping track of all the strategic initiatives made by competitors and their ultimate effectiveness. Which succeeded and which failed, and what were the apparent reasons? How well implemented were they? When organizations fail to carry out a strategy competently, some learn from the experience and do not repeat the mistakes; others make them a habit.

Organizations have a way of falling into patterns and habits in their strategic behaviors that are carried over to future strategies unless deliberate efforts are made to change. They may carefully consider their strategic decisions over a period of weeks or months, or act impulsively and reactively in a matter of days. When events occur demanding strategic action, an organization may not seem to notice until it has almost no choice, or it may jump promptly on the issues, trends, problems, opportunities, or threats as soon as they are revealed, study them carefully and quickly, and then act decisively. The formulation of strategy can be rigorously evidence-based, following a systematic, multistep process. Alternatively, the firm's strategists may believe that they have sufficient experience and judgment to make decisions intuitively.

The success or failure of previous strategies is often a function of the resources and competencies that were dedicated to them. As noted below, these strategic assets of a competitor's should be inventoried as completely as possible, with special attention to those that seem especially weak or strong, or that have changed dramatically in the past few years.

Strategic managers' background and history. A business's strategic behaviors are manifested by its strategic managers, typically on the basis of background factors that can be discovered and studied. It is good to know in what industries, companies, and functional areas a competitor's strategic decision makers have worked. The types of strategic challenges they have faced and the ways that they responded, in particular the strategy forms they have employed, may suggest what they will do in their current positions. An executive who was trained as a lawyer and previously served as vice president of planning and government relations in a large pharmaceutical company will have different strategic instincts than a research scientist who founded his own biotechnology company and made most of the strategic decisions himself.

A strategy decision maker may be more inclined to repeat the types of strategies that have worked for her in the past and avoid strategic models that have failed for her. Her strategic track record should be examined.

As a general matter, information about the educational background, formal training, avocations, and personal lifestyle of top executives in rival organizations may also offer some clues to their strategic mindsets, and their predispositions toward innovation and risk-taking.

Strategic Capabilities

An organization's resources and competencies are the assets that it has available for conceiving and carrying out any strategies. They define what it is capable of, strategically. Just as a business must catalog and assess its own resources and competencies prior to formulating strategy, so must it discover and evaluate the strategic assets that its competitors can bring to bear. The process is similar to that described in Chapter 2, with the exception that the data may be more difficult to gather. (See the section on competitive intelligence.)

The review of competitors' strategic assets can take either or both of the internal value chain, or resources and competencies approaches.

Internal value chain. Because the competitor is producing the same goods and services, its value chain will closely resemble the firm's. However, it may not be identical; there are likely to be subtle and not-so-subtle differences. By scrutinizing competing chains, a firm can identify activities in which a competitor is weak and vulnerable to attack, as well as those areas that are sources of strength and may pose a threat. It might also be assumed that the strong points in the chain will be the keys to any strategies that the competitor decides to initiate.

An important part of the value chain analysis is an activity-by-activity comparison with the firm's value chain. This comparison can be presented graphically by drawing the firm's and a competitor's value chains in parallel so that the activities match up, and specifying which activities are comparative strengths or weaknesses for the firm, in which activities it is in parity with the competitor, and which activities are entirely unique to either the firm or its competitor. The comparison can be enhanced by showing in which activities the firm has a cost advantage (i.e., is performing the activity more efficiently) or is adding more value (i.e., is performing the activity differently).

Resources and competencies. This phase of competitor analysis uses approximately the same categories as the firm employed in its own internal assessment (Chapter 2). More than an overall inventory, it identifies specific assets that may serve as strengths or weaknesses in carrying out the competitor's strategic intentions. Some summary results from such an analysis of a teaching hospital might look like this.

Technology and Innovation

- Basic EMR system, lacking many sophisticated features (i.e., preventive medicine prompts, clinical decision support, coding guidance, e-prescribing, integration with lab, pharmacy and imaging systems).
- More sophisticated management information system (MIS), measuring resource utilization and costs at the individual level.
- Information technology (IT) director knowledgeable about system architecture.
- Only mediocre computer systems support and maintenance.
- Impulse for top management to adopt proven new technologies, restrained by desire to avoid offending influential medical staff physicians.

Operations

- Highly efficient scheduling of operating room (OR) and outpatient surgeries.
- Less-effective mechanisms for controlling costs.
- Rather ineffective infection control systems.
- Above-average performance on JCAHO Hospital Quality Standards.
- Prime physical location virtually adjacent to local medical school.
- Limited physical space that offers little room for expansion.

Organizational

- Culture that emphasizes employee participation in decision making, resulting in higher morale.
- Good management relations with nurses' union.
- Average management relations with medical staff.
- Below-average management relations with private payers.
- Demonstrated effectiveness at team building and teamwork.
- Several top physicians in oncology and radiology.
- Weak physician staffing in pediatrics.

Finance

- Loyal and generous base of charitable donors.
- Good cash flow from commercialization of research discovered in hospital-based labs.
- Steady and low operating margin (1.7–2.0 percent).
- Standard & Poor's BBB bond rating.

Management

- CEO one of most highly regarded in local market.
- Executive team has shown willingness in the past to take bold strategic moves of modest proportions.
- CEO is approaching retirement age with no obvious successor in sight.
- Middle management is dedicated but weak in experience with hospitals in competitive markets.

Marketing

- Strong local reputation for patient-centric care and service.
- Excellent response to patient feedback and complaints.
- No unique or substantially differentiated clinical services.
- Weak managerial competence in advertising and promotion.
- Spends below market average percentage of revenues on marketing budget.

Using Analysis Results to Forecast How a Competitor Is Likely to Behave Strategically

The purpose of gathering this wealth of industry and competitor knowledge is to inform the firm's strategic actions. It wishes to anticipate the points at which rivals will launch strategic offensives in order to take preemptive action or at least minimize the damage. The firm also wants to know where a competitor is weakest and concentrate its own strategies there. In the end, it hopes to overwhelm any competitor resistance to the achievement of its own strategic goals.

In playing this high-stakes corporate chess match, a business will ask and answer a sequence of basic questions.

1. Initially, a firm wants to know the likelihood that a particular competitor will make any strategic move at all. Information on the timing of the move would be equally valuable.
2. If the competitor is showing signs of near-term strategic movement, exactly what form will it take? Will it sell to a new market niche, offer new products or services, or new features in existing products, charge lower fees or prices, use marketing to create new customer value perceptions, or distribute through different channels?
3. What methods will the competitor use to implement the strategy? Will it negotiate strategic alliances or partnerships with competitors, suppliers, or customers? Will it move to integrate vertically or horizontally within its industry value chain? Will it merge with or acquire other businesses in order to gain access to their resources and competencies? Will it take steps to develop new strategically potent

resources and competencies internally? Will it increase its budget for research and innovation? Has it taken steps to obtain additional debt or equity capital that might be used for strategic purposes?

4. If the strategic movement seems imminent, how much energy and resources is the rival firm likely to commit to the effort? Will it be a large-scale initiative backed by substantial financing and staff, or a modest, even tentative strategic foray? Perhaps the initiative is a pilot version of the strategy, to test the response of both the market and the competition.
5. What is the best estimate of the chances of success for the competitor strategy? A well-intentioned strategic plan may fail because it is not well designed for the existing market conditions, it is not supported with adequate resources or competencies, it is not competently implemented, or it provokes a response from other competitors that is so powerful that it does not achieve its goals.

   The "success" of a strategy also is a relative matter. A new initiative may not fail so completely that it is abandoned, but it still might not achieve its planned objectives. As a result, its competitors feel unaffected by the strategic outcome. For example, the smallest of three pharmacy chains competing in a large metropolitan area may attempt to gain market share by opening a number of smaller outlets offering only prescription medicines and herbal supplements. Its ambition is to grow its share of the market from 7 percent to 12 percent. Its two competitors would have been inclined to respond if that goal had been reached. In fact, the share increased to only 9 percent. The two rivals chose to ignore that outcome.
6. If the strategic move is successful, what kind of threat will it pose to the firm and how serious will it be? A strategy may be well conceived, well executed, and ultimately successful, yet it may not target a market that is of concern to the firm. For instance, an MCO may launch successfully a health plan tailored to the needs of baby boomers qualifying for Medicare coverage. Such a move will not threaten another MCO that has concentrated on delivering health care services to young families and their children.
7. Apart from its own strategic initiatives, to what strategic moves of the firm is the competitor most likely to respond? The firm wants to take this knowledge into account in planning those strategies. It might be inclined to focus on an area where the competitor is vulnerable—where there are weaknesses in its resources or competencies, where there is a gap in its market coverage, or where it will have difficulty retaliating. However, if that weak point or gap is nonetheless critical to the competitor's primary mission, it might feel compelled to react with considerable force, regardless of the cost.

8. If it appears that the competitor will respond, what will be the nature and intensity of its response? How damaging might that response be to the firm's initial move and the chances of successfully implementing the strategy? Can the response be prevented, preempted, defused, or simply ignored? Should the firm prepare a counter-response to the competitor's response?

The sequence of actions and reactions plays out like a chess match. To simulate the range of possibilities, some firms conduct elaborate war games or role plays.

With the knowledge gained, an organization is in a good position to make two types of strategic decisions.

- It can anticipate and prepare itself for competitor strategy moves by choosing to ignore them, responding moderately, responding vigorously, or fighting to the death.
- It can launch its own carefully crafted strategic initiatives, while simultaneously preparing for countermoves by competitors. The initiatives may aim to avoid major confrontations with competitors, focus on market niches that are of less importance to competitors, or attack them head-on at points where the firm has the resources to defeat or push them back.

It is a challenge to assess accurately the strategic potentials of a single competitor, and what its actual behaviors might be. The problem becomes immensely more complex when a firm faces multiple competitors. Not only are there more possible threats to keep track of but the actions of several different competitors are bound to interact with each other, creating even more unpredictability.

Competitive Intelligence

It is not as easy to gather information about a competitor's strategic capabilities and intentions as it is for one's own organization. To minimize the waste of time and money, and maximize the volume and quality of useful information gathered, a few guidelines are helpful.

The firm must commit to the creation of a formal and permanent competitive intelligence-gathering program, even if it consists of nothing more than the part-time efforts of a clerk in the marketing department. One-shot information on a competitor is next to worthless; its strategic possibilities are constantly evolving.

The data-gathering process must begin with clear statements from the firm's strategy decision makers about exactly *what they want to know* about their competitors. Competitive intelligence gathering should not be an open-ended fishing expedition. It may help for the decision makers to have a dialogue with the competition researchers to learn what kinds of information might be available.

The next step is to identify the *best sources* for competitor knowledge that would meet the strategists' needs and inform their decisions. A surprising variety of data are available about companies operating in the U.S. economy. Because of the close scrutiny the health care industry is under, information about its members is even easier to find. There are three broad categories of methods for collecting competitor information—accessing publicly available data, paying for privately gathered data, and conducting original field research. These are a few of the leading corporate information sources.

Publicly available data:

- Media articles—journals, magazines, newspapers
- Mandatory reports filed with public agencies—SEC filings (EDGAR), IRS tax filings, documents in lawsuits, patent and copyright filings, licensure and accreditation reports
- Speeches by top managers, especially to financial analysts, business reporters, trade groups, and shareholder meetings
- Corporate public relations announcements (PR newswire)
- Corporate statements on Web sites (Google Alerts news feeds), in promotional material and advertisements, and in annual reports
- Health care–specific Web sites:
    - National Center for Health Statistics
    - Agency for Healthcare Research and Quality
    - Centers for Medicare and Medicaid Services
    - Centers for Disease Control and Prevention
    - Health Resources and Services Administration
    - National Cancer Institute
- American Hospital Association
- American Medical Association
- The Dartmouth Atlas of Medical Care

Privately gathered commercial data:

- LexisNexis (legal filings, litigation reports)
- Hoover's, Dun & Bradstreet (private, non–publicly traded companies)
- Moody's, Standard & Poor's, Fitch (credit ratings)
- PACER (Public Access to Court Electronic Records)
- PAIR (Patent Applications Informational Retrieval)
- Consulting firms
- Market research firms

- Trade associations
- Think tank publications
- Commercial industry newsletters
- Investment banking research reports

Original field research:

- Interviews of employees who have contact with or knowledge of competitors (purchasing agents, private practice physicians)
- Surveys of suppliers who also serve competitors
- Surveys of the firm's customers who may also frequent the competition
- Contracted surveys and research on competitors

A veritable sea of information is available from legitimate sources about the operations of almost every FP, NFP, and public entity in the United States. The availability of strategy-relevant information on competitors is due to grow dramatically as the concept of "consumer-driven health care" spreads throughout the industry. There is no reason ever to employ the unsavory, illegal data-gathering methods that a few organizations have tried.

The large volume of information that will quickly accumulate must be sorted and organized to make it accessible. It will certainly be categorized by competitor, but other relevant classifications may be used as well—industry strategic groups, level of competitive threat posed, types of strategies employed.

The information is then analyzed and conclusions drawn about its relationship to the firm's strategies. One part of the analysis must be to rate the reliability of the information sources. The conclusions will be closely related to the firm's current and proposed operations. The strengths and weaknesses of each competitor should be delineated, with translation into the opportunities and threats that they present to the firm. Trends in all these areas should be plotted. An effort will be made to estimate the impact that projected competitor actions will have on the firm if they are not checked in some way. The technique of describing several likely scenarios is often an effective way of exploring future possibilities.

Ultimately, the information, in the form of some raw data and more conclusions and predictions, is compressed into reports that are sent on a regular basis to the firm's strategy decision makers. The focus of the reports may vary, depending on the strategists' needs and requests. During a period of major new strategy initiation (and certainly when the firm does strategic planning for the first time), very comprehensive studies will be prepared on the entire industry and all of its participants. At other times, periodic reports may be submitted on primary competitors or significant competitive issues. Occasionally, an executive may request a one-time summary of information on a particular organization or topic in the competitive arena.

In the end, the reports that come out of the competitive intelligence (CI) program are used by the business's managers to place the organization in the optimal strategic position vis-à-vis its competitors. If they do not have that utility, there is no point in operating such a program. A well-conceived intelligence effort that leads to strategic decisions that are more perceptive reflections of industry opportunities and threats can be a powerful competitive advantage in and of itself.

A business must make a decision about how much money and other resources to devote to its CI program. Because this activity needs to be ongoing, rather than a one-time compilation of data, it should be a regular item in the organizational budget. Two problems come up in creating these programs—giving them more resources than their output is worth to the firm's strategists and collecting more information than they can realistically digest and use. As a guideline, the largest corporations spend somewhat over $1 million a year on CI.

Corporate-Level Competition

This chapter has focused on the competition among individual businesses operating in the same industries in pursuing customers in the same markets. But, what of the competition between large corporations composed mainly of portfolios of numerous SBUs?

Whether such corporations are in competition with each other depends on the composition of their portfolios. If they are made up of the same types of SBUs competing with each other in the same markets, then it is fair to say that the corporations are also competing with each other. For instance, in a particular multistate regional market, there may be two corporate networks of a number of acute care hospitals serving the general inpatient needs of local residents. The individual hospitals are in competition, as are their parent corporations. The situation is different, and the competition would not exist, if one of the networks owned hospitals in the Southwest while the other's hospitals were located in the Northeast. The same thing would be true if one network were composed of specialty hospitals for children and the other provided primarily rehabilitation services through its hospitals.

Multi-SBU corporations do not always fall into neat categories—having either virtually identical or totally dissimilar portfolios. A corporation may own and oversee several different types of SBUs—hospitals, physician practices, pharmacies, and laboratories. The industries and geographic markets in which they operate may overlap only partially. How similar must two corporations' SBU portfolios be before it can be said that they are in competition?

When multi-SBU corporations do in fact compete, the form of that competition is quite different than the rivalry among SBUs. They are not directly vying with each other for customers to increase their revenues and profits. Instead, they aim to deliver value to their owners-shareholders by assembling portfolios of SBUs that, individually and in collaboration with each other, grow total revenues and profits better and faster than a competing corporation's portfolio. A primary source of competitive advantage for a multi-SBU is its unique, sustainable ability to gather together and sensitively manage a potent collection of SBU's.

Study Questions

1. Can you think of any other forces, in addition to the five generic forces identified by Michael Porter, that might influence the intensity of competition in an industry? Do this in the context of the health care industry. Are there forces unique to health care that influence competition?
2. One of Porter's five forces is the bargaining power of suppliers and employees. Among the members of that group for a hospital are its physicians and nurses. Looking at those professions separately, how has their bargaining power vis-à-vis hospitals waxed and waned over the past ten to fifteen years? At what points have they seemed to have a great deal of power, and at what other points have they been in weak bargaining positions?
3. How does an organization decide who its competitors are? How does it determine which of those competitors pose the greatest threat to it?
4. What legal and ethical steps would you take to figure out the strategic intentions, and even specific plans, of a competitor organization? What information would you like to have and where would you get it from?
5. Become as familiar as possible with the questions provided in this chapter for predicting a competitor's strategic moves. Whenever you read about a business announcing a change in its operations, ask yourself what this may portend about its strategic intentions or plans. It might be a layoff of a hundred employees, a change in advertising agencies, the hiring of a new vice president of finance, or the acquisition of one of its supplier or customer organizations.

Learning Exercise 1

Draw a diagram depicting the industry value chain for a teaching hospital. Take into account all the inputs that go into the hospital's operations and all the outputs that emanate from it. Trace the chain as far back and as far forward as you can. Sometimes the chain will branch; follow those branches out to their ends. When you have finished the diagram, consider the possibilities for the hospital to integrate vertically backward or forward in that chain. List the reasons for and against vertical integration by the hospital.

Learning Exercise 2

Identify a local medium-sized physician group practice. Perform a five-forces analysis of the group. Try to gain direct access to the group by offering your free services as a student consultant. Otherwise, use whatever information you can gather from general, publicly available sources. This will be a quick and dirty analysis, nothing like what the organization would do on its own. Identify and describe the factors driving each one of the five forces affecting the group.

Notes

[1] *Competitive Strategy: The Core Concepts*. In: Porter M. *Competitive Strategy.* New York, NY: The Free Press; 1998:3–33.

[2] Porter M. *Competitive Strategy*. [city]: Free Press; 1998:10.

[3] Eisenberg DM, Davis RB, Ettner SL, Appel S, Wilkey S, Van Rompay M, and Kessler RC. Trends in alternative medicine use in the United States, 1990–1997: results of a follow-up national survey. *JAMA*. 1998;280(18):1569–1575.

References

Brown SL and Eisenhardt KM. *Competing on the Edge*. Cambridge, MA: Harvard Business School Press; 1998.

Buzzell RD and Gale BT. The PIMS Principles: Linking Strategy to Performance. New York, NY: The Free Press; 1987.

Chattopadhyay P, Glick WH, and Huber GP. Organizational actions in response to the threats and opportunities. *Academy of Management Journal.* 2001;44:937–955.

Coff RW. When competitive advantage doesn't lead to performance: The resource-based view and stakeholder bargaining power. *Organization Science*. 1999;10:119–133.

Daems H and Thomas H. *Strategic Groups, Strategic Moves and Performance*. Amsterdam, The Netherlands: Pergamon; 1994.

Gordon ME and Milne GR. Selecting the dimensions that define strategic groups: A novel market-driven approach. *Journal of Managerial Issues.* 1999;11(2):213–233.

Hamel G and Prahalad CK. *Competing for the Future*. Cambridge, MA: Harvard Business School Press; 1994.

Harrigan KR. Barriers to entry and competitive strategies. *Strategic Management Journal*. 1981;2:395–412.

Hawawini G, Subramanian V, and Verdin P. *Is profitability driven by industry- or firm-specific factors? A new look at the evidence*. INSEAD; 2000.

Jennings DF and Lumpkin JR. Insights between environmental scanning activities and Porter's generic strategies: An empirical analysis. *Journal of Management*. 1982;18:791–803.

Kahaner L. *Competitive Intelligence*. New York, NY: Simon & Schuster; 1996.

McGahan AM. Competition, strategy and business performance. *California Management Review*. 1999;41(3):74–101.

McGahan AM and Porter ME. How much does industry matter, really? *Strategic Management Journal*. 1997;18(8):15–30.

Porter ME. *Competitive Strategy: Techniques for Analyzing Industries and Companies*. New York, NY: The Free Press; 1980.

Porter ME. Towards a dynamic theory of strategy. *Strategic Management Journal*. 1991;12:95–117.

Rumelt RP. How much does industry matter. *Strategic Management Journal*.1991;12(3):167–186.

Sawka K. Demystifying business intelligence. *Management Review*. October 1996:49.

Schere FM and Ross DR. *Industrial Market Structure and Economic Performance*. 3rd ed. Boston, MA: Houghton Mifflin; 1990.

Schoemaker PJH. When and how to use scenario planning. *Journal of Forecasting*. 1991;10:549–564.

Shaker SM and Gembicki MP. *War Room Guide to Competitive Intelligence*. New York, NY: McGraw-Hill; 1999.

Shamsie J. The context of dominance: An industry-driven framework for exploiting reputation. *Strategic Management Journal*. 24:199–215.

CHAPTER

6

Defining Future Direction of the Organization

Learning Objectives

After reading and studying this chapter, you should be able to:

- Explain the concept of "strategic direction" and why it is the first step in the delineation of an organization's strategic intentions.
- Distinguish between strategic direction at the level of the corporation and within its individual SBUs.
- Describe the mission statement and the purpose it serves in the strategic planning process.
- List the characteristics of a good mission statement.
- Describe the vision statement and the purpose it serves in the strategic planning process.
- List the characteristics and benefits of a good mission statement.
- Describe the values of an organization and the purpose they serve in its operational and strategic activities.
- Describe the substance of an organization's strategic objectives and the contribution they make to the strategic planning process.
- Distinguish between strategic objectives at the corporate and SBU levels.

With a good sense of what it is capable of, in terms of resources and competencies, and what it faces in the outside world, in terms of markets and customers, competitors, and general environmental factors, an organization is in a good position to begin plotting a course into the future. An organization's future is virtually limitless; there is an infinity of directions in which it can choose to steer itself. The decision needs to be reached in a thoughtful, systematic manner. Over several decades of strategic management practice by many organizations in many industries, there has developed a set of four documents that define an organization's future direction. These are a mission statement, a vision portrayal, a code of values, and a set of strategic objectives. They are usually prepared in that order. The introspective and ongoing process that creates these documents is often the first time that an organization consciously expresses its strategic intentions.

RESPONSIBILITY FOR DEFINING STRATEGIC DIRECTION

Strategic direction can be defined at the corporate, SBU, functional area, and other appropriate levels within a large organization. The direction is necessary for the strategies that are implemented at each of those levels.

The mission and vision statements created by the corporate center describe the strategic direction for the total organization. Because the corporation is often the sole legal entity capable of raising debt and equity capital for use by its various components, the essence of that direction and how well it is followed is watched closely by external stakeholders in the financial community. However, the direction of the corporation is concerned mainly with the types of businesses that will be contained in its portfolio. It is at the SBU level that the direction statements focus on the markets in which each business intends to compete and how it will gain sustainable competitive advantages there. If the entire organization consists of a single business, these will be its only direction statements; there is no portfolio strategy to explain.

The identities of the organization personnel who will be involved in defining its strategic direction is not a trivial matter. When a company is first formed, as in the case of a biotechnology startup, the founders determine that direction. They may not do it consciously; they may not think of it in terms of a "strategic direction." It often starts with the promising results of a university-based research project that shows some commercial

Table 6.1 Hierarchy of Strategy-Making Levels in an Organization

Corporate Center
↑↓
Multiple SBUs
↑↓
Within each SBU, multiple functional areas
↑↓
Within each functional area, multiple departments
↑↓
Within each department, multiple teams and task forces

potential. The lead researchers create an organization to begin that commercialization process. In another example, a group of three physicians who recently completed residencies decide to set up a practice together. Whatever direction the practice has will come from the three doctors.

If the business succeeds and grows, it usually becomes necessary eventually to formalize the strategy-making process, including making a clearer statement of strategic direction. At this point, the founders or chief executives of the business still take lead roles in the process, though they are likely to begin consulting other managers and staff within the organization.

The historical model of delegating all strategy-making responsibility to a vice president of strategic planning and his staff now seems archaic and insular. The movement is definitely in the direction of making the process much more inclusive. A key step in that direction was the use of "strategic planning retreats" to which a few more managers were invited. Now, in some organizations, almost every employee is given an opportunity to provide some input to the strategy-making process. It seems especially useful to include those people who are likely to participate in the implementation of the strategies. Occasionally, even external stakeholders are consulted.

In the midst of this democratization of strategic management, the organization's leaders remain the catalysts and guides. Their particular strategy preferences may not always dominate, but they are primarily responsible for making sure that the necessary systems are in place, the process occurs, the steps are followed, and concrete results are achieved. In the end, the top executives are responsible to the board of directors, and the board of directors in turn is responsible to the organization's owners or other external stakeholders.

■ MISSION

An organization's "mission" is the current purpose for the organization's existence. The mission statement is a concise explanation of what the firm is, what it does, and what it does not do. It describes the "business" of the firm, the domain of the firm, the areas in which it has chosen to operate, and the means by which it competes in those areas. It is a practical summary of the activities and operations of the firm, often expressed in terms of the products that it intends to manufacture and sell and the markets/customers it intends to serve. The mission is concerned mainly with the activities of the firm, and with things that it does in the present or near future.

The mission statement is the starting point for an organization's strategic decisions. It is quite difficult to plot a course into the distant future without having a good sense of where a business stands in the present.

Mission statements are prepared by parent corporations, their constituent SBUs, and independent freestanding business entities. Such statements might also serve a useful purpose for functional areas and even departments within businesses and corporations. The mission statements of individual SBUs should fit with the statements of their parents, and vice versa.

A good mission statement defines a manageable number of substantial spheres within which the company will operate and compete. Those spheres are defined in terms of industries, points along the industrial value chain, products or services, technologies and competencies deployed, customers and market segments, distribution channels, and geographic areas.

Industry. Many firms operate in only one industry. Others, particularly multi-SBU corporations, are more likely to be active in several industries. When a corporation is operating in several disparate, unrelated industries, it raises the question of whether it possesses the diversity of resources and competencies necessary to compete effectively in such different areas.

Industrial value chain. Every business must make a decision about the points along the industrial value chain at which it will operate. Will it be a supplier to other companies? Will it purchase raw materials from suppliers and manufacture products? Will it serve as a distributor between the manufacturers and retail outlets? Or will it sell directly to end users at the retail level?

Products or services. There is an infinity of products or services that a business can offer. It cannot create and sell them all. On what select group will it focus its resources and competencies?

Technologies and competencies. Some organizations are distinguished by the technologies and other competencies that they employ in their operations. This part of the mission statement specifies which of those qualities a business will emphasize.

Customers and market segments. This is a description of to whom and where an organization intends to promote its products/services and earn its revenues. It cannot be all things to all people and therefore must make choices about whose product preferences it will attempt to serve.

Distribution channels. In many cases, the same products may be offered to customers through different distribution channels. A business may prefer to become adept at reaching its customers only through selected channels.

Geographic areas. This feature of a mission statement defines the physical locations in which a business will operate, at which it will sell its products and services, or in which its customers will reside.

Some statements may also include a commitment to growth and financial soundness, an intention to be responsive to social, community, and environmental concerns, as well as an expression of the organization's beliefs, values, and ethical priorities.

In making these choices, a business's leaders will try to concentrate its energies on a limited number of opportunity areas. Companies succeed when they do not try to do too many things at once and instead apply their core competencies where they will have the greatest impact.

The primary purpose of a mission statement is to circumscribe the strategic decision-making of a business's leaders. It sends the message, "Within the limits of this defined mission, use your imagination to the fullest and compete as aggressively as you can. Do not stray outside the mission at the risk of squandering resources and competencies." It is an open question to what extent the leaders actually heed their mission statements.

Developing a Mission Statement

There are no firm guidelines on how to create a mission statement. The process certainly should involve as many employees and stakeholders as possible, in order to benefit from their knowledge of the possibilities and to encourage their commitment to the mission that emerges. They might start by reading a few selected articles on mission statements and reviewing examples of mission statements from all organizations. It probably is not a good idea to look at the statements from those firms that are similar or directly identical. The managers themselves could be assigned to prepare drafts of a statement, or they could be asked relevant questions, the answers to which would be used to compose a mission statement. The managers, other employees, and outside stakeholders might then provide their inputs before a final version is created. The critical final step in the process is communicating the statement to all relevant constituencies in a way that persuades them that the firm intends to operate fully within the terms of its mission.

Good Reasons for a Mission Statement

A well-drafted mission statement benefits an organization in several ways. It is a tool for mobilizing a unanimity of purpose throughout the organization. It offers a focal point for individual employees and stakeholders to identify with the organization's purpose and direction. It serves as a framework for translating broad strategic objectives into action plans leading to the assignment of specific tasks to individual employees. It becomes a basis for allocating organizational resources, designating where they may be committed and where they may not. The mission statement is a vehicle for an organization to present itself favorably to existing and potential stakeholders, such as suppliers who might sell to the organization, doctors who might join the medical staff, providers who might contract with a managed care organization, or employees who might take jobs with the organization. It provides motivation, general direction, an image, a tone, and a philosophy to guide the enterprise.

Changing a Mission Statement

A mission statement is not forever. If it no longer seems appropriate to the firm's circumstances, it can be modified. If the firm is having no long-term success in pursuing its existing mission, an entirely or partially new one can be selected. Frequently, when a new management team takes over a business, it wants to make adjustments to the mission. When a business feels that it has exploited all the growth opportunities available in its current areas of operation, it may choose to expand any of its mission parameters—additional market segments, products, distribution channels, or geographic areas. In contrast, a business may find itself overextended, spreading its limited resources and competencies across too many products and markets, resulting in below-average financial returns. The answer might be to narrow the scope of its mission.

It must be kept in mind that changes in missions usually lead to changes in objectives, strategies, organizational structure, activities, and behaviors. Sometimes the pressure is in the opposite direction; the overwhelming imperative to modify existing objectives and pursue different strategies compels a rethinking and restatement of the mission.

Rather than proactively managing mission statements, most companies tend to forget about them when times are good (spending the excess cash on new activities and acquisitions that depart substantially from the mission) and worry about them when they get into difficulty (and then divest the superfluous activities and businesses to return to their core competencies).

The renowned management consultant and guru Peter F. Drucker wrote an excellent article discussing the need to pay constant attention to the corporate mission and be willing to change it when necessary.[1] He used the term "theory of the business," which clearly encompasses the concept of mission, and laid out a few general rules about that theory. The assumptions behind the theory must fit reality, the theory must be known and understood throughout the organization, and the theory must be tested constantly. In the article, Drucker noted that mission statements are most likely to be revised when an organization is facing difficult times. He pointed out that it also sometimes makes sense to adjust the mission when the company is doing well.

Characteristics of a Good Mission Statement

A good mission statement has the following characteristics:

- It should be short, about 200 to 300 words, definitely no more than a single page. Drafting a concise mission statement can pose a challenge for many executive teams that are inclined to describe at length the premise of the organization.

- It should be memorable (one reason for the brevity). Key stakeholders, certainly the managers and employees, should be able to remember it, almost verbatim, and explain it to someone else without hesitating.
- It should be stated in broad enough terms to allow for the generation and consideration of feasible alternative objectives and strategies without unduly stifling management creativity. The generality of language gives the firm flexibility in adapting to changing external environments and internal operations.
- It should be expansive in a way that reconciles differences among, and still appeals to, an organization's diverse stakeholders (employees, managers, shareholders, board of directors, customers, suppliers, distributors, creditors, government regulators and payers, labor unions, competitors, public interest groups, community groups, media, and the general public). All stakeholders' claims on an organization cannot be satisfied with equal emphasis. A good mission statement indicates the relative attention that an organization will give to the interests of different stakeholders.
- It suggests where managers should be looking for future opportunity, and steers them away from other areas. It provides a basis for generating and screening strategic options, and selecting specific strategies to implement.
- It highlights the points of differentiation with other businesses, particularly competitors, and sets forth the basis for the firm's competitive advantage.
- It arouses positive feelings and emotions about the organization and an individual's role within it. It attracts and deters potential staff. It gives the impression that the firm is successful, knows what it is doing, is professionally managed, has direction, and is worthy of time, support, and investment.
- It is communicated to, understood by, and embraced by all members of the organization.
- It is more pragmatic, with a more immediate purpose, than a vision statement.

The faster the external environment is changing, the more frequently the mission should be reviewed. A successful organization will inevitably outgrow its original mission. As time passes and its operations expand, the organization will develop new competencies and a more perceptive view of available opportunities. Mission changes will seem to make sense.

Even if they are not overly concerned about their social obligations, for-profit corporate executives still have to reconcile an inevitable duality in their missions. One mission is to maximize the return to the owners of

Role of Social Obligation in Mission Statements

A major argument in the debate about the future of the U.S. health care system concerns the obligations of health care-related businesses and organizations to meet societal needs for clinical treatment of physical and mental suffering. The issue has become even more salient with the widespread movement of for-profit businesses into the health care industry. There is no better place than the mission statement for an organization to explain how it intends to balance the desire of shareholders for maximum financial performance against the demand for this basic human necessity, often under dire circumstances and with no assurance of an ability to pay. Few attempt it.

How a health care organization cares for the sick and uninsured is just one of a number of "social policies" that it must wrestle with. Other social policies may concern the religious beliefs of patients and employees, and medical treatment at the end of life. How an organization handles these policies directly affects its customers, products and services, technology, profitability, self-concept, public image, reputation, and brand identity. It is not easy to ignore these issues, especially with so much attention being focused on the delivery of health care.

Not-for-profit organizations and public agencies do not face the same stark challenge as for-profit businesses in the health care industry. Their mission statements can express an unreserved commitment to providing health care for all. In practical terms, however, they still must deal with the financial realities of that commitment.

One way of approaching this issue is to define the social obligation, whatever it is, in terms of the potential costs and benefits to the organization. Many of them will be subjective and unquantifiable. They still provide a rational basis for examining the tradeoffs that have to be made. For instance, the mission statement of a community health center may include a phrase promising to "within the limits of fiscal responsibility, meet the health care needs of everyone who visits the health center."

the business, the shareholders, on the investments that they have made in the business. The other mission concerns the substance of the organization's operations—the products and services that it creates and the customers that it offers them to. Many, perhaps most, for-profit business shareholders do not care about the substantive mission of the organizations in which they invest. Tobacco companies have never lacked for shareholders—as long as their financial performance has been above average. It is true that some investors will buy shares only in "socially responsible" businesses, although that term itself has different meanings for different people. Other investors place their money with companies whose industries they understand particularly well or whose products, leaders, management style, or geographic location they prefer.

The mission concerns felt by shareholders and the overall capital market is diffused among the individual SBUs of a multibusiness corporation. Shareholders invest in, and banks lend to, the overall corporation whose management then reallocates the funds to the SBUs in its portfolio. One of corporate management's primary tasks is regularly assessing its capacity to raise additional capital and taking steps to satisfy the demands of the investors and banks providing that capital.

■ VISION

Once an organization has established the parameters of its current existence in its mission statement, it is ready to begin thinking about where it wants to head in the future. Strategies are about moving an organization to a place different from where it is now. If it is content with all the dimensions of its mission and perceives no threats to it in the near or medium-term future, there is no need for strategies. It is doubtful that a single business in the health care industry would be content to continue operating the way it is now for the next three to five years.

One of the best ways to think about the future is to imagine the most desirable, ideal future state of the organization. If the organization, its leaders, and its employees could operate in the best possible world five years from now, what would it look like? The conditions of that world are captured in a "vision" statement. The firm then dedicates itself to implementing strategies in order to create that future for itself.

This vision is a critical, empowering concept. Many businesses allow themselves to be controlled by the world around them, virtually giving up on any sort of serious strategic management. Their attitude seems to be that the external environment is too complex and the future too unpredictable to warrant any attempts to shape it to the business's advantage. Most organizations are not quite so passive. They engage in systematic strategic planning designed to influence selected forces in their environments, or at least position their organizations to take greatest advantage of future trends. However, the ultimate step is to commit all the organization's resources and competencies literally to create—that is, to make a reality—exactly the future that the organization wants. What are the odds that a single organization can truly create all the elements of a future set of conditions? Perhaps not great. What is true is that this kind of long-term focus, this strategic clarity and passion, is likely to motivate the organization to achieve more of its desired future than a competitor taking a less ambitious approach.

Peter Senge explains a number of useful and practical guidelines on creating vision in his seminal book on learning organizations, *The Fifth Discipline*. Indeed, one of the five disciplines is "shared vision." The "shared" element adds the important dimension of participation by all organizational members in the description of the vision and, as a result, commitment to its fulfillment.

Another revolutionary approach to working out an organization's vision is an exercise called a "future search."[2] Under the guidance of skilled facilitators, an organization identifies all its primary internal and external stakeholder groups and invites sixty to eighty representatives of those groups to a three-day session at which they discover common ground and plot future scenarios for the organization. The plans that emerge have the support of not only the firm's employees, but also its suppliers, customers, and other members of the local community.

Like the mission statement, the description of a vision can be prepared at any level within an organization—from the highest levels of a multi-SBU corporation to individual employees within each SBU. Indeed, a primary prerequisite of the shared vision described in *The Fifth Discipline* is that each member of the organization have a clear idea of his or her personal vision.

Characteristics and Benefits of a Good Vision Statement

To perform its function of propelling the organization toward an identified point in the future, the vision statement should have certain qualities.

- A vision could be viewed as a kind of "dream" that motivates and drives the organization. It is definitely different from what the organization has now and appears to be a significant improvement. The difference between the current reality described in the mission statement and the idealized future described in the vision statement represents a significant "stretch" for the organization. The vision is bold and there is some uncertainty about whether it can be achieved.
- However, the vision statement is grounded in reality and it is possible. It reflects a solid understanding of the organization's resources and competencies, in the context of the opportunities and threats that exist in the external environment.
- It will be challenging for employees to accomplish the vision. They will have to develop new abilities, dedicate themselves passionately to the effort, and perform at their very highest levels. A truly shared vision gets employees excited, makes them feel proud to be part of the organization that is pursuing it. They want to tell their friends what they are doing.
- All the firm's stakeholders find something appealing about the vision, an aspect of it that serves their interests. It is flexible and

adaptable enough to allow managers and employees to display individual initiative in pursuing it. It is capable of being communicated to all interested parties.

■ VALUES

Most strategy-related documents aim to describe what the organization is doing or would like to be doing in purely business-related terms concerning matters like resources, competencies, markets, customers, competitors, opportunities, and threats. Values attempt to lay out guidelines for the behavior of employees as they go about conducting the organization's business, whether operational or strategic. Values say more than, "We will not violate antitrust laws or acquire competitive intelligence by hacking into our rivals' computer networks," although they will include such prohibitions.

Values address the beliefs and attitudes of all members of an organization. It is appropriate to say that they "dictate" how employees will conduct themselves as they go about their day-to-day activities, striving to achieve the firm's vision. Such guidelines take on greater importance when employees are operating under conditions of rapid change, heightened competition, constant deadlines, and intense job stress—all of which are prevalent within the health care industry.

Traditionally, values in a corporate setting have tended to be more implicit than explicit. The recent spate of scandals and the resulting legislation is one of the reasons why more organizations are publishing explicit statements of values. The implicit values have not gone away, though. They are still found in the organization's culture. The culture is sometimes seen as an amorphous, mysterious force by many managers, but it can be influenced and shaped. Explicitly stating management's expectations for employee behavior is a good way to start. It helps, too, if ethics and values are taken into consideration during the hiring stage, and if managers themselves model the behavior they would like to see in their subordinates.

When values are written and published, they typically address issues like this.

- Zero tolerance for even minor legal violations.
- Integrity, honesty, and ethics both within and without the firm.
- Attitudes toward and treatment of coworkers.
- Attitudes toward and treatment of customers/patients.
- Attitudes toward and treatment of suppliers and independent contractors.
- Acceptance of risk taking and failure.

- Attitudes toward innovation, and the future.
- Tolerance for change within the organization.
- Commitment by both the organization and its employees to the development of those employees.

The delivery of health care services in the United States presents some unique value challenges for top management. Some of the issues that employees must wrestle with, and that might be addressed in a statement of values, include:

- The time spent with patients, under pressures to improve productivity and patient throughput.
- The dominant role of physicians giving way to professional egalitarianism and multidisciplinary teams.
- The shift in health care organizations from the treatment of existing diseases to the outright prevention of diseases.
- The shift in organizational emphasis and priorities from the provider to the patient-consumer.
- Ideology-driven issues like abortion procedures and stem cell therapy.

An organization's values are more likely to be practiced if they match the values of employees who joined the firm. This requires raising the issue of values during the hiring process, during which it might be a good idea to show all applicants the mission, vision, and values statements. If an organization is attempting to make adjustments in its values, it may have to fire some existing employees. That contingency can be minimized and workforce buy-in maximized by involving employees in the process of developing new values.

Complications with Values

Explicitly stating and enforcing values sounds like a win-win proposition for any organization, but complications can arise.

A big problem area is the variations in values throughout an organization. Quite different values may be accepted within divisions of the same business, or within departments of the same division. There frequently are value differences among different functional specialties (marketing versus finance), medical specialties (surgery versus internal medicine), or medical professions (physicians versus nurses). In a large, multi-SBU corporation, it would not be surprising to find variations in values among the different businesses.

These dissimilarities in values create difficulties in several ways. Employees in different parts of the organization, different professions, or different specialties may feel that their behavior is being judged in a discriminatory manner. Even if they are not individually upset by the disparate standards, complications may result as the business attempts to coordinate the implementation of strategies or other forms of significant change. Sometimes the values conflicts extend beyond the organization, creating barriers when it attempts to integrate with, merge with, or acquire other organizations.

■ STRATEGIC OBJECTIVES

This next step in the strategy-making process is a move toward slightly greater specificity and practicality in describing the business's strategic direction. Strategic objectives are long-term strategic thrusts that will bring the organization closer to realizing its vision. They are a more explicit and workable statement of the broad, almost generic strategic impulses that the organization would like to follow over the next several years. Management believes that these objectives must be attained if the organization is to fulfill its mission and achieve its vision. They offer guidelines for the types of specific strategies that will be considered appropriate at this point in the organization's life. Strategies of those types are then designed and implemented to achieve the objectives.

Strategic objectives can be set at both the corporate and SBU levels. Within individual SBUs, it may also make sense to establish such objectives for each service line, market segment, or functional area. The objectives at all of these levels and in all of these areas must be consistent and aligned with each other.

Setting the objectives is normally the result of negotiations that involve consultation among units and their managers throughout the entire firm. It is an iterative, political process, with bargaining and conflict coupled with rational analysis. The process should involve both the top executives looking to create focused strategic momentum and managers lower within the organization who will be responsible for implementing the strategies intended to meet the objectives.

In setting strategic objectives, there is a particular tension between the top-down pressures of capital markets (debt and equity) and the bottom-up pressures of competitive business markets. A firm's financial managers will want to make sure to maintain creditworthiness and access to capital markets while marketing and operations managers will be thinking mainly about how to acquire and sustain competitive advantage over rivals. It is possible to maximize short-term financial objectives in a way that harms long-term strategic objectives, and vice versa. Clearly the two groups need each other; their strategic interests are not incompatible. Nonetheless, difficult tradeoffs must be made in defining the objectives for which they will be held accountable at designated times in the future.

To be useful, an objective should satisfy several criteria:

- It should describe an attribute that can be measured.
- It should designate a unit of measurement for that attribute.
- It should specify an exact level of that attribute that is to be achieved.
- It should state a time period by which that level is to be reached.
- It should identify a person who will have primary responsibility for reaching that level within that time period.

The measurement feature of the objective is essential. Without it, the objective loses most of its motivating power. For instance, if a hospital organization sets an objective of "increasing the occupancy rate" over the next three years, and the rate actually goes up from 83.1 percent to 84.7 percent, it can say that it met its objective. However, if it had set a specific target of 87.0 percent, it might have found that it could reach that level quite easily. Setting a precise numerical goal is a way of driving organizational performance to higher levels. The objectives can be financial or nonfinancial, whatever suits the organization's strategic desires.

Many firms tend to set the objectives and measure performance benchmarked against what has been achieved in previous periods. That is an insular, myopic approach. In a competitive marketplace, every business should be measuring itself against what similar, competing firms are doing. To go back to the hospital occupancy rate example just above, an improvement to the 87.0 percent rate may be quite unsatisfactory if the average for other hospitals in the local area is 91.0 percent.

A timeline for achievement of the objectives is just as important. Otherwise, employees may feel, even subconsciously, that they can take forever to reach the goal.

Assigning a named individual the primary responsibility for organizing the firm's efforts to reach the objective ensures that formal accountability lies somewhere within the organization. That one person is not likely to do all the work herself, or even most of it. She will mobilize the necessary resources—human, financial, and otherwise—and do the necessary action planning. She knows that when the time deadline is reached, top management will be looking to her to see whether the objective has been achieved.

Different types of generic strategic objectives will be set at the corporate and SBU levels. Remember, corporate management is primarily concerned with managing its portfolio of SBUs and meeting the demands of its shareholders and creditors. Top executives in the SBUs are focused on issues like market share, customer satisfaction, and costs of production. To be more specific, these are examples of strategic objectives that might be set at these two levels:

Corporate Strategic Objectives

- Improve shareholder return, as measured by the corporation's stock price.
- Increase the economic profit from the entire portfolio.
- Grow total revenues from the portfolio at a specific annual rate over the next three years. Alternatively, allow revenues to stabilize for a short period while corporate management reconfigures the portfolio, replaces the management of some SBUs, and renews operational efficiency and productivity throughout the portfolio.
- Increase the overall portfolio cash flow to a level that is able to subsidize the rapid-growth SBUs in the portfolio.
- Diversify the makeup of the portfolio into new, related industries. (This may be difficult to measure.) Alternatively, divest the portfolio of SBUs that no longer match the corporation's core competencies.
- Increase the level of sharing of resources and competencies among the SBUs. (This also will not be easy to measure.)

SBU Strategic Objectives

- Conduct a "turnaround" of the business, laying off employees, reducing the number of product lines, and enforcing cost-cutting measures throughout the organization.
- Improve the business's share of its market from 31 percent to 36 percent by four years from now.
- Develop, acquire, and deploy specific new technologies within the next three years.
- Reduce error rates in the creation of products or services from 4.2 percent to 3.8 percent in the next year, and to 3.1 percent in the following year.
- Improve the quality of the business's products or services to a specified level, as measured by an independent assessment organization or by customer surveys.
- Develop, acquire, and deploy employee knowledge/competence in narrowly defined areas that will be the basis for future strategies.

Problems to Avoid in Setting Objectives

Even when it is possible to reach a consensus within the organization on strategic objectives, there still are things that can go wrong with the objectives themselves.

Good objectives "stretch" the people assigned to achieve them. Very ambitious goals can sometimes motivate people to achieve at much higher levels than anyone thought possible—under appropriate conditions. If supporting resources, like money, space, equipment, and people, are not available to the effort, no amount of motivation will be able to reach the goal. If the steps required to reach the goal call for higher levels of risk taking by employees or new approaches to traditional tasks, their managers must be willing to allow that risk and those new approaches, as well as the failure that may come with them. Sometimes objectives are simply set at levels that cannot be achieved by any means. When employees realize this, they are likely to lose interest and motivation, reduce their work effort, and withdraw from or avoid the assignment. Little will be achieved.

An organization may agree on objectives that end up motivating the wrong employee behavior. Particularly when the objectives are accompanied by powerful incentives, employees will often concentrate their performance on meeting those objectives and give less attention to other responsibilities. In order to earn those incentives, employees may engage in practices like "gaming the system" or "manipulating the numbers." One way to minimize these distortions is to avoid emphasizing any single measure by balancing performance priorities and providing for some measurement redundancy. These kinds of employee behavior also are less likely when they have had a chance to participate in negotiating the objectives, and understand their context and the ultimate strategic aim (the vision).

■ EXAMPLES OF REAL-WORLD STRATEGIC DIRECTION DOCUMENTS

This is a somewhat random selection of strategic direction documents for a variety of health care-related organizations, including full-service tertiary care hospitals, a specialty care hospital, a hospital network, a public health care system, drug companies, an integrated delivery system, a managed care organization, a health care management consulting firm, and a public health school. They represent both good and bad examples of these kinds of documents. There is much to be learned by scrutinizing them and noticing the differences among them.

Quorum Health Group

The Quorum Health Group, a network of hospitals, ceased to exist as an independent entity when it was acquired in 2000 by Triad Hospitals. Prior to that time, however, Quorum published two consecutive mission statements that illustrate how a business's mission can expand and evolve.

This is the initial mission statement:

> Quorum Health Group, Inc., is a hospital company committed to meeting the needs of clients as an owner, manager, consultant or partner through innovative services that enhance the delivery of quality healthcare.

This is the subsequent mission statement:

> Quorum Health Group, Inc., owns and manages healthcare systems and is committed to meeting the needs of consumers and providers through innovative services that enhance the delivery of quality healthcare.[3]

What differences do you notice between the two statements? In the later version, Quorum is no longer simply "a hospital company." It is dealing in "healthcare systems." Note the use of the action verbs "owns" and "manages." It moved from meeting the needs of "clients" (a somewhat sterile all-purpose word) to those of "consumers" and "providers." Which version do you think reflects best on the company? In your opinion, is this truly a vision statement? Or are there elements of the system's mission included within it?

Province of Ontario's Health Services System

This is a description of the "vision" of the health services system for the Canadian province of Ontario. It is an interesting example of an attempt by a public health care system to explain what it is trying to do.

> Our vision is of a publicly administered health services system that provides universally available, comprehensive, accessible and portable services that meet or exceed internationally derived performance benchmarks. A provincial system organized to foster diversity among its elements and decision-making by the people affected, it is constituted of sectors that together provide the full spectrum of health services needed to promote health and provide health care for Ontario's population.
>
> We see a health services system in which regions, the sectors and their component institutions and organizations are distinctive, but committed to purposes in common. The contributions of each region, sector, institution, and organization are integrated, and complement those of all others to meet the provincially set policies, goals, objectives, and priorities necessary to achieve Ontario's vision of health.[4]

Rockcastle Hospital and Respiratory Care Center

These are the basic strategic direction documents of the Rockcastle Hospital and Respiratory Care Center in Mt. Vernon, Kentucky. They are simple and succinct, refreshing for their clarity in contrast with the sometimes overly long statements of other organizations. Are they too concise? Do they say enough about the organization and what distinguishes it from its competitors? The description of the organization as a "family-oriented team" is unique and may appeal to certain patients and other stakeholders. Delivering the "highest quality of care" seems to be a worthwhile commitment, but how many of

Rockcastle's competitors make the same assertion? Is the goal of making Rockcastle the "hospital of choice" in a county in Kentucky a sufficiently inspiring vision? In contrast, is the intention to become "the facility of choice nationwide for ventilator care" overly ambitious? The statement of values seems quite satisfying, encompassing qualities that perhaps carry some weight in Kentucky.

Mission Statement
Rockcastle Hospital and Respiratory Care Center, Inc. is a family-oriented team of healthcare professionals dedicated to delivering the highest quality of care to those we serve.

Vision Statement
Rockcastle Hospital and Respiratory Care Center, Inc.'s vision is to be the hospital of choice for healthcare in Rockcastle County and surrounding areas and to be the facility of choice nationwide for ventilator care.

Values
We value excellence, friendliness, compassion, cleanliness, and our commitment to our community.[5]

Pfizer Pharmaceutical
These are the strategic direction documents for Pfizer, one of the leading international pharmaceutical companies. Is the first sentence really a "mission" statement? The use of the future-directed term "will" makes it read more like a vision statement. In contrast, the next section, "Our Purpose," has the ring of a mission statement. Looking back on what has been said in this chapter about the purposes of mission and vision statements, do you think that the "Our Mission" and "Our Purpose" language here is detailed and specific enough to serve those purposes? Look at the list of values that Pfizer claims to practice. Are they unique? Are they inspirational? How do you imagine this list might alter the behavior of Pfizer's workforce?

Our Mission
We will become the world's most valued company to patients, customers, colleagues, investors, business partners, and the communities where we work and live.

Our Purpose
We dedicate ourselves to humanity's quest for longer, healthier, happier lives through innovation in pharmaceutical, consumer, and animal health products.[6]

Values
To achieve our Purpose and Mission, we affirm our values of Integrity, Respect for People, Customer Focus, Community, Innovation, Teamwork, Performance, Leadership, and Quality.[7]

Johnson & Johnson
Johnson & Johnson is another pharmaceutical company whose strategic direction language contrasts sharply with that of Pfizer. This is the language exactly as it appears on the Johnson & Johnson Web site.

At Johnson & Johnson there is no mission statement that hangs on the wall. Instead, for more than 60 years, a simple, one-page document—Our Credo—has guided our actions in fulfilling our responsibilities to our customers, our employees, the community and our stockholders.

Our Credo
We believe our first responsibility is to the doctors, nurses and patients, to mothers and fathers and all others who use our products and services.

In meeting their needs everything we do must be of high quality.

We must constantly strive to reduce our costs in order to maintain reasonable prices.

Customers' orders must be serviced promptly and accurately.
Our suppliers and distributors must have an opportunity to make a fair profit.

We are responsible to our employees, the men and women who work with us throughout the world.
Everyone must be considered as an individual.
We must respect their dignity and recognize their merit.
They must have a sense of security in their jobs.
Compensation must be fair and adequate, and working conditions clean, orderly and safe.
We must be mindful of ways to help our employees fulfill their family responsibilities.
Employees must feel free to make suggestions and complaints.
There must be equal opportunity for employment, development and advancement for those qualified.
We must provide competent management, and their actions must be just and ethical.

We are responsible to the communities in which we live and work and to the world community as well.

We must be good citizens—support good works and charities and bear our fair share of taxes.
We must encourage civic improvements and better health and education.
We must maintain in good order the property we are privileged to use, protecting the environment and natural resources.

Our final responsibility is to our stockholders.
Business must make a sound profit.
We must experiment with new ideas.
Research must be carried on, innovative programs developed and mistakes paid for.
New equipment must be purchased, new facilities provided and new products launched.
Reserves must be created to provide for adverse times.
When we operate according to these principles, the stockholders should realize a fair return.[8]

This is clearly a statement of mission, and an especially comprehensive and thoughtful one. Is this too much to be included in what should be a relatively memorable description of what the organization is trying to be? Several of the points in the Credo could have a profound impact on the stakeholders to whom they are directed. With regard to employees, the promises regarding the making of complaints, job security, and adequate compensation could almost be interpreted as contracts with them regarding their terms of employment. The Credo also does not shy away from the financial performance of the business, including the desire of its owners for a "fair return" on their investments.

Division of Genetics, Department of Medicine, Brigham & Women's Hospital

This is an interesting example of a mission statement for a subunit within a much larger organization. It shows that attempts to document strategic direction can make sense for smaller entities that do not appear to be operating in traditional market environments. The Division of Genetics at this hospital might even be considered to have competitors—for space and resources within the hospital, and for grants from its funding sources. It would not be inappropriate for this division to formulate and pursue strategies designed to optimize its position within the hospital and the genetics research community.

Mission

The Division of Genetics at Brigham & Women's Hospital is committed to discovery, education and scientific excellence in genetic research in a hospital-based research environment. Our mission is to attract, train and send forth the next generation of outstanding physician-scientists, armed with the knowledge to make scientific discoveries that would ultimately cure disease and alleviate suffering.[9]

Massachusetts General Hospital
This mission statement for Boston's venerable teaching hospital, Massachusetts General Hospital, is a model of lucidity. In the simplest possible terms, it highlights its three primary purposes: care delivery, medical research, and medical education. However, this statement surely would apply, without modification, to dozens of other teaching hospitals around the country. If that is true, what is its strategic value to this particular hospital? Try to imagine the ways in which Massachusetts General would employ this document in its strategic planning processes. Does this statement effectively delimit the domains in which the hospital will conduct operations and initiate strategies?

> **Mission Statement:** To provide the highest quality care to individuals and to the local and distant communities we serve, to advance care through excellence in biomedical research, and to educate future academic and practice leaders of the health care professions.[10]

DoctorsManagement
This is the mission statement of a modest-size physician practice management consulting firm. It does a rather good job of covering several key elements in the practice of management consulting—continual learning, client orientation, unstinting objectivity, and high ethics. These guidelines would appear to be useful in the conduct of the firm's everyday business.

> To strive daily to learn more about all aspects of medical management for the continuing benefit of our clients.
> To apply our knowledge and experience in a conscientious manner to enable our clients to achieve their goals.
> To be totally objective in all advice, even when that advice may be contrary to our clients' opinions.
> To adhere to the highest standards of business ethics.[11]

Blue Care Network of Michigan
These are the strategic direction documents of the Blue Cross/Blue Shield organization in Michigan, taken directly from its Web site.[12] There are several points worth noting about the language here. The vision statement is placed before the mission statement, not normally the order in which they are created and employed. Both the statements sound like mission statements. They both use the present tense. The vision statement implies that the organization already has achieved the status of the "premier man-

aged care plan in Michigan." Perhaps there is nothing left for the organization to achieve and a true vision seems unnecessary. Does the language of the two statements provide the organization's top management with direction for their strategic decision-making? Do the values offer guidance to the firm's employees in their work behaviors?

> **Vision**
> As the premier managed care plan in Michigan, Blue Care Network's purchasers, members, physicians, unions and employees are partners in maintaining and improving health.
>
> **Mission**
> People helping people to promote health and peace of mind through high quality care and service.
>
> **Values**
> Integrity and honesty
> Family and personal life
> Personal accountability
> Helping and caring
> Quality and excellence
> Diversity and inclusiveness
> Community involvement[12]

Partners HealthCare System

Partners HealthCare System is a large, well-managed integrated delivery system composed of several major hospitals in the Boston market, including the Massachusetts General Hospital mentioned above. As with a number of other organizations, there seems to be some confusion in Partners between a mission and a vision. Both the mission and vision statements use language describing current activities and intentions. True, the vision talks about "seeking" to attract top people and being an industry leader, but nothing in these documents really describes a future state to which the organization is aspiring. The language itself is rather uninspiring. What does it mean to be an "international leader in fulfilling our missions"? It is bound to be a leader in fulfilling its own missions, since every other organization is concentrating on its mission. It also is not encouraging to see the same exact sentence in both the mission and vision statements.

The list of goals is interesting. They are not in fact goals; they do not constitute practical, measurable, time-limited targets for achievement. Instead, they appear to be select operational areas in which Partners does have goals, or "tasks," which it is not revealing. The goals in some of these areas could actually be strategic in nature. Others are likely to be of more local and short-term concern.

Our Mission
Partners is committed to serving the community. We are dedicated to enhancing patient care, teaching and research, and to taking a leadership role as an integrated health care system. We recognize that increasing value and continuously improving quality are essential to maintaining excellence.

Our Vision
Partners is an integrated health care system that serves our communities by providing the full range of services from preventive primary care to long-term care. We improve our quality of care and further serve the public at large by pursuing our teaching and research missions. True to our heritage, we seek to attract the best people and to be an international leader in fulfilling our missions. We recognize that increasing value and continuously improving quality are essential to maintaining excellence.

Our Goals
Partners' goals include targeted tasks in each of these twelve areas:

Research and education
Patient care: quality improvement
Patient care: sharing across the system
Patient care: non-acute care services
Service to the community
Labor force diversity and retention
Financial stability
PCHI
Public policy and advocacy
Communications
Aligned incentives
Disaster preparedness[13]

University of South Florida Health—College of Public Health
This is a remarkable collection of strategy documents from a different type of health care organization, a school of public health. The mission statement could not be shorter. The list of values could not be much longer. They say a great deal about the school's philosophy and culture, serving in some ways as an extension of the mission statement. The vision statement is an outstanding example of a generally quite specific description of a future that the school intends to create for itself. It is easy to imagine the school's leaders referring to this document as they make their strategic decisions.

Mission
Our mission is to promote public health through research, education, and service.

Values
Commitment to Public Health—In supporting our fundamental commitment to the principles of public health we value:

- A population, culturally diverse approach to solving public health problems
- The efficacy of prevention and health promotion
- An ecological, systematic approach to public health
- Development and participation in community partnerships
- Service to underserved and vulnerable populations
- The best quality and equity in all public health services

Discovery—In upholding our commitment to discovery we pledge to:

- Be innovative in addressing public health problems
- Use the highest ethical standards
- Assure our discoveries are appropriately and widely disseminated
- Appreciate the scholarly activities and contributions of others
- Expect excellence

Collaboration—In participating in collaborative efforts we are:

- Supportive of each other's pursuits and disciplines
- Sincere in our efforts and communication to develop partnerships
- Willing to engage in positive collaborations to promote healthy communities

Collegiality—In promoting collegiality we strive to:

- Assume personal responsibility for our relationships
- Foster ethical and respectful relationships
- Support effective relationships among the wide variety of public health disciplines and settings

Lifelong learning—Recognizing that lifelong learning is essential, we are committed to:

- Foster an environment that encourages a continuous pursuit of knowledge and skills

- Constantly improving educational methods and outreach to students and the public health workforce
- Assure skills and knowledge learned are relevant to public health.

Vision

A College that will be the leading authority in public health education, research, policy and practice in Florida.

A growing national and international reputation that is the product of our collective efforts.

A scholarly environment that attracts the best people to freely explore their intellectual interests.

A passion for learning and scholarship in public health to create healthy communities.

A superior and diverse learning community seeking excellence.

A supportive culture that fosters personal and professional development.

An environment that values interdisciplinary collaboration within the College and across the Health Sciences Center, the University and the community.

A school of first choice for those who want to pursue creative public health solutions.

Accountable to each other for co-creating the College's destiny.[14]

Study Questions

1. Obtain the mission and vision statements for two hospitals that you are aware of, perhaps in your city or where you have received care. After reading them, what image/impression do you have of the hospitals? Compare them. If you or a family member needed health care and had to choose one of them, which would it be? If you were offered similar attractive jobs by both hospitals, which would you accept?
2. Choose a health care organization in your town with which you are somewhat familiar. Without learning its actual mission statement, write a mission statement for it.
3. Imagine two absolutely identical hospitals—except for the fact that one is for-profit and the other is not-for-profit. What differences would you expect to see in their mission statements?
4. Think of an organization you currently work for or have worked for in the recent past, even at a relatively low level. Imagine yourself as the CEO of that organization. Ask yourself and answer these questions about the organization:

What is the mission of that organization? Specifically, what types of operational activities are encompassed by the mission and what activities would be considered outside the scope of the mission?

Does the organization appear to have a vision for the future? Does it seem to have a clear, explicit idea of where it is headed?

The organization has a value system, whether it wants it or not. The question is, has it expressly chosen a set of values that its employees will follow in performing their jobs? Are the other values written down and promoted to all employees?

Does the organization ever talk to its employees about its strategic intentions? Are the employees aware of grand strategic objectives or specific plans that the organization is pursuing? Is any attempt made to help each employee understand the connection between her job and accomplishment of the organization's long-range goals?

Learning Exercise 1

Choose a company or an industry in which you have worked or would like to work. It could be a hospital, physician practice, MCO, government health agency, health care consulting firm, or a health-oriented NGO.

- Identify all the important stakeholders for the entity.
- Determine the primary aims/objectives of each stakeholder.
- Assess the power of each stakeholder to affect the company's strategic plans, and how it might apply that power.
- Explain how the company might respond to the possible actions of each stakeholder.
- Recommend tradeoffs that company managers could make to accommodate the stakeholders in a way that optimizes the company's own performance.

Learning Exercise 2

The following is a generic mission statement for a primary care physician group practice. You have been hired as a consultant by the group to review the statement and make suggestions for revising it. Before you begin any revisions, what information do you want about the group and its environment? From where will you get that information?

"Serving all patients in need of care, Riverside Family Care Associates, Inc., a private physician group practice, provides the highest quality health care services to our patients and their families in a compassionate and caring environment. Riverside Family Care constantly strives to provide care in a cost-effective manner and to continuously improve customer satisfaction and patient care."

Make some assumptions about the group and its environment, and prepare a draft of a new mission statement, including explanations for all your proposed changes. Be sure to take into account the growing trend toward consumer-driven health care.

Learning Exercise 3

This exercise asks you to create a personal vision for your own life. Start by finding a comfortable chair in a quiet place. Close your eyes, relax, and imagine yourself on the beach, in the mountains, or some other place you would go to get away from it all. Gradually, begin thinking about your life five years from now. In your mind, create the ideal life situation. If you could have everything that you wanted out of life, what would it look like? What kind of job would you have? Where and how would you live? Who would be your friends and acquaintances? What knowledge and skills would you have acquired? What would be your self-image and how would others view you? What contributions would you make to the world around you? Mentally explore every dimension of the life you would like to have. Take out a piece of paper and begin describing that life. Write in the present tense, as though it is five years from now and you already have built the life you desire. "I am the effective CEO of the Neighborhood Health Plan, a rapidly growing, highly respected managed care organization serving the health care needs of low income people in the city where I live. I earn $150,000 a year. I am writing a book on my experiences running a community-focused health care organization. My spouse and I live with our two children in a suburb of that city. I am an esteemed member of several community organizations. I commute to work by bicycle and am of above average fitness for my age."

That is your vision for the future of your life. You can see that a part of your vision intersects with the vision of the organization for which you work. To realize your vision fully, you need to make certain things happen in your workplace. Imagine the motivational power of a group of employees all of whom see in their jobs not just a source of income, but also a means of satisfying many of their life's desires.

Notes

[1] Drucker PF. The Theory of Business. *Harvard Business Review.* September-October 1994.

[2] Future Search Web site. http://www.futuresearch.net.

[3] Quorum Health Web site. http://www.quorumhealth.com/HomePg4.nsf. Accessed July 6, 2007.

[4] Ontario's Health Services System Web site. http://www.health.gov.on.ca/hsrc/vision.htm. Accessed July 6, 2007.

[5] Rockcastle Hospital and Respiratory Care, Inc., Web site. http://rockcastlehospital.org/frame.php?section=AboutUs. Accessed July 6, 2007.

[6] "Our Mission" and "Our Values" from Pfizer, Inc., Web site. http://www.pfizer.com/pfizer/are/mn_about_mission.jsp. Accessed July 6, 2007.

[7] Pfizer, Inc., Web site. http://www.pfizer.com/pfizer/are/mn_about_vision.jsp. Accessed July 6, 2007.

[8] Johnson & Johnson Web site. From http://www.jnj.com/our_company/our_credo/index.htm. Updated November 14, 2005. Accessed July 6, 2007.

[9] Division of Genetics, Department of Medicine, Brigham & Women's Hospital Web site. http://genetics.bwh.harvard.edu/genetics/philanthropy.html. Updated December 6, 2006. Accessed July 6, 2007.

[10] Massachusetts General Hospital Web site. http://www.massgeneral.org/about.html. Accessed July 6, 2007.

[11] DoctorsManagement Web site. http://www.doctors-management.com/DM+Mission+Statement/4. Accessed July 6, 2007.

[12] Blue Care Network of Michigan Web site. http://www.mibcn.com/home/blue_care_network_michigan/visionMissionValues.shtml. Updated February 2, 2007. Accessed July 6, 2007.

[13] Partners HealthCare System, Inc., Web site. http://www.partners.org/about/about_mission.html. Accessed July 6, 2007.

[14] USF Health Web site. http://health.usf.edu/publichealth/mission.html. Accessed December 26, 2007.

References

Abell DF. *Defining the Business: The Starting Point of Strategic Planning.* Upper Saddle River: Prentice-Hall; 1980.

Baetz MC and Bart CK. Developing mission statements which work. *Long Range Planning.* 1996;29(4):526–533.

Bart CK and Baetz MC. The relationship between mission statements and firm performance: An exploratory study. *Journal of Management Studies.* 1998;35:823–853.

Bartkus B, Glassman M, and McAfee RB. Mission statements: Are they smoke and mirrors? *Business Horizons.* 2000;43(6):23.

Campbell A and Yeung S. Creating a sense of mission. *Long Range Planning.* 1991;24(4):10–20.

Collins J and Porras J. Building a visionary company. *California Management Review.* 1995;37:80–100.

Collins JC and Porras JI. Building your company's vision. *Harvard Business Review.* September-October 1996:65–78.

Cummings S and Davies J. Brief case—Mission, vision, fusion. *Long-Range Planning*. 1994;27(6):147–150.

Drucker P. *Management: Tasks, Responsibilities, Practices*. New York, NY: Harper & Row; 1973.

Gratton L. Implementing a strategic vision—Key factors for success. *Long Range Planning*. 1996;29(3):290–303.

Ireland RD and Hitt MA. Mission statements: Importance, challenge and recommendations for development. *Business Horizons*. 1992;35(3):34–42.

Kerns CD. An entrepreneurial approach to strategic direction setting. *Business Horizons*. 2002;45(4):2–6.

Kim W and Mauborgne R. Charting your company's future. *Harvard Business Review*. 2002;80(6):5–11.

Langeler GH. The vision trap. *Harvard Business Review.* March-April 1992:46–55.

Larwood L, Falbe CM, Kriger MP, and Miesing P. Structure and meaning of organizational vision. *Academy of Management Journal.* 1995;38(3):740–769.

Lissak M and Roos J. Be coherent, not visionary. *Long Range Planning*. 2001;34(1):53.

McTavish R. One more time: What business are you in? *Long Range Planning*. 1995;28(2):49–60.

Oswald SL, Mossholder KW, and Harris SG. Vision salience and strategic involvement: Implications for psychological attachment to organization and job. *Strategic Management Journal*. 1994;15(6):477–490.

Pearce JA II and David F. Corporate mission statements: The bottom line. *Academy of Management Executive*. 1987;1(2):109–115.

CHAPTER

7

Formulating Corporate-Level Strategy

Learning Objectives

After reading and studying this chapter, you should be able to:

- List and describe the functions by which a corporation adds value to its constituent SBUs.
- Understand the concept of corporate portfolio management and describe a model process for performing that function.
- Explain the three basic generic corporate portfolio strategies—growth, stabilization, and retrenchment.
- Describe the primary strategies by which a corporation may choose to grow its portfolio—concentration, related diversification, and unrelated diversification.
- Explain the different forms that diversification may take, as well as the means by which it may or may not be "related."
- List and explain the traditional tools for carrying out a growth strategy.
- Suggest the circumstances in which a stabilization strategy might make sense.
- Describe the circumstances in which retrenchment becomes necessary and the several different ways in which it can be carried out.
- Understand and apply the two most popular tools for portfolio analysis and management.
- Identify the ways in which the corporate center may facilitate synergy among its SBUs.

When most people think of the organizations that they encounter in the U.S. economy, they presume that they are in one "business" or another. In fact, this is true only for the smaller and more narrowly focused organizations. An example might be a company that manages the parking structures at all the hospitals in a city. It manages nothing but parking structures, it does it only for hospitals, and it does it only for hospitals in one particular city. Another example is a startup biotechnology company engaged in developing and commercializing a drug based on early research of its founder at a local university. The company is working on one drug and has not begun to think about the customers to whom it might sell the drug.

Most organizations of even modest size or larger are composed of several "businesses," often referred to as strategic business units or SBUs. Together, they constitute the "business portfolio" of the organization. The corporate "center" or headquarters is usually quite small by comparison with the SBUs. For instance, a hospital network corporation might rely on a corporate staff of 200 people to oversee its 23 facilities in 10 states employing a total of 11,000 people. The corporate center produces no goods or services and competes in no markets; its primary function is to assemble, manage, and cultivate the collection of businesses. Typically, the corporation is the sole legal entity capable of entering into contracts, such as those involved in issuing bonds, borrowing money, or selling equity shares. Occasionally, the SBUs in the portfolio will be legally independent with the corporation holding a controlling ownership interest.

VALUE-ADDING FUNCTIONS OF THE CORPORATE CENTER

As the parent for multiple SBUs, the corporate center deserves to exist only if it adds value to the operation of the individual SBUs. It can do this by performing a variety of functions that fall into three broad categories. Initially, it assembles and manages the portfolio of SBUs that make up the total corporation. This determines which businesses will and will not be part of the corporation's operations. Second, it may provide resources and capabilities directly to individual SBUs to support them in conducting their operations and implementing their strategies. Lastly, the parent may encourage and facilitate the sharing of resources and capabilities among the SBUs. This chapter describes the specific ways in which the center can add value to the overall corporation.

I. MANAGE THE PORTFOLIO OF SBUs

The dominant function of a corporate parent is portfolio management; without a portfolio of SBUs, the corporation does not exist. This begins with the creation of a comprehensive, unifying vision for the corporation that provides the basis for the specific types of SBUs that will be brought into the portfolio. This vision guides the parent executive team in selecting new SBUs to acquire and in choosing SBUs currently in the portfolio to drop. When the corporation is for-profit, the vision expresses some clarity of corporate purpose to shareholders, lenders, and financial analysts. It conveys to the individual SBUs that they are part of a larger whole and contributing to a grand strategic purpose. The vision may inspire employees to see how they can realize their personal goals through achieving the organization's goals.

- To fulfill that corporate vision, the center acquires, merges with, or otherwise absorbs new businesses. In some cases, the corporation may develop new businesses internally. As that vision evolves and external factors change, the center may choose to divest businesses from the portfolio. Much as a private investor buys and sells shares of company stock to maintain a desired mix of industries and risk, and maximize the returns in his investment portfolio, corporate leaders move businesses in and out of their SBU portfolios in an effort to achieve a grand strategic vision while balancing risk and returns. They do not acquire and divest companies as quickly as a day trader buys and sells stocks. An SBU usually remains in a corporate portfolio for several years and, if it is performing satisfactorily, for decades. Corporate managers also can and do intervene to varying degrees in the management and operations of their SBUs; individual shareholders do not have that opportunity.
- The parent will frequently set performance standards and goals, and measure the SBUs and their executives against them. The standards are normally of a strategic nature, such as profitability, sales growth rate, and market share. In some cases, corporate management will propose, encourage, negotiate, and even mandate specific strategic directions for an SBU. The corporate center may be counting upon each SBU to perform a unique strategic function. While it is investing significant funds in one SBU on a steep growth curve, it may look to another, more mature SBU to be a source of cash. Furthermore, its grand vision for the type of corporation it wishes to become may depend on the SBUs moving in particular strategic directions.

  Parent management has the authority to dictate which products and services will be offered and which market segments will be targeted, as well as any other aspect of SBU operations. However, at a certain level of parental intervention, the business is no longer an independent SBU. The value of maintaining separate SBUs with relatively autonomous managers is that they are presumed to have specialized competencies in the SBUs' industries and markets. It is unlikely that the corporate managers of a diversified portfolio would have the ability to direct operations effectively in several different markets.

- Corporate management can choose to apply pressure to the SBUs to resolve problems, meet objectives, and improve performance. When it feels that SBU leadership is not meeting its expectations, it has the option of replacing the heads of individual SBUs. The extent to which the corporate center dictates strategy to SBUs and intervenes in its implementation will depend on the parenting style it adopts. This activity in some ways parallels the approaches that supervisors may take with their subordinates. Some corporate leaders do their best to hire top-notch SBU managers, succinctly explain their strategic expectations for the SBU, and give the managers almost complete discretion in satisfying them. Other corporate parents are less trusting. They provide much more detailed direction to their SBU heads, even down to the operational level, and very closely monitor their performance, being ready to jump in if the managers stray too far from the objectives set by the corporate center.

Model Process for Corporate Portfolio Management

After defining an overriding vision for the corporation, parent management might follow a systematic process something like this for assembling and maintaining a portfolio of businesses:

1. At any given point in time, parent management must make a fundamental decision about the overall strategic thrust of the corporation. Filled with optimism about opportunities in the marketplace and its unique abilities to exploit them, the organization may set off on an aggressive *growth* path. Content with developing its current strategies and strengthening some competency gaps, the organization might opt for *stability* for a few years. Or, because it has been out-strategized by the competition for several years or just poorly managed on its own, the organization might feel compelled to engage in *retrenchment*. As strategies succeed or fail, the direction of the thrust will change. Two or three years of retrenchment may enable the corporation to embark on a new growth initiative.
2. On the basis of the grand corporate vision, parent executives make choices about the geographic areas in which the corporation will operate, the markets that it will serve in those areas, and the products and services that it will deliver to those markets. Taken together, these decisions set the mission of the organization.
3. Within the defined mission, the corporate center next decides how many businesses (SBUs) will make up the organization portfolio and exactly which businesses those will be. Making these decisions is not like going to the supermarket and picking products off the shelf. The com-

Are Multi-SBU Corporations Obsolete?

Some strategy scholars argue that the concept of portfolio creation and management is obsolete and should be phased out. No organization should consist of more than one full-blown strategic business unit. Top executives should focus on what they know best—the management of businesses, not portfolios. Investors interested in owning packages of related businesses can assemble them by purchasing individual company shares in the stock market, in the mixes that they prefer, rather than shares of large multi-SBU corporations. If there are good synergy reasons for businesses to collaborate and share resources and competencies, they can do so through arm's-length transactions—contracts, alliances, joint ventures, and the like.[1]

position of the portfolio will depend upon the corporate resources (primarily financial) available for investment, and on the existing businesses available for acquisition or merger. It also is possible for a corporation with the right resources and competencies to develop new business units internally.

4. Finally, there is a golden rule about portfolio management that is observed by few organizations. In making the decisions about the SBUs that will be gathered into the corporate portfolio, it should be established that each and every one chosen for inclusion is better off within the corporation than it would be outside on its own. This is critical to the efficiency of the overall organization.

Corporate-Level Strategic Options

After corporate management makes an initial general decision about whether to grow, retrench, or stabilize portfolio activity at its current level, it must choose among several specific portfolio strategies.

Growth—*Expand the Portfolio*

The most common corporate-level strategy direction is growth. There are several reasons for this.

- If the corporation's SBUs compete in expanding industries or markets, they will have to grow simply to maintain their market shares. Stagnation in a dynamic industry leads to decline and eventually death.
- By growing the size of its operations, the corporation may be able to achieve economies of scale and scope that allow it to reduce costs and either lower prices or increase profits. In an expanding industry, the increased economies may be necessary just to keep up with the competition.

- In addition to economies of scale, expanded operations allow an organization to increase its experience, which in turn can lead to improved operating efficiency and lower costs.
- Sometimes, the egos of top executives compel them constantly to take action and move forward. Anything else seems like an admission of weakness or failure.

Remember, a corporate-level strategy of growth and expansion in a portfolio means adding new businesses to the portfolio. Increases in revenues, profits, and cash flow result from actions taken at the level of the SBU.

Growth strategies are categorized by the types of products/services that the new businesses offer and the markets in which they compete, and the relationship of the products and markets to those of the businesses currently in the portfolio. When a corporation expands by acquiring businesses that are similar to its existing businesses, it is pursuing a concentration strategy. It is *concentrating* on the products and markets it already understands. A strategy to acquire or develop businesses offering different products/services to different markets is one of diversification. The degree of diversification can vary by how closely related the new businesses are to the current ones.

Growth by Concentration

This is the least complicated of the corporate-level strategies. All businesses start with a concentration strategy—dedicating all their resources and efforts to a single, or a very few, products or services. A biotechnology startup is an excellent example. On the basis of its founders' lab research, it sets out to develop a single drug product that it can sell or license to a large pharmaceutical company. For several years, the pursuit of that one objective fully occupies the business and its employees.

Concentrated growth occurs by one of three basic means. A business can increase the sales of its current products in its current markets. It can create new products for sale in its current markets. Or it can sell its current products in new markets. Anything involving the creation of new products for sale in new markets is some form of diversification, not concentration.

It is possible for a business to stay concentrated for a considerable period of time—growing by adding new products, new product features, expanding into adjoining market areas, but remaining in the same general sphere of business. As long as growth opportunities continue to be available, there is no reason to consider another strategy.

Advantages of a concentration strategy: It permits a corporation to specialize, to become highly competent in the management of one type of business. In the process of doing that, it acquires and develops sophisticated knowledge and unique competencies that are especially attuned to that kind of business. This focus makes it much more likely that the corporation will be effective in directing those businesses. There will be little confusion throughout the corporation about the strategic direction in which it is headed. All this concentrated, refined effort may help the organization achieve a sustainable competitive advantage.

Disadvantages of a concentration strategy: Through this strategy, the corporation essentially "puts all its eggs in one basket." When changes occur in the single industry, markets, or product line that is the basis of the strategy, there can be damaging effects on the corporation. If revenues simply increase and then decrease at regular intervals (as in the case of seasonal sales), it may be challenging for management to maintain efficient operations and ensure a steady cash flow. The chosen product line is likely to have a life cycle that eventually reaches a maturity stage in which further revenue growth becomes virtually impossible. At some point, the products may simply become obsolete. There is no longer a market for them or revenues for the corporation—at least until it can develop or acquire replacement products.

Eventually most businesses reach the point where:

- they have captured as large a market share as they are likely to be able to do,
- their current market is stagnating, maturing, shrinking, or otherwise lacking in growth potential,
- they have excess cash on hand that needs to be invested productively, or
- management has greater ambitions for further achievement, which typically leads the business to expand into products and markets beyond its initial core activities. A strategy in that direction is called *diversification*.

Growth by Related Diversification

In this strategy, a corporation moves beyond its existing markets and product lines but continues to apply the competencies that it has developed as a concentrated business. Those competencies may exist in any of the corporation's functional areas. The research and development department may be able to create a different, yet profitable set of new products. The marketing function may have the skills to promote those different products to its current markets. It may be possible to distribute them through the same channels. The new products may be similar enough to the current ones to be able to leverage the brand image they have created.

The *relatedness* of the diversification implies that the new businesses are likely to have rather close connections to the existing businesses. A good way to appreciate this is in terms of the industrial value chain (discussed in Chapter 5) of those existing businesses. The relatedness or connection

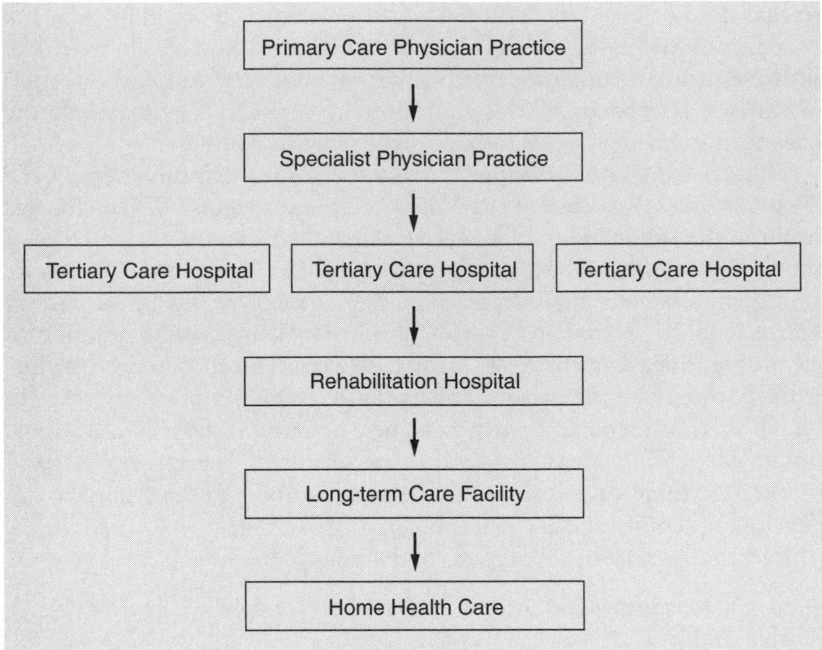

Figure 7.1 Health Care Industry Value Chain (With Vertical and Horizontal Dimensions)

may be in either a vertical or horizontal direction from the location of the existing businesses in that chain. Consider the example of a single tertiary care hospital in Figure 7.1.

If its parent corporation decided to pursue a strategy of growth through related diversification, it could move in one of three directions with relation to that chain. If it chose to acquire or develop physician practices, it would be vertically integrating backward along the chain. If it acquired a rehabilitation hospital or long-term care facility, it would be considered vertical integration forward along the chain. Horizontal expansion would occur if the parent began to acquire additional tertiary care hospitals, most likely in other geographic market areas.

Forms of relatedness. The relationship between the existing and the acquired businesses can occur with regard to their products, services, processes, systems, markets, or other significant aspects of their operations. It is an important criterion in a growth strategy because of the synergies that it permits. The relatedness may be either tangible or intangible. It might involve sharing manufacturing facilities, distribution channels, marketing media, and support services (e.g., purchasing, inventory management, maintenance, housekeeping, human resource management). It can also be based upon more subtle factors like a brand image, a corporate-wide reputation, skills in creativity and innovation, or general managerial expertise.

The presence of relatedness between two businesses does not necessarily mean that synergies will result when they are brought within the same portfolio. There are several reasons why that desired outcome may not occur. There may not be a "strategic fit" between the organizations. This means that their strengths and weaknesses do not mesh with each other. They are strong in the same areas and weak in the same areas, rather than having strengths offsetting weaknesses. They also may lack the capabilities for sharing and communication that are necessary if resources and competencies are to pass back and forth between them. Sometimes, corporate management simply may not work hard enough to coordinate the two businesses.

Vertical integration. The vertical integration form of related diversification is a natural one and particularly popular in the health care industry. An organization either acquires existing businesses or develops its own business at other points along its industry value chain. In doing so, it is effectively integrating under a single umbrella entity several or all of the entities along that value chain. When an organization expands in the direction of its suppliers, it is said to be integrating "upstream" in the value chain. Expansion toward the organization's distributors is called "downstream" integration. In the case of a typical community hospital, upstream integration would involve acquiring, merging with, or developing a primary care facility or a physician group practice (either of which is responsible for admitting patients to the hospital). To integrate downstream, the hospital might purchase a rehabilitation hospital or home health care business, which typically accepts patients after they have been discharged from a community hospital.

This growth strategy was very popular in the health care industry during the 1990s. In one initial form, hospitals purchased the physician practices of many members of their medical staffs to create physician-hospital organizations (PHOs). Their stated goal was to create a single legal entity that could offer most of the medical services that an average population of patients might require and then contract with Managed Care Organizations (MCOs) to provide those services to their members. They believed that the MCOs would prefer this sort of one-stop shopping rather than having to contract separately with individual hospitals and physicians. Furthermore, it was felt that the sheer size of the PHO and the number of providers that it represented would give it greater bargaining leverage in the contract negotiations with MCOs.

The PHO concept failed for several reasons. While the sponsoring hospitals may have had competence in managing hospital operations, this ability was not transferable to physician practice operations. The productivity of the now-salaried physician employees of the PHOs declined. Some MCOs in the early 1990s actually tried to avoid dealing with larger provider entities because of their greater negotiating power. Perhaps the greatest problem with PHOs was that none of the participants—hospital or doctors—changed their operating practices as a result of the new affiliation.

A second form of growth strategy through integration was far more successful. Another group of hospitals, some of which had gone through the unsatisfying PHO experience and some of which were trying dramatic growth strategies for the first time, partnered with other hospitals, with existing physician group practices, and with a variety of ancillary organizations (labs, pharmacies) to create integrated delivery systems (IDSs) or networks (IDNs). These had several characteristics that contributed to their greater success. The IDSs took immediate steps to truly "integrate" the operations of their various components with a view toward managing the cost and quality of the care provided. This forward-looking businesslike attitude was appealing to potential MCO partners. The systems and networks were based less on outright ownership of the components and more on linking them through contracts. This less capital-intensive approach has been referred to as "virtual integration." In addition, the attitude of MCOs toward their contracted providers had matured; they had come to realize that they needed to think in terms of building long-term partnerships with them rather than adversarial relationships.

In a few cases, once the IDS was well established, it took a further step in upstream vertical integration by developing its own managed care products, taking over the health care insurance function through creation of HMO or PPO health plans.

One of the earliest truly integrated systems is also one of the most all-encompassing—Kaiser Permanente, founded in 1945 in California. It owns its own hospitals (Kaiser Foundation Hospitals), contracts exclusively with its own physicians (Permanente Medical Groups), and offers its own insurance plans (Kaiser Foundation Health Plan). An integrated system may or may not include both delivery and insurance components. Managed-care organizations today are integrated systems, though most of them contract only nonexclusively with hospitals and physician groups and exercise care management through the terms of these contracts.

In choosing the strategy of vertical integration, an organization must make several key decisions in the tradeoff between producing and managing the goods or services internally and purchasing them externally.

- It must determine whether it has the resources and competencies to manage the new business operations as an in-house unit as well as it could be managed as an independent entity.
- It must choose a form for the integration—complete ownership, partial ownership, a joint venture or strategic alliance, or simply a long-term contract.

- It must consider the impact of the integration move on its other stakeholders. If a hospital acquires a partial ownership interest in its linen laundry, will the laundry's other hospital customers take their business elsewhere?
- It must keep in mind the overall proportion of all its operations that it is bringing in-house.

The opposing trend to vertical integration is outsourcing. This involves contracting with an outside organization to take over the performance of a function or activity previously conducted in-house. A good example of this is the use by physician practices of outside billing and collection services and medical transcription services. As more and more clinical and financial health care information becomes computerized and digitized, the opportunities for outsourcing various aspects of hospital and physician practice operations will grow.

Good reasons for vertically integrating. There are several good arguments in favor of the business integrating either backward or forward in its industrial value chain.

- By eliminating overlap and redundancy throughout the value chain, total costs can be reduced.
- There is better coordination at the interface between components in the value chain, which creates efficiencies leading to cost savings.
- When the integration is achieved through outright acquisition, profit-taking at several levels in the chain can be eliminated, further reducing costs.
- The overall corporation has greater control over essential inputs (resources) and outputs (distribution channels).
- Intimate connections throughout the value chain open up a broad network of sources of competitive intelligence.
- Participation in a greater stretch of the value chain gives the corporation access to more points and activities at which to create unique value.
- A corporation that controls a major portion of the value chain may choose to totally redesign or reengineer the way it functions.
- Forward-directed vertical integration brings a business closer to its end users and gives it a better chance to understand and satisfy their needs.

Things that go wrong with vertical integration. It is not a simple matter to bring together several related, but still somewhat different, businesses and coordinate their operations to produce a line of goods or services efficiently. The resulting integrated entity should do at least as good a job as the value chain did when its component businesses were connected by

Owned Versus Virtual Integration

When vertical integration was all the rage in the health care industry during the late 1990s, when a variety of health care providers took steps to create integrated delivery systems capable of meeting all the health care needs of a given population of patients, the first impulse of the catalyst organization often was to purchase and own the other components of a system. When the Partners HealthCare System began to take shape in Boston following the merger of Massachusetts General Hospital (MGH) and Brigham and Women's Hospital, it initially bought outright some physician practices that used these hospitals. Around the same time, many hospitals sought to secure their flows of patients by acquiring, owning, and managing the practices of the physicians on their medical staffs. The Partners System quickly realized that it did not need to own the physician practices to achieve the integration objectives it had in mind for them. In the other cases, the hospitals discovered that they had no competencies in managing physician practices, which function quite differently from hospitals. They found better, non-ownership ways of binding medical staff physicians to the hospital.

Instead of owning physician practices, or any other business in the industrial value chain, it frequently is possible for a corporation to enter into contracts or other types of strategic agreements that commit it and a supplier or customer to collaborate in synergistic, mutually beneficial ways. The legal control that comes with ownership is not necessary to achieve those ends. The contracts create a sort of "virtual integration."

market forces and arm's-length contracts. The new integrated system can fail in a number of ways.

- Excessive costs may be incurred in managing both the newly acquired businesses as well as their interfaces with the existing business and with each other.
- The business that initiated the integration process may not be able to use the full capacity of the suppliers or customers that it has acquired. In that case, in order to maintain operations at maximum capacity, the system may find it necessary to sell to its competitors—if they are willing to buy. For instance, physician groups that contract with managed care organizations often prefer to retain the right also to provide services to other non-system organizations.
- The question arises whether the business must deal exclusively with its new integration partners. It may find that better deals can be negotiated with other suppliers and customers outside its system.

- Once a business is committed to working closely with the components in a longer, more complex value chain, its strategic flexibility becomes constrained. It now must take into account the effects of any proposed strategies on all the new businesses in its integrated system.
- That inflexibility may also tie it into inefficient processes, poorly managed units, and obsolete technologies.
- Ultimately, if the business cannot coordinate effectively the larger section of the value chain, it may end up increasing its costs of operation and limiting its opportunities to provide unique value to its customers.

Horizontal expansion. The corollary of vertical integration is horizontal expansion. Instead of growing by moving forward or backward along the industry value chain, an organization moves sideways. It normally does this by acquiring or merging with other organizations similar to itself, though it may also turn to other integration options like self-development of new entities, partial ownership, and long-term contract relationships.

The aim of many horizontal growth strategies is to serve the same markets with the same products/services, often facing the same competitors, but in different geographic locations. This is the basis for the formation of the several networks or chains of health care organizations over the past two decades. Typically, an organization in one geographic area acquires or merges with a comparable organization in another area. Quite often the horizontal expansion involves deals with direct competitors.

An organization may move into an area not currently served by anyone at all by creating a new entity there. This rarely happens in health care delivery as most parts of the country are reasonably well populated with hospitals and other provider organizations.

An interesting example of a horizontal expansion leading to a vertical integration was the formation of Partners HealthCare System in Boston mentioned earlier. It originated in 1994 with the merger of Brigham and Women's Hospital and Massachusetts General Hospital (MGH), two major teaching hospitals located three miles apart. This was a horizontal expansion involving two direct competitors. This initial move was followed over the next several years by mergers, acquisitions, and affiliations with a mix of community hospitals, specialty hospitals, community health centers, a physician network, home health and long-term care services, and other health-related entities. These vertical integration steps created an IDS that is a major force in the health care delivery industry in Massachusetts.

There are numerous examples of horizontal expansion in the health care industry—multistate hospital networks, nationwide systems of health plans, and large nursing home chains.

In certain situations a horizontal expansion strategy makes particular sense.

- A good time for horizontal growth is when the market in which the organization competes is growing. Because the "pie" is getting larger, there will be a need for greater capacity to meet the growing customer demands for products. Acquiring an existing entity is a quick way of expanding capacity. Antitrust enforcers may also be less concerned with industry concentration during a time of rapid market growth. Certainly, an organization in an expanding market will have to grow simply to maintain market share.
- Another appropriate moment to absorb a competitor in the market is when the competitor is doing poorly because it lacks resources or competencies possessed by the acquiring firm. Not only will there be a natural synergy between the two organizations, but the struggling firm may be more open to being acquired. Consider two small, even startup, biotechnology research firms working to develop similar new pharmaceutical products that are based on analogous technologies. One is making good progress toward developing a marketable product and is thinking ahead to its next area of research. The research of the other firm has been slowed by its lack of access to a researcher with a particular expertise and a unique piece of laboratory equipment. The first firm possesses both the necessary equipment and someone with the necessary skills. It would make good strategic sense for the first firm to acquire or in some other way affiliate with the second firm.
- Horizontal growth is appealing when the greater size of the expanded organization enables economies of scale that give it a competitive advantage. A medium-size physician group practice that acquires or merges with similar groups in another area of its city can realize several benefits—serving the billing and claims processing needs of more physicians in numerous locations through a single office (or receiving a larger volume discount from an outsource claims processing firm), receiving larger volume discounts from outside suppliers of the products and services that a physician practice purchases, earning considerable cost savings on the acquisition and upkeep of single EHR and other IT systems, and spreading the fixed costs of basic practice functions (like staff recruitment, benefits management, patient scheduling and contact, coordination with laboratories, pharmacies, and referral physicians) across more physicians in more offices. In addition, the costs of raising capital may be reduced when it is done in larger amounts with the risks spread across a wider range of operations. The resulting economies may win the group more contracts with MCOs on the basis of its ability to accept lower reimbursement fees or capitation rates.

- Sometimes an organization can merge with or acquire another similar organization competing in the same area to create a dominant position in the market without incurring the disapproval of antitrust enforcement authorities. It all depends on the size of the entities, the size and importance of the market, the share of the market they will then control, and the enforcement priorities of the antitrust officials. When the Partners merger between Brigham and Women's Hospital and MGH described above was proposed, the Massachusetts state attorney general scrutinized the arrangement closely before giving his approval.

Even with these good reasons for a horizontal expansion, it is essential that the expanding firm feel confident that it has the financial and other resources, the managerial competence, and the time and energy required to take over a second organization and give it the attention it deserves.

Advantages and benefits of related diversification. When implemented competently, related diversification strategies deliver a number of benefits to the parent corporation.

- The primary argument for related diversification is to create synergies among the existing and acquired businesses.
- Related diversification strategies reduce the overall risk of the corporation by acquiring businesses facing different threats and uncertainties in different markets and industries. The corporation can balance high-risk businesses with low-risk businesses.
- It is possible to assemble a portfolio of businesses at different life cycle stages, permitting cash flow cross-subsidization and replacement of dying businesses with infant businesses.
- The corporation may have managed its existing portfolio businesses so well that it has excess cash flow and debt capacity that deserve to be employed productively in additional business areas.
- It is certainly expected that the acquired businesses will be managed competently and generate additional revenues, profits, and overall growth for the corporation.
- The greater size of the expanded corporation gives its various businesses greater market power vis-à-vis competitors, suppliers, and customers.
- Despite the similarities between the existing and acquired businesses, there often is an opportunity to acquire new knowledge, competencies, and technologies from the new businesses.
- Although the parent corporation is not likely to mention it, a related diversification growth strategy may enhance the status, power, and compensation of its top executives.

- The consensus of the variety of research that has been done on the performance of different types of growth strategies is that related diversification produces results superior to both concentration and unrelated diversification.[2]

Common forms of inter-SBU synergy. The types of synergy that are possible among businesses in the corporate portfolio will depend on the nature of their operations. These are some generic examples:

- When businesses employ similar processes, systems, and equipment, they can share their solutions to problems and ideas about improving operational efficiency.
- Businesses with similar facilities may be able to exploit any slack capacity to achieve economies of scale.
- By combining their purchasing of similar input needs, the businesses can earn volume discounts and enjoy greater negotiating power with suppliers.
- Related businesses can integrate their computer systems, sharing knowledge of the most effective systems, of problem solutions, and of methods for improvement.
- As their employees are likely to be performing similar tasks, combined personnel development programs will be possible.
- By sharing R&D facilities, the businesses can reduce their innovation costs and spread the research risks across more projects. Transfers of relevant technology can occur faster, with lower costs of adoption. Researchers in related businesses can engage in joint learning and share their knowledge and best practices in research methodologies. It may even be possible to move research scientists between the businesses.
- There may be opportunities to share distribution channels, sending greater volumes of product through the same distributors. This can give the businesses greater bargaining power with the distributors, leading to lower per-unit costs of distribution.
- The businesses may be able to leverage the use and application of influential brand names and images. They may choose to conduct joint advertising and promotional campaigns. Their sales and marketing departments can cross-sell and bundle products and services.
- Economies of managerial scope may be available. The expert managers of one enterprise can easily apply their skills to several related businesses.
- There is a wide variety of opportunities for knowledge transfer—techniques, principles, practices, policies, methods, procedures, solutions, approaches, strategies, tactics, processes, and structures.

There can be problems in the implementation of related diversification strategies. Corporate management must invest a significant amount of time and resources in ensuring that the possible synergies are actually realized. Sophisticated expertise and diplomacy may be required to facilitate the exchange of resources and competencies among the SBUs in the portfolio. Individual SBU managers may be reluctant to participate in the sharing if there appears to be no payback to them or their respective businesses. Competent management at the corporate and SBU levels easily overcomes these challenges.

Growth by Unrelated Diversification

A corporation composed of unrelated businesses is sometimes called a conglomerate. There are virtually no similarities or commonalities among the businesses. They operate in different industries or markets, serve different customers, and face different competitors. There are no opportunities for sharing resources or competencies. One might wonder what value the corporation adds to the individual businesses, or what value the businesses bring to the corporation, by collecting them within a single portfolio.

As with related diversification, the acquisition of diverse businesses operating in different industries and markets may spread the risk of poor or fluctuating performance. This may be comforting to corporate management, but the argument does not carry much weight with some investors. They frequently prefer to make their own decisions about risk spreading and diversification by buying stock in different companies of their own choosing.

One of the most powerful cases against unrelated diversification is that it is difficult, if not impossible, for a single team of executives adequately to understand the operations, technologies, cultures, and contexts of multiple businesses in distinctly different industries and markets. The result is likely to be a series of management miscues (misdirections to SBU executives, inappropriate allocation of financial resources) that degrade the performance of the businesses below what it would be if they were independent and autonomous. The acid test of any diversification strategy is whether a particular business is better off being part of a large corporation rather than a freestanding entity.

A handful of corporate executives are a sort of "renaissance manager" with sophisticated, almost universal management talents that are applicable to many different kinds of businesses. Warren Buffett is a current example of such a manager. The corporation he leads to very high levels of performance, Berkshire Hathaway, includes a brick company, a candy company, a jewelry business, and a fast food chain. Perhaps some conglomerate CEOs persuade themselves that they have Warren Buffett-like managerial skills.

One unreservedly positive reason for an unrelated diversification strategy is its avoidance of antitrust legal problems. Such problems usually result when businesses either collude with competitors or acquire monopoly power in a particular market. Prohibited collusion or monopolies are not possible when multiple distinct markets are involved.

Growth strategies should not really be viewed as three distinct options—concentrated, related diversification, and unrelated diversification—though that is how they are described here. The degree to which the businesses that a corporation adds to its portfolio are similar or different from those already in the portfolio is a continuum. They range from being absolutely identical (that is, selling the same products and services to the same customers in the same markets, and facing the same competitors) to being totally dissimilar from each other (that is, offering different products/services to a different set of customers in different markets, competing against different competitors).

Real-Life Examples of the Generic Growth Strategies

A physician group practice might grow by developing or acquiring the following three new businesses, reflecting the generic growth strategies:

Concentrated horizontal expansion. Open a second office to serve better its patients located on the other side of town. The new office would provide the same services, using some of the same physicians from the first office, to some of the patients who previously traveled to the first office for their care, as well as to others. Most of the patients at both locations are members of health plans paid for by their employers.

Related diversification. Open a second office in an area of town with a large elderly population not currently treated by the group. It would hire new physicians in different specialties to deliver services aimed at the diseases and conditions unique to the elderly. Most of the patients at the new location are covered by Medicare.

Unrelated diversification. Purchase the building in which the current office is located and lease space to a primarily professional clientele, some doctors, but also lawyers, engineers, and architects. The services provided (maintenance, security), the customers served (professionals rather than patients), and the competency required (building management) are completely different from the group's current areas of core competency.

Tools for Implementing Growth Strategies

There are several established methods for carrying out a growth strategy—that is, bringing new businesses into the corporate portfolio.

Internal development. The parent corporation can assemble resources from its own asset pool and from the existing businesses in its portfolio to create the desired new business from the ground up. The advantage of this approach is that corporate management can configure the new business to fit precisely the position it would like to fill within the portfolio. The disadvantage is the considerable time it can take to get a brand-new business up and running. Furthermore, there is no assurance that the business, as designed by the corporation, will be successful.

Internal new venture creation. This is a variation of the first method. Individual SBUs can encourage entrepreneurial endeavors within parts of their organizations, starting off as pilot projects or test marketing initiatives that, if they prove successful, are spun off as independent businesses. Their chances of ultimate success are greater because they emerge from existing businesses intimately in touch with the market. They also are not expanded to full-blown companies until the business concept has been proven on a trial basis.

Investments in new ventures. One way for a corporation to get its foot in the door of a new business is to make an investment in a new venture or startup. It can start off with a minority interest. Through its ownership, it will have a first look at new technologies that the venture may be developing. It also will be in a prominent position perhaps to take a controlling interest when the venture needs additional financing.

Acquisition. The corporation identifies an existing business that closely approximates the type of organization that it has in mind to fill a slot in its portfolio. It then purchases the entire business outright. There are several variations of the purchase arrangement. The corporation may acquire only its assets, or it may avoid assuming the business's liabilities. The advantage of this approach is that in a relatively short period of time, the corporation can own a fully operational new business. That business also will have a track record, demonstrating how successful it already is or can be in the future with some fine tuning by its new parent. The disadvantage is that the business may not exactly satisfy the criteria that the corporation has for the new business it would like to add.

Merger. The difference between a merger and acquisition is often in the legal details of the process by which two businesses become one. In a pure merger, it is not necessary for any money to be exchanged between the businesses. The management and owners of each business all decide that they can be more successful in achieving their respective goals if they combine their resources and competencies under a single leadership team.

Joint venture/strategic alliance or partnership. These arrangements do not actually bring a new business into a corporation's portfolio. However, they may achieve the same end purposes. Through formal contracts, agreements, or other legal writings, two businesses commit themselves to joint decision-making and cooperation on a variety of operational and strategic issues. There is likely to be extensive sharing of resources and competencies. It is possible for an alliance or partnership to be so close as to be indistinguishable from an actual merger. The advantage of these devices is that the businesses can collaborate in any ways that they wish without having to surrender their individual legal autonomy.

Stability—*Maintain the Portfolio*

The vast majority of for-profit corporations seek to be constantly growing, if for no other reason than that their stakeholders (shareholders and debtors) demand it. Most of the growth will come through increased revenues and profits in the SBUs already in the portfolio. Over time, there is an expectation that significant growth also will be created by adding entirely new businesses to the portfolio. Occasionally, however, a corporation may decide to pause for a few months or a year or two in an aggressive growth strategy. There are several possible reasons for this.

The corporation may have simply grown too fast, outstripping its financial and managerial resources. Its ability to raise additional debt or equity capital for acquiring new businesses may have been exhausted. It will be necessary for the businesses currently in the portfolio to improve their performance sufficiently to expand the corporation's debt capacity or allow it to issue additional stock. Corporate management may also require some time to hone its abilities to oversee the existing collection of businesses in the portfolio before it takes on the responsibility of administering other businesses with different product lines in new markets. The corporation may have run into problems assimilating some recent additions to the portfolio; several existing SBUs may have encountered serious financial or operational problems. A reassessment of the composition and direction of the entire portfolio may seem in order.

Sometimes, the reason for the pause may be more benign. Corporate management cannot think of anything better to do. It may have some portfolio growth objectives in mind, but the new businesses that would help meet them are not currently available for acquisition. Perhaps it is waiting out some imminent environmental change—for instance, the growing likelihood of some form of national health care reform. After catching its breath for a period of time, the corporation eventually may resume its growth strategy or decide to cut back or dramatically reconfigure the portfolio.

Some businesses continue in this stable non-growth state interminably. Family-owned small businesses that are content with the present level of financial returns often see no need for growth. That lack of ambition is acceptable as long as the external environment is not changing and there is no vigorous competition.

Retrenchment—*Cut Back the Portfolio*

Quite often, a corporation needs to do more than just pause and rethink. It becomes necessary to regain control of inefficient operations, rebuild resources and competencies, and reconsider strategic direction. In the process, the corporation may change shape dramatically and actually shrink. These are the most common options that a corporation has in such situations.

1. *Getting back down to fighting weight— "lean and mean."* When times are good, revenues are growing, profit margins are above average, and the overall portfolio management strategy seems to be succeeding, undisciplined corporations sometimes get fat. Overconfident in their ability to assemble and oversee one good collection of SBUs (usually in a concentrated or related diversification strategy), corporate management may begin to believe that it can manage any combination of SBUs.

   They acquire new SBUs whose market focus is on the fringes of the stated mission of the corporation; their controls over the performance of individual SBUs grows lax. Every part of the corporation accumulates excess, value-inefficient resources and competencies, as well as too many and the wrong kind of SBUs, products and services, and employees. Revenue growth slows, margins dwindle, free cash flow dries up, and credit ratings are downgraded.

   Before pursuing any further growth strategies, the firm chooses to pause to rid itself of resources and competencies that are not essential to the conduct of current operations. The goal is to make itself as lean as possible while continuing to do business. This process may be referred to as a "turnaround" from the firm's declining fortunes to a state of relative stability from which new, more carefully considered growth strategies might be launched. Such corporate recovery efforts are a not uncommon occurrence in American industry.

   The specific tactics of a retrenchment strategy are substantial layoffs of employees, closing of the least efficient production facilities (hospitals in a hospital network, retail outlets in a drugstore chain), across-the-board cuts in operating budgets (salaries; supplies, equipment, and service purchases), and institution of new processes and procedures aimed at greater cost effectiveness.

   The orchestration of a turnaround strategy is a fine art. Misconceived, it can result in cutting beyond the fat of the organization, into the muscle. One possible negative outcome is the departure of the best employees (taking advantage of incentive retirement plans to leave a declining business), leaving behind demoralized staff functioning at lower productivity, perhaps resulting in higher unit cost of lower-quality products.

   A select few executives have built reputations around their ability to execute a corporate turnaround successfully. They usually do it by paying inordinate attention to the needs of their human resources, starting with detailed planning for what will happen to employees at all levels and in all categories. Other expedients are employed before resorting to large-scale layoffs: reducing hours, limiting overtime, switching from full-time to part-time status, wage and salary cuts, prohibiting new hiring, retraining and cross-training workers, new job assignments, job-sharing opportunities, and incentive retirement schemes. When layoffs become unavoidable, they are managed with sensitivity for the concerns of those leaving and those left behind. Outplacement services and career counseling are offered to departing employees, while programs are conducted to maintain the morale and productivity of the remaining staff.

2. *Returning to core businesses and competencies.* Sometimes, during the good years, a company does more than just put on weight in terms of excess businesses, functions, products, and people. It strays from its chosen strategic path by acquiring businesses that do not fit its defined mission or move it toward realization of its vision, and attempting to perform activities that are not based on its core competencies. These major strategic diversions can lead to substantial declines in financial performance that do not go unnoticed by the sources of debt and equity capital. The solution to this state of affairs is for the corporation to return to the businesses that it knows best, getting rid of those that are outside its range of unique, more highly developed competencies. There are several proven methods for doing this: selling the unwanted businesses to other corporations, selling the businesses to its current executives through a leveraged buyout, and spinning the business off so that current shareholders also get a proportional interest in the new freestanding business. Whenever a corporate refocusing like this becomes necessary, the inevitable question is, what sort of strategic self-discipline could have averted it?
3. *Seeking a "white knight" to take over.* In a situation where a corporation encounters serious, but not life-threatening, problems that could be resolved through better management and an injection of resources, particularly capital, it can choose to surrender its independence voluntarily to another carefully selected company. It is an amicable coming together, a form of rescue merger. Steps are taken to protect the interests of current debtors and shareholders, but otherwise no money need change hands.
4. *Selling the entire organization.* When no white knights are forthcoming, the corporation may choose to offer itself for sale on the open market. This is a desperation move. The organization is usually in such a weakened financial condition that the potential sale price is quite low. Nonetheless, enough money is earned to satisfy the creditors and owners. There also is the possibility that the new owner will be able to resuscitate the corporation.

5. *Divesting pieces of the corporate portfolio.* As environmental conditions change and the corporation shifts its strategic direction, corporations frequently get rid of some businesses while they are acquiring new ones. This divestment strategy can also be a good approach when corporate management feels that it has too many SBUs in its portfolio to manage effectively or wants to raise additional capital to support more promising businesses by divesting a few less-attractive businesses. Divestment may occur through an ordinary sale of the business or by a spinoff in which existing shareholders receive shares in the now-independent business. Another variation is a "leveraged buyout" by the existing managers of the business.
6. *Voluntarily filing for bankruptcy and reorganization.* Sometimes, a corporation's financial ills are so serious and the pressure from its creditors so great that the only solution is for it to make a voluntary filing for protection from the creditors and subsequent reorganization under Chapter 11 of the U.S. Bankruptcy Code. When such a filing is accepted by the bankruptcy court, the creditors are held at bay while the corporation makes a last-ditch effort to resolve its financial difficulties through radical reengineering of its operations. It does this all under the supervision of the court, which must approve all major management decisions. The price of attempting a Chapter 11 reorganization is high—in terms of fees to lawyers, accountants, and investment bankers. The outcome is not at all certain—only about one-fifth of the corporations that file under Chapter 11 are able to put together a plan that satisfies the court overseers and revives its financial fortunes sufficiently to bring it back to profitability.
7. *Voluntarily or involuntarily filing for bankruptcy and liquidation.* This is the strategic dead end for a business. At a certain point, the business's financial condition may become hopeless, beyond repair, and the only option left is to terminate operations and liquidate the assets. Since the debts normally exceed the assets by a wide margin, the allocation of the limited funds to the creditors is administered through a filing for Chapter 7 bankruptcy. The filing may be initiated by either the business or its creditors. No attempt is made to salvage the business as a going concern.

Tools for Portfolio Analysis and Management

It is not a simple matter for corporate strategists to keep track of the numerous SBUs in their portfolios, follow their performance relative to each other and to the corporation's vision, allocate the correct resources to each SBU, and recognize gaps in the portfolio that might be filled by acquisitions or internal development. Several useful graphical tools have been developed to assist in those tasks. They take the form of matrices that portray two or more variable factors that are considered key to strategic portfolio decisions. Each SBU is placed on the matrix at the point where its two factor values intersect. The symbol identifying each SBU may also contain information about it. The models below are two of the most popular matrices.

BCG (Boston Consulting Group) Growth-Share Matrix

This matrix model, devised by Bruce Henderson at BCG in 1970, contrasts the market growth rate (MGR) of the industry in which a firm competes (or the several industries in which all a corporation's SBUs compete) with its relative market share (RMS) in that industry. The "market growth rate" is the annual percentage increase in total industry sales. It is viewed as a rough indicator of the external threats and opportunities faced by the SBU and the cash that is needed to address them. "Relative market share" is defined as the business's absolute market share divided by that of its other largest competitor. It is assumed to be a general indicator of a business's internal strengths and weaknesses, and its ability to generate cash (Figure 7.2).

Each axis in the figure is divided into two segments. The midpoint on the growth rate axis is the growth rate for the industry in which all the firms on the matrix compete. If the matrix is used to assess a portfolio composed of businesses in several industries, the midpoint might be the average growth for the economy as a whole. The midpoint on the relative market share axis is usually set at between 1.0 and 1.5. By definition, only the top firm in a market will have a relative market share over 1.0.

The result is a matrix with four quadrants. The businesses are located on the matrix at the intersection of their growth rate and relative market share scores, using circles whose size corresponds to the firm's size (measured by sales revenue or as a share of overall corporate revenues). The businesses located in each quadrant have come to be described as follows:

Stars—Have a high market share in a growing market. These are usually market leaders at the top of their life cycle growth curves. They are generating enough cash to support that growth. When the grow rate of their markets slows down, so does the business's growth rate and it becomes a "Cash Cow."

Cash Cows—Have a high market share in a mature, slow, or no-growth market. They generate more cash than is needed to maintain their market share, so are "milked" to support businesses earlier in their life cycles—typically "Question Marks."

Question Marks—Have a small market share in a growing market. These are usually recent startups with products at the beginning of their growth curve that require far more cash than they can

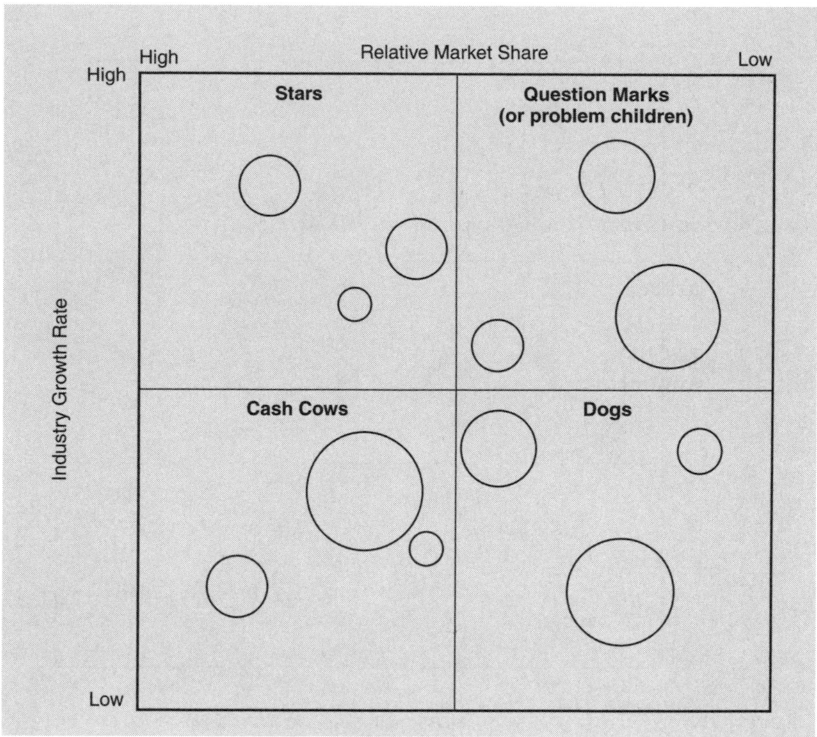

Figure 7.2 BCG Growth-Share Matrix

generate. In a corporate portfolio, they rely on "Cash Cows" to subsidize them.

Dogs—Have small market shares in stagnant or declining markets. These might be businesses approaching the end of their productive life cycles. They should be dropped from the portfolio rather promptly.

GE (General Electric) Business Screen

The popularity of the BCG analytical tool drew attention to the matrix concept for portfolio management. During the 1970s, McKinsey & Company consultants devised a nine-cell matrix to assist their client General Electric in screening its large portfolio of SBUs. Like the BCG matrix, the GE/McKinsey model places SBUs on a grid with two axes, one representing industry attractiveness, the other business strength.

"Industry attractiveness" and "business unit strength" are calculated by first defining criteria for each variable, assigning a weight to each criterion reflecting its importance, determining the business's score for each criterion, and multiplying that value by the weighting factor. The result

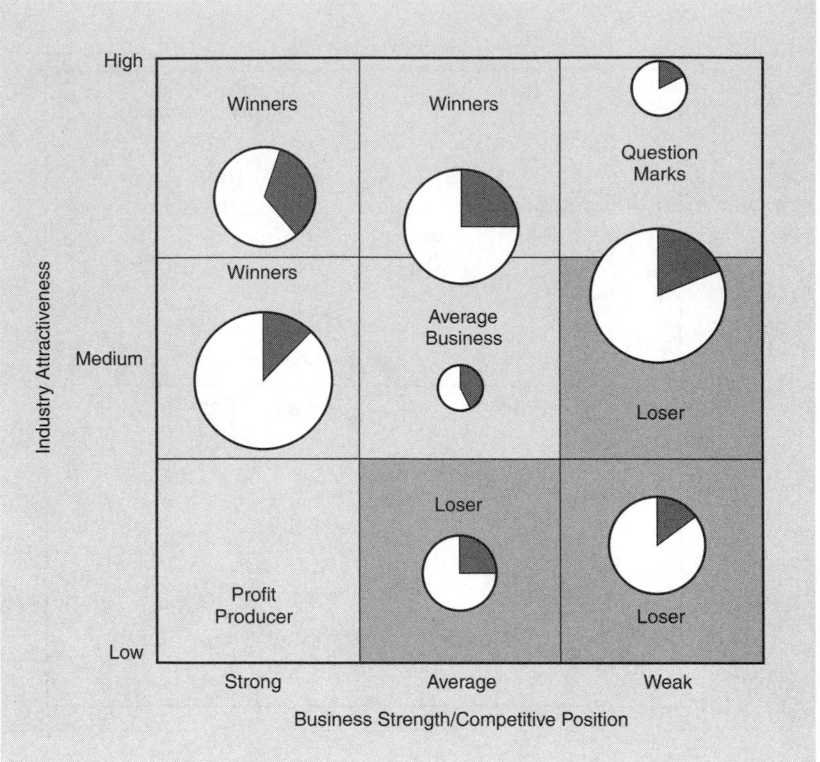

Figure 7.3 GE Business Screen

is a quantitative measure of industry attractiveness and the business unit's relative performance in that commercial sector. The current business is then placed on the nine-cell grid, along with other businesses in the portfolio, in order to portray the composition of the portfolio at a single glance (Figure 7.3).

The vertical axis on the grid or matrix represents the industry attractiveness. Such factors as the bargaining power of the buyers and the suppliers, the internal rivalry, and the threat of new entrants and substitutes are weighed and considered. The horizontal axis represents the firm's strength or ability to compete in the industry. The competitive strength includes an analysis of the value and quality of the products or services it offers, the market shares they have garnered, the sustainability of the firm's position, and similar factors.

The circles on the matrix represent the various businesses. Both axes are divided into three segments, yielding nine cells. The nine cells are grouped into three zones:

The green "Go" zone consists of the three cells in the upper-left corner. If an enterprise falls in this zone it is in a favorable position with relatively attractive growth opportunities. This indicates a "green light" to invest in this product/service.

The yellow "Caution" zone consists of the three diagonal cells from the lower left to the upper right. A position in the yellow zone is viewed as having medium attractiveness. Management must therefore exercise caution when making additional investments in this product/service. The suggested strategy is to seek to maintain share rather than growing or reducing share.

The red "Stop" zone consists of the three cells in the lower-right corner. A position in the red zone is not attractive. The suggested strategy is that management should begin to make plans to exit the industry.

Portfolio analysis matrixes have several benefits in the strategic planning process. In a single graphic they can portray the comparative performance of all SBUs in a single unified portfolio. This information is helpful in deciding where new SBUs should be added and which existing SBUs should be prodded or divested. It reveals the interrelationships and dependencies among the SBUs, along with the different roles that each one of them plays in the portfolio. The act of preparing a matrix compels the incorporation of external data into the strategic portfolio management decisions. It is important that the matrixes be employed as analytical tools and not as rigid guides to specific strategies.

■ II. RAISE FINANCIAL CAPITAL FOR ALLOCATION TO THE SBUs

If it does nothing else, the corporate center must raise the capital required by its several SBUs to finance their strategies and operations. If the SBUs are simply components of an overall parent organization, they lack the separate legal existence that would permit them to raise capital by issuing stock or borrowing money. It is a primary function of the parent to obtain the necessary capital and allocate it among the SBUs according to some rational formula that maximizes the total return to the corporation. The principles of corporate capital financing are discussed in Chapter 11.

■ III. ALLOCATE RESOURCES AND SERVICES TO THE SBUs

By their nature as independent, self-governing entities within a larger corporation, SBUs are generally responsible for managing their own resources. However, there are several ways in which the corporate center can assist in this process. The primary example is the raising and allocation of financial resources, as just discussed. The corporation may also have developed or accumulated within its center other resources and competencies that can be made available to the SBUs. For instance, there may be located at the corporate-level human resource management services, a research and development function, a technology assessment capability, information technology support, and a corporate legal department, all of which could be useful to individual SBUs.

IV. FACILITATE SYNERGIES AMONG THE SBUs

The raison d'être for most multi-SBU corporations is the synergies that are possible among the businesses. The corporate center plays a key role in fostering the sharing of resources and competencies. It can assist the synergistic sharing process in several ways. It can watch closely the direction of each SBU's operations and strategies, notice areas where it lacks critical resources or competencies, regularly inventory the resources and competencies possessed by all the SBUs, match up a deficient SBU with an SBU that already owns the required asset, and encourage the actual sharing. If necessary, it may assure the sharing SBU that it will not suffer for its good deed in any performance assessment by the center.

These are some of the specific forms facilitation may take:

- Disseminating specific knowledge and best practices among the SBUs.
- Facilitating and transferring knowledge assets and services throughout the corporation (as in a "learning organization").
- Encouraging collaboration and coordination across SBUs in the portfolio.
- Arranging the transfer of skills and capabilities among the businesses.
- Coordinating the activities of shared unit functions (i.e., centralized purchasing) to attain economies of scope.
- Cultivating the ability of the SBUs to carry out effective strategic planning and management.
- Providing appropriate continuing education, training, and coaching to SBU personnel.
- Building a central database of resources, skills, and competencies to which all SBUs have access.
- Temporarily assigning a specialist from one SBU to another for the purpose of transferring her knowledge.
- Sponsoring regular meetings of inter-SBU groups to share information or jointly solve common problems.

■ V. CHOOSE A PARENTING STYLE FOR SBU INTERACTIONS

Corporate management can interact with the SBUs in its portfolio in a variety of ways. Over a period of time, it will be seen to have a certain "style" in its treatment of them. The possibilities lie along a continuum from almost complete detachment from SBU operations as long as it meets agreed-upon targets to very close involvement in the strategic and operational management of the SBU. It is an important decision. Without enough guidance from the center, SBUs might veer off course from the strategic direction plotted for the overall organization or simply mismanage their individual strategies and operations. In contrast, a center that is overly intrusive may stifle the creativity, spontaneity, and entrepreneurial impulses that are the essence of the SBU concept. It is a good idea for the center to make a conscious decision about its style and regularly monitor its effectiveness in generating maximum value from all the organization's components.

One of the criticisms of a center's deep involvement in SBU operations is that it cannot understand well the strategic challenges faced by the SBUs—their customers and competitors, their unique external environments, and even the resources and capabilities they can bring to bear. The corporate center does not deal with those issues on a day-to-day basis and it would be virtually impossible to keep in close touch with what is going on in several different SBUs. If the corporate center grasped these issues as well as the SBUs' management, perhaps there would be no need for the SBUs.

■ VI. PARTICIPATE IN THE SBU STRATEGIC PLANNING AND MANAGEMENT PROCESS

One aspect of the parenting style of the corporate center is the degree to which it involves itself in the strategic planning and management carried out by the individual SBUs. Because corporate management has certain strategic expectations for each SBU that it has chosen to include in its portfolio, it may be tempted to intervene to make sure that their strategic decisions are consistent with those expectations. When it does that, of course, it takes the risk of stifling the spontaneity and entrepreneurial impulses of the SBU managers. The assumption behind the parent-SBU arrangement is that relatively autonomous SBU executives, acting on their own instincts and in their own interests, are likely to produce superior performance. The challenge for the parent is to keep the businesses in its portfolio headed in a generally positive direction without inhibiting them. At a minimum, corporate management usually insists upon negotiating with SBU executives over the strategic broad objectives that they will pursue.

VII. OVERSEE AND MONITOR THE PERFORMANCE OF THE SBUs

Regardless of the degree to which corporate management participates in SBU-level strategy making, it will want to follow closely the performance of each of the businesses. It needs to be kept informed of their progress in meeting strategic objectives and the general financial health of their operations. The parent normally would like to know about developing problems before they become so serious that crisis intervention is necessary.

VIII. MANAGE THE CORPORATION'S RELATIONSHIPS WITH EXTERNAL STAKEHOLDERS

A large multi-SBU corporation must deal with a variety of external stakeholders. Some are unique to individual SBUs and can be handled by their managers. Others are of primary concern to the overall corporation and come within the responsibility of top management. Then, there may be other stakeholders who are important to many or all of the SBUs. It may make more sense for the corporate center to tend to them.

HOW THE CORPORATE CENTER CAN REDUCE THE VALUE CREATED BY ITS SBUs

As noted above, there is some doubt that corporations that are little more than collections of unrelated businesses can add much value to those businesses beyond what they could achieve independently. There are some other ways as well that the corporate center can actually destroy, rather than enhance, the value created by its SBUs.

- The parent corporation can add costs with systems and hierarchies that delay decisions and hinder market responsiveness.
- Its role as a source of capital insulates SBU executives from the realities of the financial market. Comments from corporate executives and their decisions on the allocation of internal capital resources do not provide as powerful feedback as stock prices do for publicly traded shares.
- Some corporations are so large and diverse that it is hard to see a common thread or overriding strategic thrust to what they are doing.
- The corporate center may develop a wieldy, bloated headquarters staff that delivers relatively little value to the SBUs yet must be paid for by them out of their revenues.

The challenge for the top executives of a large corporation is to find ways to overcome these dysfunctional, value-negating patterns.

Study Questions

1. As you walk down a city street, noticing stores and businesses along the way, and as you read or watch news reports about businesses, think about whether each of them is an independent, freestanding company, an SBU in the portfolio of a large corporation, or simply a unit, outlet, store, or facility in a medium-sized corporation. If you wanted to know for sure, where would you go to find out?
2. What are the reasons that corporate executives believe that they must constantly grow their organizations? What would happen if they chose not to pursue growth aggressively, but instead allowed the business to expand or contract naturally?
3. What are some of the problems that are encountered in assembling and managing the integrated health care delivery systems that are so popular? List seven principles that should be followed to ensure the successful operation of such systems.
4. Imagine that you are a corporate "turnaround" specialist who has been hired to save a 400-bed hospital in a large metropolitan area. It faces competition from two well-managed teaching hospitals, has experienced declining occupancy rates, and has been losing money for six years. Common sense and good business thinking says that the hospital should simply be closed. Political considerations will not allow that to happen. Suggest ten steps that the hospital could take to ensure its survival for the next five years.

Learning Exercise 1

Identify a corporation in the health care or biotechnology industries that manages a portfolio of multiple strategic business units (SBUs). Some examples are health care delivery systems, multistate hospital networks, nationwide MCO systems, and international pharmaceutical companies. Conduct some library or Internet research to learn the company's basic strategy. Visit the corporation's Web site, as well as general-purpose business Web sites (*Wall Street Journal, Business Week, Hoovers, Forbes,* SEC), and look for business news about the company over the past year. Get answers to these questions about the company.

1. Determine the number of SBUs in the portfolio and their type, in terms of product/service line, market segment served, geographic area of operation, and so on.
2. Identify the ways in which the SBUs are related to each other, if at all. Describe commonalities among the businesses—in terms of markets targeted, distribution channels employed, or resources

and competencies shared. Look for evidence of ways in which the SBUs take advantage of their relatedness. Are there particular resources and competencies that they share with each other? Imagine additional ways that the SBUs could support each other.

3. Determine the specific ways that the SBUs benefit from their presence in the corporate portfolio. Identify the types of value that the corporate center provides to the SBUs. Would any of these businesses compete just as effectively, or more so, if it operated independently, on its own?
4. By researching the history of the corporation, determine when each of the SBUs was added to the portfolio and the means that were used—merger, acquisition, internal development, and so on.
5. On the basis of your research, the current makeup of the portfolio, and the history of its accumulation and growth, make a best guess at the generic strategy (as described in this chapter) that the corporation seems to be following.
6. Assume that you have been hired as a consultant by this corporation to advise it on its future growth strategies. Make specific recommendations for the management of its portfolio.
   - How rapidly should it expand the portfolio?
   - What types of new SBUs should it add to the portfolio?
   - By what means should it bring them into the portfolio?
   - What should be the relationship of the new SBUs to the existing SBUs?
   - Should any existing SBUs be divested from the portfolio, and for what reasons?

(Optional) Identify a second corporation of the same general type. Compare the second with the first in terms of apparent strategies and comment on how well they are being implemented.

Learning Exercise 2

Research two multistate hospital or health plan corporations. Describe in detail the composition of their portfolios. Where do the portfolios overlap and where are they unique? Gather available information on the portfolio management strategies that each seems to be following. In what future directions does the strategy seem to be headed? Over the next five years, what mergers, acquisitions, and divestments of SBUs do you predict that each corporation will carry out? Alternatively, offer your own recommendations for changes that you think should be made in the two corporate portfolios.

Learning Exercise 3

A matrix is a powerful instrument for succinctly capturing a lot of information about a complex situation. Employing the adage that "a picture is worth a thousand words," its graphic simplicity permits a person to comprehend in one brief look the interplay of a number of factors. It can be used for almost any multifactorial analysis task. Try it.

Pick a health care-related industry or market for which some interesting data are available. It might be all the major drug companies in the United States, all the HMOs in a particular state, or all the hospitals in a particular city. The data might come from annual reports available on the Internet or directly from the companies, from industry directories in a local or university library, or from a government agency that regulates the industry or market. Pick two variables from the data that seem to say something about how well each business is doing. It might be percentage of revenues devoted to R&D and stock price trends (for drug companies) or number of members and Healthcare Effectiveness Data and Information Set (HEDIS) ratings (for MCOs). Array the variables along the two axes of the matrix. At this point, formulate a hypothesis about what the matrix will reveal. For instance, high R&D expenditures predict steadily rising stock prices, or large MCO memberships are associated with high HEDIS ratings. Place a symbol at the appropriate point on the matrix to represent each company. Use the symbol to depict additional information. The size of a circle symbol might indicate the company's total revenues with a pie slice to show its share of market.

Study the resulting matrix. Does it confirm the original hypothesis? What other conclusions can be drawn about the industry or market, and about individual participants? How could the matrix be refined to reveal more, perhaps to support a strategic decision that a firm on the matrix needs to make? For what other applications would a similar matrix analysis be useful?

Learning Exercise 4

Research business news reports for the past three to five years. Identify at least two health care organizations that filed for Chapter 11 reorganization. There have been several—hospitals, hospital networks, health systems, and physician groups. In the reports at the time of the filing and subsequently, try to determine what measures the organizations employed in their efforts to regain financial solvency. Then, check the news further to learn the eventual outcome. Did the organizations survive in some form or finally go out of existence?

Notes

[1] Williamson OE. Strategy research: Governance and competence perspectives. *Strategic Management Journal*. 1999;20(12):1087–1108.

[2] Palich LE, Cardinal LB, and Miller C. Curvilinearity in the diversification-performance linkage: An examination of over three decades of research. *Strategic Management Journal*. 2000;21:155–174.

References

Aggarwal RK and Samwick AA. Why do managers diversify their firms? Agency reconsidered. *Journal of Finance*. 2003;58:71–118.

Bowman EH and Helfat CE. Does corporate strategy matter? *Strategic Management Journal*. 2001;22:1–23.

Brush TH, Bromiley P, and Hendrickx M. The relative influence of industry and corporation on business segment performance: An alternative estimate. *Strategic Management Journal*. 1999;20:519–547.

Burgelman RA and Doz YL. The power of strategic integration. *MIT Sloan Management Review*. 2001;42(3):28–38.

Chandler AD Jr. *Strategy and Structure: Chapters in the History of the Industrial Enterprise*. Cambridge, MA: MIT Press; 1962.

Collis DJ. Corporate strategy in multi-business firms. *Long-Range Planning*. 1996;29:416–418.

Collis D and Montogomery CA. Competing on resources: Strategy in the 1990s. *Harvard Business Review*. 1995;73(4):118–128.

Douglas TJ and Ryman JA. Understanding competitive advantage in the general hospital industry: Evaluating strategic competencies. *Strategic Management Journal*. 2003;24:333–347.

Goold M. Parenting strategies for the mature business. *Long-Range Planning*. June 1996:359.

Goold M and Campbell A. Desperately seeking synergy. *Harvard Business Review*. 1998;76(5):131–143.

Goold M, Campbell A, and Alexander M. Corporate strategy and parenting theory. *Long Range Planning*. April 1998:308–318.

Gupta D and Gerchak Y. Quantifying operational synergies in a merger/acquisition. *Management Science*. 2002;48:517–533.

Harper NWC and Viguerie SP. Are you too focused? *McKinsey Quarterly*. Mid-summer 2002:29–38.

Harrigan KR. Formulating vertical integration strategies. *Academy of Management Review*. 1984;9:639.

Harrison JS. Alternatives to merger: Joint ventures and other strategies. *Long-Range Planning*. December 1987:78–83.

Hedley B. Strategy and the business portfolio. *Long-Range Planning*. February 1977:9.

Henderson BD. *Henderson On Corporate Strategy*. Cambridge, MA: Abt Books; 1979.

Hill CWL. Diversification and economic performance: Bringing structure and corporate management back into the picture. In: Rumelt RP, Schendel DE, and Teece DJ. *Fundamental Issues in Strategy*. Cambridge, MA: Harvard Business School Press; 1994:297–321.

Hill CWL and Hansen GS. A longitudinal study of the cause and consequence of changes in diversification in the US pharmaceutical industry. *Strategic Management Journal*. 1991;12:187–199.

Hill CWL, Hitt MA, and Hoskisson RE. Cooperative versus competitive structures and related and unrelated diversified firms. *Organization Science*. 1992;3:501–521.

Hitt MA, Harrison JS, and Ireland RD. *Mergers and Acquisitions: A Guide to Creating Value for Stakeholders*. New York, NY: Oxford University Press; 2001.

Hoskinson RE and Hitt MA. Strategic control and R&D investment in multiproduct firms. *Strategic Management Journal*. 1988;9:605–621.

Kwak M. Maximizing value through diversification. *MIT Sloan Management Review*. 2002;43(2):10.

Lauenstein MC. Diversification: The hidden explanation of success. *Sloan Management Review*. Fall 1985: 49–55.

Markides CC. To diversify or not to diversify. *Harvard Business Review*. 1997;75(6):93–99.

Markides CC. Corporate strategy: The role of the centre. In: Pettigrew A, Thomas H, and Whittington R. *Handbook of Strategy and Management*. Thousand Oaks, CA: Sage; 2002:98–112.

Marks ML and Mirvis PH. Managing mergers, acquisitions, and alliances: Creating an effective transition structure. *Organizational Dynamics*. 2000;28(3):35–47.

Matsusaka JG. Corporate diversification, value maximization, and organizational capabilities. *Journal of Business*. 2001;74:409–432.

McCann JE III. The growth of acquisitions in services. *Long-Range Planning*. December 1996:835–841.

Paine FT and Power DJ. Merger strategy: An examination of Drucker's five rules for successful acquisition. *Strategic Management Journal*. 1984;5:99–110.

Park C. The effects of prior performance on the choice between related and unrelated acquisitions: Implications for the performance consequences of diversification strategy. *Journal of Management Studies*. 2002;39:1003–1019.

Pearce JA II and Robbins DK. Retrenchment remains the foundation of business turnaround. *Strategic Management Journal*. June 1994:407–417.

Porter ME. From competitive strategy to corporate strategy. In: Hussey DE. *International Review of Strategic Management*. Vol. 1. Chichester, England: John Wiley & Sons; 1990:29.

Prahalad CK and Hamel G. The core competence of the corporation. *Harvard Business Review*. May-June 1990:79–91.

Reimann BC and Reichert A. Portfolio planning methods for strategic capital allocation: A survey of Fortune 500 firms. *International Journal of Management*. March 1996:84–93.

Robins J and Wiersema ME. Resource-based approach to the multibusiness firm: Empirical analysis of portfolio interrelationships and corporate financial performance. *Strategic Management Journal*. 1995;16:277–299.

Rumelt RP. *Strategy, structure, and economic performance*. Cambridge, MA: Harvard Business School; 1974.

Stuckey J and White D. When and When Not to Vertically Integrate. *Sloan Management Review*. Spring 1993:71–83.

Wright P, Kroll M, Lado A, and Van Ness B. The structure of ownership and corporate acquisitions strategies. *Strategic Management Journal*. 2002;23: 41–53.

CHAPTER

8

Formulating SBU-Level and Functional Area Strategy

Learning Objectives

After reading and studying this chapter, you should be able to:

- Identify and explain the strategic responsibilities of top management of SBUs.
- Understand the relationships regarding strategic matters between the corporate center management and the managers of the SBUs in its portfolio.
- Lay out the generic methods by which a business can grow its revenues and profits.
- List the major types of growth strategy.
- Explain the concept of "sustainable competitive advantage."
- Compare and contrast the four generic business strategies defined by Michael Porter.
- Discuss the pros and cons of "hybrid" strategy and how to achieve it.
- Distinguish functional area strategies and how they interact with SBU-level strategies.
- Describe the several basic strategic postures a business may adopt toward its competitors.

In contrast with corporate-level strategy that deals primarily with management of a portfolio of several or many SBUs, strategy at the level of those individual SBUs is concerned with developing resources and competencies, competing in product and service markets, confronting competitors in those markets, creating and sustaining a competitive advantage, and responding to other changes in the external environment. These are approximately the same duties that the managers would have in a freestanding, autonomous business that is not a component of the portfolio of a larger corporation. This is competitive, market-oriented strategy, the sort that most people imagine when they think of business strategy.

There is a definite trend toward consolidation in the health care industry, gathering small physician practices into large multi-specialty group practices, hospitals and nursing homes into large multistate networks, a variety of providers into integrated delivery systems, and health plans and MCOs into regional and national aggregations. It is increasingly important to discuss the strategic behavior of businesses within the context of the larger entities to which they belong. Top management of SBUs have strategic responsibilities that are different from, but complementary to, those of the executives in corporate headquarters.

At the same time, there remain a great many health care-related businesses that are freestanding and autonomous. New independent businesses emerge within the industry every time a recent medical school graduate opens a practice or a university researcher forms a biotechnology startup. Most health-related public agencies and many not-for-profit health care organizations will remain self-governing entities and never grow into multi-SBU corporations. The managers of such self-governing establishments face strategic challenges similar to those of executives in SBUs.

To a certain degree, and depending on the size of the organization, functional areas within SBUs or independent businesses also have significant roles to play in strategic planning and management. Their strategic efforts must be coordinated with those at the SBU executive level. They will be narrower in scope and perhaps have shorter time horizons.

STRATEGIC DUTIES OF SBU MANAGEMENT

The top executives of each SBU in a corporation's portfolio have strategic as well as operational responsibilities. Some of their strategic duties are similar to those at the corporate level, while others are unique to their being in direct contact with customers and competitors.

Define Strategic Direction

Top SBU management sets the strategic direction for the entire unit. This includes creating and disseminating statements of mission, vision, values, and strategic objectives, as laid out in Chapter 6. Those statements for the SBU must be consistent with the counterpart statements for the corporation. If the corporate mission describes operations in particular markets or industries, the SBU mission should fall within one of those markets or industries. The SBU vision can be more freewheeling and idiosyncratic but still cannot be a radical departure from the future envisioned by the corporate center. There should be close parallels between the corporate and SBU values sets, though an SBU might aspire to a more risk-taking environment than the corporation. The strategic objectives will be unique to the SBU as it pursues its vision.

Conduct Internal and External Environmental Assessments

It is an ongoing strategic responsibility of an SBU's managers to continuously monitor and assess the business environment in which it operates and competes, while simultaneously keeping an eye on its own resources and competencies for taking actions within that environment. In doing this, they will follow the principles laid out in Chapters 2–5.

Negotiate Strategy with Corporate Parent

A regular preoccupation of SBU executives are the negotiations with their colleagues at the corporate center regarding the fit of the SBU's strategic objectives with the corporate objectives, the achievability of the strategic metrics by which SBU management will be evaluated, and the availability of capital and other resources that the corporate center is in a position to provide. The corporation's strategic objectives will describe the composition of the SBU portfolio that it intends to build, and will include assumptions about the strategic direction of each of the SBUs. Corporate managers will be unhappy if an SBU that was acquired for its emphasis on certain approaches to certain markets decides to move off on a very different strategic course. The SBU managers will want their performance to be evaluated on the basis of metrics over which they have control, that reflect the areas in which they are focusing their energies, and that are set at achievable levels. The corporate center will try to use those same metrics to push the SBU managers to perform in areas and at levels that will contribute to the realization of corporate goals. At the very least, the SBU executive team will look to the corporation for the financial capital they need to fund their strategic aims. If there are other assets that are available and would be helpful (e.g., centralized purchasing or R&D), the SBU would like to have access to them as well.

Adopt a Generic Strategy

On the basis of their environmental assessments and consistent with the strategic direction they have adopted, the SBU managers will adopt one of four broad generic strategies:

- "low-cost leadership" targeted at the entire market,
- "differentiation" targeted at the entire market,

- low-cost leadership targeted at a segment of the market, or
- differentiation targeted at a market segment.

Formulate Action Strategies

Within the scope of the chosen generic strategy, the next step is to *formulate* action strategies specific to the SBU, its resources and competencies, and its markets and competitors. This is usually the second most complex, time-consuming phase of all the strategy work that a business must do; the *implementation* of the action strategies should be and normally is the most demanding. These strategies are what determine an organization's success or failure in competing against other firms in its industry, in winning the hearts and dollars of its customers, and in achieving its long-range vision.

Develop Needed Resources and Competencies

A business's strategies cannot possibly succeed, or even be implemented, unless they have a foundation in its resources and competencies. Those resources and competencies are not, and should not be, static. Existing resources will be consumed or become obsolete. New strategies for a changing environment will demand the deployment of new capabilities. One of management's responsibilities is to develop or acquire the additional or new resources and competencies that may be required by the strategies that it formulates, adopts, and pursues. That task in itself requires a forward-looking attitude on the part of managers.

Negotiate with Financial Markets for Needed Capital

When the business is autonomous and freestanding (not part of a larger corporation), management must assume the responsibility for negotiating with the financial markets for the debit or equity that it needs to fund its operations and strategies. This task requires sophisticated strategic financial management skills (discussed at greater length in Chapter 11) that are conveniently provided by the corporate center in a multi-SBU organization. SBU managers in such organizations need to negotiate with parent management for allocation of the financial capital they need.

Negotiate with Functional Area Managers for Strategy Implementation

Once each SBU's executive team has formulated strategies that are acceptable to its corporate parent, they must negotiate with their respective functional managers (e.g., operations, marketing, human resources) for short-term, more operational objectives and action plans designed to carry them out. Preferably, those managers will have participated actively in the formulation process so that functional area implications will have been incorporated into the strategies. At the very least, the strategy demands on their areas should not come as a surprise to them.

Appoint and Evaluate Functional Area Managers

Top SBU management is also responsible for appointing and evaluating the performance of the managers of the several functional areas. They will be assessed on their ability to maintain existing operations at peak levels while simultaneously contributing to the successful implementation of new strategic initiatives.

Monitor and Control Strategy Implementation

It is the duty of the lead executives in a business to institute monitoring and control systems to follow the progress of strategy implementation and make adjustments as necessary. The best systems constantly compare actual strategy achievements with the original plan goals, concurrently taking into account unanticipated changes in the firm's environment. The greatest challenge with such a system is deciding when a correction is called for and what it will be.

THE ROLE OF THE CORPORATE CENTER IN SBU STRATEGY

How an SBU goes about formulating and implementing its strategies can be influenced both positively and negatively by its corporate center. The center may be dictatorial regarding the objectives and specific strategies that it wishes SBU management to pursue. At a certain point, as the SBU's discretion and autonomy are more and more constrained, it will cease to function as a true SBU.

Even when allowing SBU managers substantial discretion, the corporate parent may hold them to standards, goals, and criteria that are difficult to meet. This may be because the corporate center itself feels pressure from financial markets to perform at certain levels. It may also reflect the center's lack of understanding of the market and competitive realities of the specific SBUs in its portfolio.

The center may be more or less generous with the financial resources that it allocates to the SBU. An SBU will probably never have all the investment capital it would like from the corporation. The corporate managers must take into account a variety of needs and priorities among the SBUs to which they will allocate the limited capital funds available to them.

The center also may be more or less effective at facilitating sharing and other synergies among the SBUs in its portfolio. One advantage of being an SBU in a larger corporation's portfolio is the possibility of borrowing or using resources and competencies possessed by sibling SBUs. The chances that such complementarities will exist are greater when the strategic logic of portfolio management is "concentration" or "related diversification" rather than "unrelated diversification." The process of inter-SBU sharing is abetted if the corporate center has a desire and the necessary skills to facilitate portfolio synergies.

FORMULATING STRATEGY IN SBUs AND INDIVIDUAL BUSINESSES

In planning strategies, individual businesses have two objectives in mind. One is to grow their revenues and profits as rapidly as reasonably possible. The other is to build sustainable competitive advantage over other companies in their industry. If it is fortunate enough to operate in an industry or field where there is no real competition, it can concentrate on growth. Where rivals do exist, it would be disastrous to ignore them.

Strategies That Grow Revenues and Profits

For many organizations, particularly the for-profit ones, the primary measures of success are financial. Their leading stakeholders—equity owners and debt holders—are most interested in organizational performance that results in maximum return on equity investments and maximum assurance that debts can be paid. This inevitably requires a constant pursuit of increase in revenues and the profits earned on those revenues.

There are only a few basic ways in which a business can grow its revenues and profits:

- Sell more units of a product/service to existing customers.
- Sell more units of a product/service to new customers.
- Sell the same number of units at higher prices, which will result in higher revenues and, perhaps, higher profits.
- Sell the same number of units at the same price, but produce them at lower cost, which will result in higher profits.

These outcomes can be achieved through several types of "growth strategy."

1. *Increase market share*. Under this strategy, the firm increases production capacity, expands its marketing activities, and sells more aggressively with the intention of winning more customers in its existing market segments. The product is the same, the price is the same, the sales volume is higher.
2. *Enter new markets*. In this case, a business aims to sell additional units of its products to new customers in different segments of the market. The customers may be in a different geographic area, a different demographic group (age, gender, ethnicity), or a different industry (nursing homes, hospitals). The key feature of the strategy is that the customers, regardless of their other dissimilarities, con-

sume or use the products in the same ways as the current customers do. No alteration in product design is necessary. This strategy usually requires market research to ferret out the best new segments, coupled with adjustments in advertising, sales, and perhaps distribution suited to the segment targeted.

3. *Identify new uses.* If new uses for existing products can be found and promoted, a firm will be able to sell more of those products to both current customers and new customers in other market segments. An example of this strategy is a pharmaceutical company that develops, obtains FDA approval for, and begins to market a drug designed to treat one clinical condition, and then subsequently discovers that the drug also is effective in treating another condition. The company now sells the drug to the market segment composed of patient-customers with the second condition. For this strategy to work, a company must do some market research on relevant, untreated medical conditions (unmet needs) and be prepared to use different marketing tactics in reaching the customers with those conditions, but, more than anything, it must be capable of the research and testing necessary to demonstrate the drug's secondary functionality.
4. *Create new products.* Once a business has squeezed all the revenues and profits that it can out of its present product lineup, the only option for further growth is the development of entirely new products for sale to either the existing or new market segments. When current products and markets are put behind, the directions for possible future growth are almost limitless. The chances of success are much greater if the firm concentrates on new products and segments that leverage the resources and core competencies that it already possesses. Pursuit of this strategy is sometimes tantamount to founding a new venture. It must combine identification of substantial unmet customer needs in market segments within reach of the firm, development of products with features that respond to those needs, design of new processes for manufacturing the products, and the launch of marketing campaigns that successfully convince the prospective customers that the new products meet their value demands.
5. *Acquire new businesses.* An organization may reach the point where it knows that it must create new products and enter new markets in order to grow, but lacks the resources and competencies to make that happen. In such a situation it has two alternatives. One is to acquire another business that already manufactures the desired products, operates in the target market segments, or has the resources and competencies to do either or both. In effect, the organization buys an established share of the market or buys an established line of products or services. This strategy has been popular in the health care

services industry (hospitals and health plans, for instance), producing a general consolidation trend. One occasional impediment is that the most appropriate acquisition targets are often near-competitors of the firm and this can present antitrust legal problems.

6. *Collaborate with others.* To gain access to new drug products they otherwise cannot develop internally, large pharmaceutical companies have taken to contracting with much smaller biotechnology research firms for the output from their often single-drug research efforts. The pharmaceutical giant may partially fund those efforts or simply pay to license the manufacturing and marketing rights to the drug. This collaborative strategy is a second way for a business to come up with the new products it needs to keep revenues and profits growing. Arm's-length contracts are one form of collaboration; others are joint ventures, strategic partnerships or alliances, multi-firm coalitions, resource pools, and short-term single-project combinations. Antitrust implications must be watched closely.

Strategies That Build Sustainable Competitive Advantage

Pursuit of growth strategies is often a zero-sum game. There is a finite number of customers and customer dollars that a business can try to attract. An increase in revenues and profits for one company means a decrease for other companies—the firm's competitors. The only exception is when the entire market is growing so rapidly—adding new customers and spending power—that all competitors can increase their sales volumes simultaneously.

In the majority of businesses, the presence of competitors must be taken into account when planning strategy. Quite simply, a successful business must find ways to position itself more positively and distinctively in the eyes of its customers than any of its competitors. When it has accomplished this, it has gained a "competitive advantage" over them. When it can keep this advantage for an extended period of time, months or even years, it is said to have a "sustainable" competitive advantage.

There is a continuum of generic strategies by which this advantage may be achieved. To choose the optimal strategy for an organization, its managers should understand the full range of possibilities.

■ SELECTING A GENERIC BUSINESS STRATEGY—À LA PORTER

When a business has a full, up-to-date appreciation of its own resources and competencies, and the threats and opportunities that it faces in the marketplace, it is in a position to formulate appropriate strategies that will carry it forward toward its vision. Some businesses simply plunge into the infinite variety of strategic alternatives available to them and do their best to fit a few of them to the business's unique circumstances. Experienced strategists can become quite accomplished at this approach to strategy-making. For executives and managers just beginning to take on strategic responsibilities, it is helpful to have a structure for thinking about possible strategies. It is hard to do better than the classification described by Michael Porter.

The ultimate aim of a business strategy is to give a business an advantage over its competitors, preferably one that can be continued as long as possible—a "sustainable competitive advantage." Any advantage must be measured in terms of what it does for the customer, what benefits or value the SBU is able to deliver that are not available from any of its competitors. (If competitors offer the same value, there is no advantage, only parity.)

There is a finite number of variables in the products and services that a business sells to its customers, the vehicles by which it provides them with value. In a basic competitive sense, business-level strategies have three variables to play with. One is the cost of creating the products or services to be sold in the market. When this serves as the basis for a business's dominant strategy, it is called a "low-cost leadership" strategy. Another variable is the features of the products and services, with the term "features" defined very broadly. It includes products' appearance and performance, their delivery or distribution, the marketing (advertising, promotion, image) of the products or services, and the before and after-purchase service that accompanies them. These characteristics and any others that the SBU might imagine can become the basis of a generic "differentiation" strategy. The features must make the products or services different from those of the competition in a way that matters to the customers.

The third variable is the range of prospective customers to whom the products and services are marketed. Either of the first two generic strategies (low-cost leadership or differentiation) can be targeted at the full breadth of the market in which the business operates or focused on a narrower segment of it, resulting in a total of four possible generic strategies:

- full market low-cost leadership
- full market differentiation
- segment low-cost leadership
- segment differentiation

There has been a lot of discussion about businesses that are pursuing (deliberately, by default, or because they cannot think of anything else to do) a combination of differentiation and cost leadership. Porter called these companies "stuck-in-the-middle" and, at first glance, it would seem to be a losing position. To be an absolute cost leader requires offering a basic, plain-vanilla product; any added, differentiating features could only add to the cost of production. Yet, the firm nonetheless wants to appear somewhat unique in its customers' eyes, so it attaches a few distinguishing features. The result is that the business is at a cost disadvantage to a competitor pursuing a rigorous cost-leadership strategy and a feature disadvantage to a competitor that is implementing a multi-faceted differentiation strategy. Traditional logic said that such a strategic position could never succeed.

In a marketplace filled with aggressive, enterprising competitors, however, a good rule of thumb is to "never say never." What seemed impossible or unworkable yesterday may be a plausible road to competitive advantage tomorrow. In fact, a number of businesses in different industries have been able successfully to pursue both strategies simultaneously. Health care is one of them.

A combination or hybrid low-cost/differentiation strategy has been virtually forced upon health care organizations. The consumers (not to be confused with the payers) of health care services in the United States have become accustomed to receiving the highest level of full-featured care from hospitals and physicians. This is partially due to the fact that in the past they have not personally paid for the services. Furthermore, until recently, there were few accurate measures of the quality or performance of most medical services and products. At the same time, the payers (not to be confused with the consumers) for health care services have been applying unrelenting pressure on health care providers to hold down the costs of the services they deliver. Those provider organizations and individuals have struggled to balance these often conflicting demands. To satisfy their payers, they must pursue a form of low-cost leadership strategy; to satisfy their consumers, they must emphasize the features of their products and services. They are truly stuck in the middle. This market dynamic is likely to change with the growth of consumer-driven health care in ways that will pose both opportunities and threats to health care organizations.

Low-Cost Leadership

"Low-cost leadership" means what it says—the business aims to have the lowest production costs of any competitor in the market. Not just lower costs, but the lowest costs. There are several routes by which a business may offer its products/services at the lowest cost. Firms pursuing this strategy will have to determine whether they are in a position to take advantage of these approaches.

1. A fundamental first step is to define and analyze the business's internal value chain with the intent of identifying points at which process modifications might produce cost savings. The concept of the internal value chain is explained more fully in Chapter 2. Besides being a

sequential process for value accumulation, it is a complex system of activities that consume costly resources. The current configuration of a business's value chain is not the only possible way to create its products and services. The existing activities could be performed better than they are. The existing activities could be replaced by different activities performing the same function. The sequence in which the activities are performed could be rearranged. Activities could be moved to different points in the chain or performed simultaneously. The interface between activities could be improved, resulting in tighter integration throughout the chain. Activities currently performed in-house could be subcontracted to outside firms. (See number 5 below.)

2. An organization can minimize its per-unit costs by fully utilizing every one of its fixed cost resources. Every business incurs both variable and fixed costs in creating its products and services. The variable costs increase or decrease in relation to the volume of products/services created. The fixed costs must be paid regardless of the volume, and even if there is zero volume. Consider the example of a medical imaging unit in a hospital or physician practice—perhaps an X-ray machine or CT scanner. The organization must pay for the space the unit occupies, the salaries of the technicians who must always be available if a picture must be taken, and the other supplies, utilities, and services necessary to keep the unit operational. All those costs are fixed. It is in the hospital's financial interest to utilize the imaging unit as much as is medically necessary in order to spread the costs across as large a number of images as possible. The result of high utilization is lower per-image cost. Another example is a hospital's bed capacity. There are very large fixed costs involved in maintaining, say, a 150-bed hospital in an operational state ready to accept patients at all times. All those costs are incurred—whether there are patients in all 150 beds or in only one bed. The hospital will make every effort to keep as many of those beds full as possible—to spread the fixed costs over the maximum number of patients. This is why one of the most important hospital performance metrics is the bed occupancy rate.

   It helps to be able to predict the demand for products and services in order to take steps to maximize utilization. In hospitals, this may involve redesignating beds from one underutilized service to another that is in greater demand. When the decrease in demand is more persistent, entire groups of beds may be taken out of service in order to eliminate at least some of the associated fixed costs.

3. Another method of achieving cost leadership that is related to high utilization is "economies of scale." This is the principle that—for some production processes—the larger the facility, the lower the cost. For instance, it does not cost twice as much to build, and operate, a

200-bed hospital as it does a 100-bed hospital. The challenge is to select the optimal size facility for the hospital's level of operation, when that level is unpredictable and constantly changing.

Once a hospital is built, it is not easy or inexpensive to make it a little bit larger as patient demand grows. In some cases, however, there is an option of increasing capacity by increments. The question is by how much and when. Assume that a pharmaceutical company has developed a very promising new drug that it expects to receive FDA approval in six months. It is planning to construct a new facility for the manufacture of the drug for retail sale and is wondering what the initial capacity of the facility should be. It projects that during the first six months after introduction, monthly sales will grow 100,000 units each month, so that sales in the sixth month will be 600,000 units. In the year after that, monthly sales will grow at the rate of 200,000 units a month. Manufacturing capacity can be added only in 500,000-unit chunks. Should the company begin with a 0.5 or 1.0 million-unit facility, and at what points should it expand capacity still further? Keep in mind that the sales projections may be high or low, that the per-unit cost will go down as total capacity increases, and that costs will be lowest when production volumes are closest to 100 percent of the existing capacity.

4. New technologies in the production of goods or services also have the potential to lower costs. Installing such technologies frequently requires substantial capital outlays. The key question is whether the initial expenditure is more than offset by the production cost savings that it allows. There are numerous examples in the health care industry of new technologies that it is claimed will reduce the soaring costs. EMR systems will eliminate the salaries of medical transcribers and medical record file clerks. Some systems include a capability to code the services provided automatically and more accurately. Electronic claims filing will further reduce the likelihood of coding errors and speed their eventual payment.
5. One route to a cost leadership position is to find the best location for the performance of every activity in a business's value chain—whether that location is inside or outside the business. When the business moves to an outside source a task previously conducted inside, it is "outsourcing". When the business pulls into the organization a task previously performed by an external source, it is "insourcing". In both the pharmaceutical and health care industries, a great deal of attention is being given to outsourcing—contracting with external suppliers—functions previously performed by businesses in-house. Examples are a large pharmaceutical company contracting with a small biotechnology firm that does nothing but initial discovery work,

and a managed care organization that contracts with overseas firms to handle claims processing. These actions are done in the interest of placing these tasks in the hands of someone who specializes in that kind of work and can do it more efficiently, at lower cost.

6. As an organization and its employees carry out the same work processes repeatedly over many months and years, they gain experience that enables them to create products and services faster, at lower cost, and with higher quality. This phenomenon is called the "learning curve" or the "experience curve." One example of this is the principle that physicians, such as surgeons, who perform the same procedure more often, in greater volumes, will do it faster and with higher quality results. An organization will move more rapidly along this curve, ideally faster than the competition is moving, if it has nurtured an environment in which employees are inspired to accumulate and share knowledge. Peter Senge described in great detail this concept of a "learning organization." The efficiencies that come with progress along the learning curve are one reason that companies in a new market often go to great lengths, even cutting prices drastically, to capture a large market share as quickly as possible. If they can reach the top of the curve first and enjoy the lower costs that exist there, they have more flexibility in fending off other competitors coming along behind them.

The Pros and Cons of Achieving a Low-Cost Leadership Position

A business has three fundamental choices of what it can do when it successfully implements a cost leadership strategy. First, it can lower its prices to a level commensurate with the lower cost structure while still earning a reasonable profit margin. Because the competition cannot match the lower prices without losing money, the business will be able to sell more of its products and services, increasing its revenues and profits. The second option is to leave prices at the same level as the competition's. With the lower costs, the business will enjoy even greater profits. Third, the business can keep prices at the higher level and use the greater margin it earns to add differentiating features to the products or services. If carefully selected, those features should produce higher sales, profits, and market share.

There are some negatives to a cost leadership strategy. A company can become so fixated on its efforts to maintain low-cost manufacturing processes that it fails to notice that customer preferences for its type of products or services have changed. In fact, the changes may require manufacturing methods different from those that the company has developed and refined. All its cost-cutting innovations become irrelevant. Even if they remain relevant, competitors may be able easily to imitate them.

Successful strategies create competitive advantages that last for some time, that are sustainable.

Keys to Success of a Low-Cost Leadership Strategy

There has been enough accumulated experience and research with low-cost leadership strategy initiatives to reach some conclusions about what makes them successful.

- The business must start with sufficient funds to cover working capital requirements until the low-cost leadership position has been attained, and to finance the strategic initiatives needed to move the organization to that position.
- It must possess the technical, operational, engineering, and process skills needed to carry out value chain modifications that result in lowest-cost production.
- The business must exercise close, tight control of all processes and personnel involved in creating the products and services, with an emphasis on their efficiency and cost.
- Compensation and other performance incentives must be aligned with the low-cost operational strategy.
- It is essential that executive leadership be experienced in managing low-cost operations and committed to doing so in this organization.
- It helps greatly if there exists a corporate culture that is comfortable with and capable of contributing to a low-cost operating model.

Differentiation

A firm differentiates by creating product value for customers in any unique way that they are willing to pay more for than it cost the firm to create it. Just because the firm is not pursuing a low-cost leadership strategy does not mean that it can assume the customer will pay any amount for valuable differentiating features. The price cannot be more than the "difference" is worth to the customer, nor can it be less than the firm paid to create it. To strike this delicate balance, the firm must create differentiating features as economically as possible while simultaneously keeping all other costs as low as possible.

The form that the differentiation takes depends also on what the firm is capable of creating and delivering. The best way to ascertain what differentiation is possible is by scrutinizing the internal value chain to see what activities can be performed differently in order to create new value for the customer. Differentiation opportunities can be found at almost any point.

By purchasing different ingredients for its drug products, a pharmaceutical company may be able to improve the purity and effectiveness of the final product. By using a different grade of steel, a manufacturer of hospital beds might be able to increase the strength and durability of the beds, while also reducing the need for maintenance. The R&D efforts of a company selling medical devices may design products that function more reliably at higher levels of performance, have more useful features than competitive versions, look more attractive, or can be manufactured less expensively, leading to lower prices. Unique collaboration techniques among surgical team members in a hospital could result in lower infection and repeat surgery rates, and shorter hospital patient stays. The process by which a consultant specialist returns a patient, with recommendations and updated medical record, to her primary care physician speeds the patient's treatment and recovery, and wins the referral loyalty of that physician. The customer support function of an EMR system vendor can take steps to provide better training for buyers and quicker response to tech support requests, resulting in less system downtime for the customer.

Almost any aspect of the product purchase experience can be differentiated; these are some generic examples.

- More product features
- New, appealing product features
- Product features tailored to individual customer preferences
- Better product performance (both alone and in combination with other products)
- Easier to use and operate, by less-skilled personnel
- Costs the customer less to use and operate
- More reliable, durable, and long-lasting
- More attractive appearance
- More convenient purchase locations
- Speedier delivery
- Friendlier customer service at all stages
- More prompt after-purchase repair and maintenance service
- Heightened reputation and image
- Regardless of the concrete differences, the customer perceives that it is receiving greater value

To be an acceptable basis for a differentiation strategy that culminates in a sustainable competitive advantage, a difference must satisfy four criteria.

1. The customer must notice it and want it. He must want it more than the product without the difference.
2. The customer must be willing to pay more for a product with the difference than it cost the business to create it.

3. The business must be capable (possess the necessary resources and competencies) of creating the product at a cost less than the price the customer is willing to pay for it.
4. It must be impossible for a competitor to create a product with the same difference at the same cost within the near future.

If a business can meet these criteria, substantial benefits can come its way.

- For as long as it can sustain a meaningful differentiation, the firm is, to a degree, insulated from the competition going on in the marketplace.
- Through differentiation, the firm in effect defines an entirely new product in a new market segment in which it is the only competitor.
- By definition, buyers of differentiated products are less sensitive to price, and even to price increases. Once a customer gets hooked on a differentiation feature, she will be willing to accept higher prices to keep enjoying it—up to a point.
- The attraction of a carefully conceived differentiation feature engenders customer loyalty that often leads to automatic repeat purchases of the product.
- That same customer loyalty makes it hard for new competitors to enter the market. The customers will be reluctant to switch to a new product source, even though that product may be virtually the same.

However, a differentiation strategy is not a surefire route to competitive advantage and above average profitability. The strategy can go wrong in several ways.

- There is no reason why a competitor cannot differentiate the product even further, finding a different combination of distinguishing features, perhaps created at lower cost, that are more appealing to customers.
- Similarly, a rival may successfully carve out a narrower segment of the market, based on a subset of even more unique product features. If enough segments are separated from the primary market, the original differentiator may be left with a much diminished customer base.
- If several competitors pursue differentiation with multiple products, customers may become confused by the variety and complexity of choices.
- Eventually, differentiated product features may no longer hold interest for consumers. This can happen as the buyers become better informed about the true value of the added features, especially in comparison to the higher prices charged for them. Will patients con-

tinue to prefer treatment at the Mayo Clinic if they discover, from objective clinical outcome indicators, that they can receive comparable quality care at a local community hospital?

- Once a firm commits to a differentiation strategy, it develops a specialized, often higher-cost manufacturing process that may come back to plague it if lower-cost versions of its products are introduced by rivals or new market entrants.
- If enough competitors copy the original differentiating features, they become commonplace, customers expect them as basic characteristics of the product, and the product becomes a commodity.
- Because most differentiating features can eventually be copied by rivals, a firm committed to this strategy must be able continuously to innovate new features that are unique, cost-effective, and valued by customers. As soon as it falls behind in innovation, the strategy begins to fail.

Hybrid

Most firms do not have the strategic discipline to dedicate themselves fully to low-cost leadership or differentiation strategies; they wind up somewhere in between, trying both to distinguish their products in some ways from the competition and to keep their prices reasonably low. As mentioned earlier, Michael Porter thought that this was an undesirable position to be in, calling it "stuck-in-the-middle." The products of these firms were not different enough from those of their competitors to draw away any customers and their costs were not low enough to attract price-conscious consumers. It appeared that such businesses were getting the *worst* of the two extremes.

In the past decade, however, a countervailing attitude has emerged—businesses that artfully pursue strategies that are a combination of low cost and differentiation may be able to enjoy the *best* of the two strategy extremes. This third strategy choice, a hybrid of the other two, aims to offer the best "value" to the customer. Not the lowest price, but one that is reasonable, not exorbitant. Not a product with all the bells and whistles, but some interesting, useful features that raise it above the bare-bones category.

It is a difficult balance to find and maintain. It requires understanding the subtleties of customer value preferences, plus possessing the resources and competencies that enable a firm to pick just the right product features, not too few, not too many, and create them at a cost that allows prices the customers are willing to pay while also returning an acceptable profit to the firm. Just a few misjudgments and the firm is truly stuck in the middle, selling products with more (or the wrong) features than customers want that are created at costs that do not allow profits.

When the strategy works, the relatively low costs of the relatively unique and appealing products generate profits that can be reinvested to make the products still more distinctive. As the products grow in popularity, their sales volume increases. This can lead to economies of scale, which allow lower prices or greater profits at the same prices. In addition, the way in which a business deploys its resources and competencies to offer products at a "sweet spot" in the market is usually so complex and hard to understand, and therefore imitate, that it gives the business a sustainable competitive advantage.

Focus

There are well over 300 million potential customers for health care in the United States and they are not all interested in exactly the same products and services. Some health care organizations do attempt to "be all things to all people" by trying to meet the needs of virtually every conceivable customer or patient. The alternative is to concentrate on doing an especially good job of satisfying the customers in only one or a few segments of the total market. This is what Porter calls a "focus" strategy.

Under a focus strategy, an organization concentrates on:

- selling to a particular group of customers,
- operating in a particular section of the industrial value chain,
- creating and selling only a few of all possible products and services in its industry, or
- selling in a particular geographic market.

By definition, a focus strategy can not possibly achieve the same sales volume as a whole market strategy. What the focused business hopes to do, however, through its focused attention to the needs of a narrow segment, is earn greater profits.

The "focus" strategy for competing applies to a smaller piece or segment of the market the same strategic concepts described above (low-cost leadership, differentiation, hybrid) for the overall market. It starts with identifying a subset of customers who may currently be purchasing the products offered in the larger market because nothing else is available. However, they have product value preferences that are somewhat different from the mainstream products. They would gladly purchase products that satisfy their more specific preferences, and might even pay a price premium for them. Through market and product research, the firm determines whether it has the resources and competencies to create the products that the narrower segments want at a cost that, combined with the price that the customers are willing to pay, allows the firm to earn above-average profits.

A focus strategy makes most sense when the overall market is in fact composed of a number of customer segments that vary significantly in the types of features they would like to see included in the basic, mass-market product. This is not always the case. Sometimes, the total market is quite homogenous and no segments can be discerned. Other times, the differences in product feature preferences are so slight that it is not economically worthwhile for a business to concentrate on satisfying them. The same thing is true when the segment is quite distinctive, but made up of relatively few customers. The firm may also choose to avoid segments in which a competitor already is operating.

In planning a strategy of this sort, a business will use the information that it gathered through the external assessment it conducted of its market and consumers, as described in Chapter 4.

It is possible to describe a few prerequisites to success in carrying out a focus strategy.

- There must be at least one definable segment of the larger market.
- The product needs or value preferences of the segment must be substantially different from those of the larger market or any other segment of that market.
- The segment is made up of enough customers to generate revenues and profits worth the effort of serving them.
- The firm must have a clear understanding of the unique product features that the segment's customers seek.
- The firm must be capable of manufacturing such a product.
- The segment customers must be willing to pay a price that allows the firm, given its cost structure, to earn an acceptable profit.
- The competitive intensity in the segment must be so low that the firm believes that it can establish a competitive advantage there.
- There must be a correlation between the purchase criteria of the customers in the segment and the resources and competencies of the business.
- As it proceeds with a focus strategy, the business must resist the impulse to broaden the market segments served or to try to serve additional segments in the pursuit of increased sales revenues.

For some organizations, a focus strategy is the only option because they lack the resources to compete on the main stage of the overall market. In fact, a single firm may be able to compete successfully in several market segments simultaneously without ever entering the total market.

There are downsides to a focus strategy.

- Almost inevitably, if the firm succeeds in making a profit in a market segment, it will draw competitors into the segment.

- Companies operating in the market as a whole may find ways to tweak their product offerings to appeal to a segment as well.
- A competitor may identify and focus its energies on even narrower sub-segments, taking customers away from the firm.
- The specialized customer preferences of the segment may shift, causing it to transform into a totally different segment. Or, they may shift back to those of the broader market, making the focus strategy irrelevant.

FUNCTIONAL AREA STRATEGIES

The major functional areas of the business must have strategies just as surely as the SBUs of which they are a part. They are large enough in terms of employees and budgets, and they play major roles in the implementation of the SBU strategies. It goes without saying that the functional area strategies must be integrated with and supportive of the strategies of their SBUs. Imagine a situation in which the SBU had decided to pursue a differentiation growth strategy, while its operations function was aggressively looking for ways to reduce manufacturing costs.

The strategies in each functional area also must be integrated with the strategies of the other functional areas in the SBU. An example of a possible problem here is an aggressive advertising campaign launched by a large physician group practice that is so successful in attracting new patients that clinical operations, whose strategy is focused on quality improvement, is unprepared to handle them. Finally, the functional area strategies must be consistent with operational activities currently being carried on by the functional area. For instance, if a health plan's marketing department is promoting the comprehensive, holistic package of services available to its members, it might seem contradictory to begin developing plan-sponsored "quick care" clinics in retail malls and drug stores.

There are certain types of activities that are most likely to be the elements of strategies pursued in traditional functional areas. These are health care-related variations of those activities.

Clinical Operations

Capacity—What is the anticipated demand for services under the strategies being implemented? Will the business have the facilities to meet the demand? How will the expansion of facilities be synchronized with demand growth?

Location—How important is facility location to patients in choosing which health plan/physician practice/hospital to visit? Is the current facility, and are future planned facilities, located most proximately to the market being targeted and served?

Organizational Structure—Does the current structure of the organization serve its strategic and operating needs? If it is currently based on medical specialties, would a service-line structure, based on patient demographics or common disease groups, work better?

Quality Assurance and Improvement—Is the level of care quality offered by the organization commensurate with its mission and strategies? Are there systems and procedures in place to maintain quality at its present level and improve it if necessary?

Reporting and Control—What kinds of clinical and cost information does the business require to support the formulation, implementation, and monitoring of its strategies? What steps must be taken to develop or acquire the systems necessary to gather, analyze, and report such information?

Marketing and Promotion

Because it is the functional area most attuned to the firm's external environment, particularly its markets and customers, marketing sometimes takes the lead in moving a firm toward formal strategic planning and management. Eventually, however, it must assume a role in support of strategies determined by collective efforts throughout the organization, finally approved by top management, and implemented through activities in all functional areas.

Market Research—What information does the firm's strategic planning require about the product/service needs, value preferences, and buying behaviors of its existing customers? On what bases might the firm segment the total market, and then choose those segments on which to concentrate its competitive energies?

Advertising and Promotion—What media and channels are best suited to the promotion necessary to advance the business's strategies? How can the business's reputation as an entire organization, as a brand image for its products and services, their quality and other characteristics, and the customer service that accompanies them, best be promoted?

Product and Service Offerings—Within the scope of the organization's strategies, what products and services should be offered, with what characteristics, at what prices, through what distribution channels?

Human Resources

Staffing—Are there functional strategies in place to assure that the requisite number of staff, in appropriate professional categories and with the needed experience, credentials, and skill sets, will be available at the designated times to perform the new activities resulting from the proposed strategies?

Motivation and Incentives—Does the business employ compensation and performance management methodologies designed to maximize productivity and other desired work behaviors? Are incentives in place to ensure that appropriate effort is devoted to strategic initiatives in general, as opposed to operational duties, and to specific strategies being implemented?

Culture and Working Conditions—What efforts are being made to develop an organizational culture that is supportive of strategic values like patient-focus and innovation mindsets? Is everything possible being done to attract and retain competent nursing staff? Is the organization cultivating its relationships with medical staff physicians in the interest of gaining their loyalty and shaping their clinical decision-making to fit strategic goals?

Employee Development—In consideration of organization-wide strategies planned for the future, what new skills, knowledge, and values need to be developed in existing employees? Are appropriate development programs in place to accomplish this?

Information and Clinical Technologies

Information Systems—What new information technologies are available for monitoring the performance of the firm's operations and emerging strategies?

Communication Systems—Is the firm using the most capable technologies available for communicating information among its employees (such as nurses), between the firm and its suppliers (such as physicians), and between the firm and its customers (such as payers and patients)?

Clinical Medical Technologies—What is the organization's policy on the adoption of new medical technologies? Does it employ a process for rigorously evaluating the technology proposals to which resources are allocated?

Financial Resources

The strategic role of financial management is the topic of Chapter 11.

Availability of Investment Capital—Will there be sufficient investment capital available to fund all the highest priority strategy initiatives proposed for implementation?

Capital Structure and Creditworthiness—Do the plans for generating, raising, and allocating capital funds result in a capital structure that inspires the confidence of financial analysts and the financial community, including creditors and investors? Will the organization's overall financial management practices earn it a credit rating that ensures access to maximum levels of external capital?

Financial Controls—Are policies and procedures in place that enable the firm to measure and control its financial metrics, such as free cash flow, economic profit, and return on strategic investments?

■ RESPONDING TO COMPETITORS' STRATEGIC MOVES

The planning and implementation of SBU strategies is not carried out in a vacuum. Most businesses operate in a competitive arena that is constantly in motion. Competitors are either launching their own strategic initiatives or reacting to the firm's strategy maneuvers. The firm must have them clearly in mind when planning its strategies. In this swirling environment of moves and countermoves, a business can adopt several basic strategic postures.

Full-bore aggression. The firm deploys all its strategic assets in an unrestrained attack on competitors. It complies with all legal limits on competitive behavior, but otherwise employs any conceivable strategy or tactic to overwhelm a competitor. If it is immediately successful, it may cause serious market and financial damage to an opposing business. Even if utter destruction is not the result, a more mild-mannered rival may be so intimidated by the onslaught that it moderates its own strategic initiatives for fear of offending the aggressor and settles for a lesser, but tolerable, position in the market.

Why don't all competitors in an industry take this attitude toward strategic action? In most industries, there is a relative equilibrium in strategic assets among competitors, and no single firm is well enough endowed to overwhelm any of the others. Furthermore, the outcome of such strategic hostility is highly unpredictable; it has the potential to destabilize the industry. Unspoken rules of acceptable competitive behavior may develop.

Seize the initiative. In this case, the firm jumps on every opportunity to gain the slightest competitive edge on its rivals. Whether it is a new production technology, a new clinical diagnostic tool, or a newly emergent market niche, it will be there first. If the new opportunity turns out to have enduring value, the firm will have a head start on every competitor in the market. In contrast, if the potential was misjudged or ineptly exploited, other organizations may learn from the mistakes of the initiator or "first mover" and take better advantage of it. The business that moves second or third may actually come out on top.

Counterattack—actual or latent. Here, the firm hopes to forestall a competitor from launching its strategic initiatives by communicating its intention to respond with an overwhelming counterattack. The communication may be openly expressed or implied by the gathering of appropriate resources and competencies. To make the threat, as well as future threats, credible, the firm must be willing to follow through. As an example, a rival hospital may be considering the expansion of its current oncology capacity by converting twenty underused beds in an adjoining unit. The other hospital, for whom cancer care patients are a major source of revenue, feels threatened by even this relatively modest move. In an attempt to ward off its rival's expansion plans, it announces its own intentions to build a new freestanding 50-bed oncology facility within the next three years, coupled with the hiring of two well-known oncology specialists from other parts of the country. Worried that it may not be able to fill its twenty new beds, the rival postpones its expansion plans indefinitely. The other hospital may never actually construct the new 50-bed unit, at least within three years. The mere threat to do so achieved its purpose.

Evasion strategies. One option for a firm is to operate only in those segments of the market where competitive intensity is low or nonexistent. It does not have to worry about threats from competitors launching their own strategies in the same market space or retaliating against the firm's initiatives there. Of course, competitors may be ignoring the segments because they are not attractive—they are not large enough to generate the revenues they seek or they present difficulties in earning above-average returns. Perhaps the firm can be satisfied with the revenue levels and has found ways, through innovation, to turn acceptable profits.

Adaptability. When competitive intensity in a market segment rises to an intolerable level or the size of the segment begins to wither, some firms may feel the impulse to flee. But, high exit barriers may compel them to continue operating in the segment at diminished revenue and profit levels. A firm can escape this situation when it has developed a degree of strategic adaptability—the ability to overcome the exit barriers and shift its strategic assets into new product/service lines, new market segments, or new distribution channels, all on short notice. The likelihood that a firm can accomplish this is dictated to a large extent by the industry in which it competes. For instance, hospitals have little choice but to invest in expensive operating assets like buildings and diagnostic equipment. Even in such cases, however, it is possible to design bed units so that they can be readily converted from one clinical service (postoperative surgery) to another (maternity).

Defend/preempt. One very effective way to deal with competitor strategy initiatives is to make them difficult or impossible to carry out. By preemptive measures, a firm can discourage competitive assaults on its market domain. By building market share rapidly, a firm can reach a level of sales volume at which economies of scale kick in sooner than it does for its rivals, allowing it to pursue a low-cost leadership strategy that gives it an unassailable market position. It can acquire the best locations that customers are likely to frequent when they wish to find and buy the products that the firm is offering—whether the locations are in the physical world (real estate) or the digital world (Internet domain names). In a multitude of ways, it can acquire or develop all sorts of unique, hard-to-copy resources and competencies (intellectual property, relationships with suppliers and customers, strategy-enhancing organizational culture, synergistic combinations of competencies) that effectively build walls against competitive assaults.

Study Questions

1. Imagine yourself as the head of an SBU in a large corporation. What are some of the ways in which the corporate headquarters could interfere in your running of the business, preventing you from accomplishing your strategic objectives? What steps could you take to minimize that interference and establish a more supportive relationship between the corporation and the SBU?
2. What are some ways in which a primary care group practice of four or five physicians could differentiate what they offer to their customers/patients from the offerings of competing physician groups? Who are the true "customers" of the group practice—the patients to whom it provides medical services or the health plans with whom it contracts to gain access to those patients?
3. Think back to the discussion about markets and customers in Chapter 4, particularly about market segments. Be aware of the importance of carefully selecting specific market segments if the business has decided to pursue a focus growth strategy. If such a strategy is to be successful, what are the necessary characteristics of the segment at which it is targeted?
4. Briefly describe the situations in which a business would be well advised to pursue a low-cost leadership, differentiation, or focus strategy.
5. What can an organization's functional areas contribute to the formulation of organization-wide strategy? What problems can occur if the functional areas are not included in the strategic planning process?

Learning Exercise 1

The argument has been made on several occasions that higher-quality health care is lower-cost health care. As a member of a health care management consulting firm, you have been asked by one of your clients, a large multistate managed care organization, to research this question. If the assertion can be substantiated, the client is interested in pursuing a hybrid growth strategy. Your assignment is to gather relevant information, either in support of or in opposition to the argument. Look for the most authoritative sources possible—evidence-based surveys and analyses. Draw conclusions and make a recommendation about the viability of this strategy for the client. If you believe that the client should proceed with such a strategy, prepare a detailed proposal about the steps that the client should take to ensure that it is offering the optimal mix of low cost and high quality in its services to customers. In particular, describe a possible internal value chain for the managed care organization and specify points in that chain where the organization has the best chance of reducing costs and enhancing quality.

Learning Exercise 2

A hospital located in the downtown area of a large city has decided to open satellite outpatient clinics in suburbs of the city, one within a year from now and the other two years after that. Describe in some detail the roles that the hospital's functional areas will have to play in establishing those clinics.

References

Barney JB. *Gaining and Sustaining Competitive Advantage*. 3rd ed. Upper Saddle River: Prentice Hall; 2006.

Campbell-Hunt C. What have we learned about generic competitive strategy? A meta analysis." *Strategic Management Journal*. February 2000:127–154.

Christensen CM. The past and future of competitive advantage. *Sloan Management Review*. 2001;42(2):105–109.

Covin J, Slevin D, and Heeley M. Pioneers and followers: Competitive tactics, environment, and growth. *Journal of Business Venturing*. 1999;15(2):175–210.

D'Aveni R. *Hypercompetitive Rivalries: Competing in Highly Dynamic Environments*. New York, NY: The Free Press; 1995.

David FR. How do we choose among alternative growth strategies? *Managerial Planning*. 1985:33(4):14–17,22.

Douglas TJ and Ryman JA. Understanding competitive advantage in the general hospital industry: Evaluating strategic competencies. *Strategic Management Journal*. 2003;24:333–347.

Faulkner D and Bowman C. *The Essence of Competitive Strategy*. Upper Saddle River: Prentice Hall; 1995.

Gale BT. *Managing Customer Value*. New York, NY: The Free Press; 1994.

Ghemawat P. Sustainable advantage. *Harvard Business Review*. September–October 1986:53.

Greaver MF. *Strategic Outsourcing*. New York, NY: American Management Association; 1999.

Hall WK. Survival strategies in a hostile environment. *Harvard Business Review*. 1980;58(5):75–87.

Hill CWL. Differentiation versus low-cost or differentiation and low cost: A contingency framework. *Academy of Management Review*. 1988;13:403.

Insinga RC and Werle MJ. Linking outsourcing to business strategy. *Academy of Management Executive*. 2000;14(4):58–70.

Ketchen DJ Jr, Snow CC, and Street VL. Improving firm performance by matching strategic decision-making processes to competitive dynamics. *Academy of Management Executive*. 2004;18(4):29–43.

Kim WC and Mauborgne R. Value innovation: The strategic logic of high growth. *Harvard Business Review*. 1997;75(1):103–112.

Lei D and Slocum JW. Strategic and organizational requirements for competitive advantage. *Academy of Management Executive*. 2005;19(1):31–45.

Miller D. The generic strategy trap. *Journal of Business Strategy*. 1992;13(1):37–42.

Porter ME. *Competitive Strategy: Techniques for Analyzing Industries and Competitors*. New York, NY: The Free Press; 1980.

Porter ME. What is strategy? *Harvard Business Review*. 1996;74(6):61–78.

Prahalad CK and Hamel G. The core competence of the corporation. *Harvard Business Review*. May–June 1990.

Sanchez R. Strategic flexibility and product competition. *Strategic Management Journal*. Special Issue. 1995;16:140.

Sharp B and Dawes J. What is differentiation and how does it work? *Journal of Marketing Management*. 2001;17(7/8):739–759.

Shimizu K and Hitt MA. Strategic flexibility: Organizational preparedness to reverse ineffective strategic decisions. *Academy of Management Executive*. 2004;18(4):44–59.

CHAPTER

9

Implementing the Strategy

Learning Objectives

After reading and studying this chapter, you should be able to:

- Understand how critical and unappreciated is the implementation phase to the success of a strategy.
- Show how an organization's resources and competencies must be matched to the strategies that it chooses.
- Discuss the role of organizational structure in strategy implementation, and the different forms of structure possible.
- Explain how each functional area contributes to the implementation of the overall organization-wide strategy.
- Describe in some detail the basic action steps that must be taken to turn a strategic plan into operational reality.
- Discuss how an organization goes about allocating resources, particularly financial resources, to its strategic initiatives.
- List some of the problems that can arise during strategy implementation.

It is not enough to formulate an excellent strategy that takes full advantage of a firm's strengths and weaknesses to exploit opportunities and resist threats that arise in its industry, markets, and general environment. To produce value for the firm and give it a competitive advantage, the strategy must be competently implemented. The disappointment that many organizations and individuals have had with strategic management probably stems more from the implementation than the planning phase of the process.

Implementation is the process by which strategies are put into action in order to achieve their desired outcome. It consists of an integrated series of substrategies, programs, action plans, policies, procedures, resource allocations, budgets, authority/responsibility delegations, teams and task forces, reward and control systems, and individual assignments. These are the same kind of initiatives that an organization would employ to accomplish any end result. In this case, the result is strategic in nature.

Each organization has its own way of assembling this series of interrelated initiatives. However, it is possible to talk about some generic components of a good strategic implementation effort and how they fit together. This is one approach for implementing strategy.

Perhaps the initial question is how carefully implementation is considered during the planning stage. It helps greatly if the planners have a reasonable belief that the organization possesses the resources, competencies, and other attributes needed to carry out the strategy. The strategic plan may itself suggest some of the steps that the planners think appropriate for its execution. But, it is not worth spending a lot of time and energy going into great detail about implementation since most of the mid- and lower-level managers with knowledge of what will have to be done are not participating at that stage.

There are three broad categories of managerial concern in implementing strategy. One is the *resources and competencies* of the firm that will be called upon to support implementation. Another is the substrategies within the firm's *functional areas* that are designed to put into practice the firm-wide strategies. Third is the mix of specific decisions and *actions that will carry out* the substrategies.

■ SUPPORTIVE RESOURCES AND COMPETENCIES

Common sense says that a strategy will not succeed if it depends upon resources and competencies that the firm does not possess. The strategy may require money in certain amounts; physical space of certain dimensions; particular types of equipment; specified numbers of people, certain skills, capabilities, and competencies; control and reporting systems; and more subtle qualities like attitude, intuition, or imagination. The availability of these elements should be considered, even if cursorily, during the strategy formulation stage. During implementation, they are the practical tools that turn the strategic plan into an operational reality. This chapter describes the major categories of resources and competencies in health care organizations and their importance to strategy implementation.

Systems

"Systems" are collections of policies, procedures, and protocols, combined with people who understand them and their purposes, often supported by dedicated electronic information processing and communications equipment, that simplify and regularize the performance of routine, high-volume tasks. Systems ensure that tasks are carried out as efficiently as possible with results that are as uniform and predictable as possible. Modern business organizations cannot function without them.

Accounting and budgeting system. If this system is not well conceived with a solid base of historical data, it may not match up either with the new strategy or with the new organizational structure that it requires. When many hospitals and physician practices embarked upon strategies that embraced managed care, utilization control, and capitation, they discovered that their accounting and control systems that worked so well under fee-for-service (FFS) reimbursement were ill suited to the new compensation arrangements. The existing budgeting system also may be incompatible with the strategic investment decisions now required. For instance, in physician groups it has not been the traditional practice to set aside funds on a regular basis for strategic capital investments.

Management information system. The entire health care financing and delivery industry is undergoing a revolution in the use of information to control resource utilization, costs, and quality of care, to manage the performance of employees, suppliers, and contractors, and to track information on patients and members. The essence of "managed" care requires the deployment of sophisticated and versatile information systems. This is complicated further by the need for systems throughout the health care industry, even among competitors, that can communicate with each other. Any new strategy initiative in the health care industry must be based on a modern, compatible management information system. It needs to integrate financial, clinical, control, administrative, and performance data. And it must do this while the underlying technology is simultaneously evolving. Such a system allows management to monitor progress in implementation of the strategy and make adjustments when necessary. In fact, the creation of a system that facilitates measurement of clinical outcomes and development of practice guidelines, responsible control of resource utilization, and pay-for-performance mechanisms is often the focus of a strategy all by itself.

Compensation and reward system. The management information system must be tied in with a reward structure that gives incentives to employee behavior that advances the purposes of the strategy. Without thoughtfulness, it is possible unconsciously to encourage conduct that is contradictory to the strategic intent. For at least two decades, there has been an ongoing debate about the best way to compensate physicians to achieve the desired effect on the delivery of medical services. Fee-for-service reimbursement encourages the provision of too many services; capitation arguably leads to the underprovision of care, with negative effects on quality. Physicians paid straight salaries are less productive. The pressure to develop a functional reward system is just as great for other employees. One of the hot trends in health care delivery is "pay-for-performance." The challenge is determining how much pay for what kind of performance.

Planning system. The preparation that goes into a strategic plan and its implementation cannot be an incidental, casual responsibility of employees who are primarily concerned with the day-to-day operations of the business. It must be the product of a formal and rational evidence-based process that is applied rigorously to the making of strategic plans. This is the competency that enables the deployment of all the firm's other strategic assets. Managers and employees must see it as fair, reliable, and serving the best interests of the organization. If this system is nonexistent or does not work properly, the business will formulate inappropriate plans that are poorly implemented.

Some businesses perform no meaningful strategic planning at all. Others do make some strategic decisions, but in a sporadic, ad hoc fashion that produces unpredictable results. A few organizations have adopted systems of planning that are ineffective, obsolete, biased, and easily manipulated, or unsuited to the current market and competitive conditions that they face. There is no single model of a good planning system. Each firm must develop methods and procedures that work best for it, and these methods must be organized into a genuine system.

Human Resources

Human resources are doubly critical to strategy implementation in health care organizations. In any organization, it is the people who manifest its valuable competencies and are responsible for putting strategic plans into effect. In most health care organizations, personnel costs represent about two-thirds of the operating budget. Strategic intentions profoundly affect, and are affected by, the value-creating activities of large numbers of people. Strategy implementation begins with making sure that there are enough human resources, with the necessary skills, available at the right times to perform the tasks and activities that will make the plan a reality. Their efforts must be choreographed by competent managers following action plans that support the strategic plans. One of the challenges in people management is enabling them to take on strategy implementation duties while continuing to work on day-to-day operations. Often the process involves retraining followed by a transition to performing new activities or old activities in new ways.

Organizational Structure

In planning long-term, business-wide strategies, the organizational structure is often taken as a given. For most managers and executives, it is hard to imagine or even be aware of other possible organizational structures, or the contribution or detriment they might make to operational and strategic effectiveness. Even if a different structure appeared to make some strategic sense, it involves a major change that takes considerable time to carry out and can cause upset and disruption throughout the organization. Nonetheless, if well selected and implemented, the structural change can transform an organization, giving it a powerful sustainable competitive advantage.

An organizational structure might be defined as a formal framework of departments, units, divisions, task forces, and groups into which people, the communication lines and reporting relationships that connect them, and the activities they perform, are organized. The alternative to a formal structure is a milling mass of humanity—unlikely to be very efficient or productive. Furthermore, some organizational structures are better than others at conducting a business's operations and carrying out its strategies. Strategy planners must be sensitive to this and recognize when a strategy to which the business is committed requires a change in organizational structure.

Functional Area Structure

The challenge is to describe and adopt a new structure that meets the organization's needs better than the current one. There are a few established organizational models that have proven popular and effective for numerous firms under a variety of circumstances. The most common is the one seen in many graphical organizational charts—the structure based on the major functions that most businesses perform in producing their goods and services. Those functions include manufacturing, marketing, research and development, financial management, and personnel, among others.

This is a good organizational arrangement for a firm that produces a relatively small number of goods and services and sells them to just a few distinct market segments, whose needs and preferences are fairly stable. There is sufficient time and sales volume for each functional area to become especially adept at its activities. As the firm concentrates on producing more and more of the same items, powerful learning curve effects and economies of scale come into play. It works best in support of a market-penetration growth strategy.

For those benefits, there are tradeoffs. Because of the deep hierarchy and centralized control, decisions must travel a long distance up and down the bureaucracy. This limits flexibility, responsiveness, and spontaneity, slowing the organization's reaction to sudden changes in the market and the environment, or by competitors. The myopic focus on developing the expertise within each functional area also inhibits coordination among the areas.

Product/Market Divisional Structure

When the market is characterized by many different segments and products/services that are constantly in flux, a more appropriate organizational structure replaces the functional areas with departments or divisions based on market segments, products or services, or geographic regions. Each of those divisions has its own set of functional activities (i.e., marketing, production, R&D). Decision-making authority is more decentralized down to the product/service level. If a product division becomes substantial in terms of sales volume, showing promise of considerable future growth, it may be developed into a more autonomous SBU.

The benefit of a market area or product line structure is that it can build exceptional competencies in serving the individual areas or creating and selling the individual products. The firm becomes better attuned to its markets and the customers in them, delivers products that more precisely meet their needs, and complements them with better service. As market forces and customer needs change, it can respond more quickly and appropriately. The sometimes awkward relationship among functional areas in the first organizational structure model is replaced by a much enhanced coordination among the functions in each market or product division.

The primary disadvantages of this structural variation are its relative inefficiencies—the economies of scale possible when operational activities and functions are combined is lost, some functional activities are actually duplicated from one division to another, and the several, separate functional areas are inevitably less competent.

The product/market division organizational structure is particularly suited to the implementation of strategies designed to deliver multiple products and services to numerous market segments. This is doubly true if those products and segments are constantly evolving. When new products become necessary or new segments are to be targeted, it is not difficult to create a new division to focus on them, a division that can grow into an SBU if appropriate.

Matrix Structure

The matrix structure is one of the most puzzling for a layperson to grasp and sometimes the most frustrating for employees to work within. It starts as a traditional functional area structure that is then crossed with a structure based on "projects."

If the projects are especially long lasting or successful, they may vault into separate product or service lines; the structure then begins to resemble the product/market structure described earlier. For instance, a biotechnology firm initiates several research projects. Each project has its own manager. The personnel assigned to the project also report both to the project manager and to their respective functional area managers (in lab research, data analysis, and equipment maintenance, for instance). Hypothetically, if the project results in a drug discovery with commercial potential, the project could be transformed into a separate division to manufacture, market, and distribute the drug. Manufacturing and marketing functions would replace the research and data analysis functions.

While it is still in the matrix stage this structural form offers several benefits. It is highly flexible and responsive to rapidly changing demands on the firm's resources. People and equipment can be more readily moved among projects. Learning and knowledge from one project is naturally spread to the others.

A matrix structure works well in an environment of intense competition, employees with transferable skill sets, and abruptly shifting work pressures. The price paid for this adaptability is greater difficulty with control and communication among the personnel participating in the projects. Technically, each person has two superiors—project and functional. It takes well-developed people management skills in those two managers and a sophisticated scheduling and coordination system to avoid conflicting assignments, priorities, and objectives. It is not impossible to operate a matrix organization; when managed effectively, there is nothing better for a turbulent market environment.

These are three very basic forms of organizational structure. There are a number of other variations (divisions, groups, network). If the firm's management can conceive a type of organization that better fits the strategies it wishes to implement, it can and should be created.

Organizational Culture

An organization's "culture" is sometimes referred to as its personality. Just as individuals with unique personalities are best suited for certain kinds of assignments and not at all for others, so too must an organization's strategies match its culture. If a physician group practice makes a strategic decision to differentiate itself as a particularly patient-friendly place to receive medical care, it is not likely to succeed with a culture that views patients with suspicion and cynicism. A medical device manufacturer will have difficulty implementing a strategy to put greater emphasis on innovation in product design and boldness in marketing tactics if managers traditionally have discouraged risk-taking and punished mistakes. If conflicts like this exist, they must be recognized well in advance, as it can take many months or even years to transform an organization's culture. A business may have to postpone a desirable strategy until it can develop a supportive culture.

■ FUNCTIONAL AREA SUBSTRATEGIES

The activities that go into creating and delivering products or services are usually organized into a few traditional functional areas. In a conventional manufacturing business, the major areas are finance, marketing, production, human resources, and research and development. The functions vary somewhat from industry to industry. In an average hospital, the key function areas or departments could include:

Clinical Services/Medical Affairs
Support Services
Non-Clinical Operations
Patient Care Services (Nursing)
Finance/Budgeting/Control
Strategic Planning/Business Development
Clinical Performance/Quality Assurance
Medical Staff
Human Resources
Legal

A research-oriented biotech or pharmaceutical company might be organized into the following sections:

Research
Development
Manufacturing
Distribution
Finance/Strategy
Human Resources
Public Affairs and Policy
Legal and Regulatory Affairs

Compliance and Actuary Services functions are likely to show up on the organization chart of a managed care organization or health plan.

Strategies are carried out not by strategic planning committees or by members of top management, but by the front-line personnel in the functional areas that constitute the organization. Functional area staff can contribute to the strategy-making process in three ways:

- They can provide information that is a background to the initial thinking about the kinds of strategies that might be appropriate and necessary.
- They can propose specific strategies to address the opportunities or threats that have been identified, and comment upon the viability of all the proposals made.
- After strategies have been approved, they will perform tasks that put them into practice.

To do this work, representatives from all functional areas must be intimately involved in the strategic planning and management process. It is not enough simply to take into account the strategy implications for each function or to inform function personnel of their strategy-related responsibilities after the plans have been formulated. Those people must participate in the planning meetings and in the decisions about which plans to approve. The possible roles of each functional area are different.

Marketing

When an organization has been doing no strategic planning and management at all, it often is the marketing area that takes the lead in pushing for greater attention to the external environment in which the organization operates, particularly customers and competitors. This is because the marketing personnel are in closer regular contact with the players in the outside world; they are perhaps the most outward-looking of all the functional areas. In fact, the marketing department may begin carrying out an abbreviated form of strategic planning on its own by focusing on particular segments of the broad market served by the organization, or by communicating features of its products that distinguish it from its competitors. To be fully effective, these marketing efforts must be backed up by activities in other functional areas to ensure that the segments are being uniquely served and to develop the distinctive product features. Eventually, the entire organization must be drawn into a sophisticated systematic strategic planning and management process.

At the beginning of the planning process, marketing will provide key inputs in the form of knowledge on market segments (currently served and prospective targets); customers' wants, needs, and preferences; the firm's perceived reputation and market position; competitor intelligence; threats and opportunities in the market; industry and general environment; and trends in all these areas.

As strategies begin to emerge in the form of specific proposals, marketing will have specific suggestions—depending on the broad strategic momentum. If the firm is committed to growth, marketing will have ideas about new products or services, enhancements of existing products or services, new customers who might be served, customers' needs that are not being met, new technologies that would be well received by the market, ways that customer service could be improved, or new distribution channels for reaching market segments. If the firm feels the need to retrench or even shrink, it might turn to marketing for advice on economy measures with the least impact on sales revenues or customer loyalty, such as cuts in the number of market segments served or the products offered.

Once strategies are agreed upon, marketing will have many possible roles to play. When a strategy is based upon new innovations, it is the job of marketing to make customers aware of them through various publicity media. When a strategy creates new product or service features to differentiate the firm from its competition, marketing will work to explain their value to prospective customers. Sometimes, a strategy intended to boost demand for a product will lean heavily on unique marketing tools like aggressive advertising, price promotions, personal selling, and direct marketing. In its routine promotion efforts, marketing will be expected to support the public image of the firm required by its strategies. Whatever the strategy, it will be the responsibility of marketing to fill out the details of the marketing mix to be employed, particularly pricing and promotion.

Operations

In most firms, operations represent the core of the business. This is where its products and services are created for delivery to customers. In traditional businesses, this area might also be called production or manufacturing. In a hospital, it would include clinical services, support services, and nursing services. In a pharmaceutical company, it would encompass manufacturing or production, though it might make sense also to bring in R&D since it is the primary focus of the drug business and the largest factor in its cost structure. The operations of a small biotechnology company consist almost exclusively of some form of research whose output is sold or licensed to larger pharmaceutical companies that take over the manufacturing and distribution.

The operations functional area is a major component in a firm's strategies. If the plan is to do nothing more than increase volume in current market segments, operations must have the capacity available to deliver the demanded quantities of products or services at the time they are demanded—not too soon and not too late. This often requires finding additional space, acquiring new equipment, and hiring more or different employees. A strategy based on new products or new features for existing products assumes that operations is capable of creating those products. When a firm is retrenching or trying to move toward a lower-cost position in the market, much of the burden for reducing costs is likely to fall on operations to choose which employees to lay off and which facilities to close. A competitive skill that is as vital in health care as other industries is management of a firm's supply chain. This is naturally the responsibility of operations.

Research and Development

The research and development (R&D) function can be extremely broad and diverse, or virtually nonexistent, depending on the type of business. In large pharmaceutical, medium-size biotechnology and medical device, and very small startup biotechnology companies, R&D is virtually the entire business. In a physician practice, a rural hospital, or a small health plan, no R&D will be conducted. When the R&D function is more modest, it sometimes is folded into operations.

Pharmaceutical companies tend to concentrate their R&D efforts in a few select disease areas. It would entail a major strategic shift for a company to move into a new area or end research in an existing one. If such a choice were made, for sound strategic reasons, the R&D managers would have to agree that the discontinued area was no longer viable and that they had, or could acquire, the resources and competencies to conduct promising research in the new area. They would have to plan for the purchase of necessary new equipment and the hiring of new scientists with appropriate skills.

Any organization that contemplates strategies based on new products or product features would have to be assured that it already had, could readily acquire, or could easily develop the desired product offerings. In fact, in research-driven entities, like drug companies, the outcomes of R&D function efforts may be the primary source of new strategy ideas.

Information Systems

The existence of a functional area dedicated to information systems is more likely in health care than in many other industries. Most modern businesses are using computers to administer their cost accounting, inventories, human resources and employee benefits, customer relationships, and corporate communications. The information systems in health care provider organizations have greater and more critical responsibilities that are becoming more complex all the time. These are some of those responsibilities:

- Tracking every service and product delivered to each patient to permit the filing of claims for reimbursement with the appropriate payer.
- Managing that claims submission and collection process.
- Receiving and acting upon orders from treating physicians for medications, tests, procedures, and other patient services and interventions (e.g., CPOE—computerized physician order entry).
- Maintaining a permanent and accessible record of each patient's condition and the treatments that she has received (e.g., EMR, EHR—electronic medical or health record).
- Gathering clinical outcomes data and correlating them with treatments and procedures to facilitate the development of practice guidelines.
- Correlating data on costs of treatments and their efficacy to determine their cost effectiveness.

- Gathering data on resource utilization and clinical outcomes for the purpose of evaluating individual physicians.
- Enabling the transmission of all these data, plus scanned clinical images, among departments and individuals within the provider organization, as well as physicians, pharmacies, laboratories, payers, and even patients external to the organization.

There are similar unique applications of information systems in MCOs and biotechnology research organizations.

Because the health care industry is at a juncture where many of these information systems capabilities are in the early stages of their implementation, an organization's decision to adopt, for instance, a comprehensive EHR system linked with the members of its medical staff may be considered a significant strategy initiative unto itself. A physician group practice that is the first in its market to install a system that permits it electronically to submit and reconcile reimbursement claims with payers, or a system for communicating test results, appointment and medication reminders, and other messages to patients, may be seen to have gained a competitive advantage.

The information systems function is relevant to strategy planning in a multitude of ways. It may be a mechanism for differentiating a firm from its competitors. If a planned strategy will increase the volumes of sales or customers, it is important that information systems have sufficient capacity to handle them. This function may have an important role to play in cost-cutting strategies, by streamlining processes for creating products or delivering services, by identifying points of cost inefficiency, or by integrating purchasing decisions with suppliers.

Human Resources

Health care provider organizations sell relatively few products; they are largely a service industry, and services are delivered by people. It is a highly labor-intensive industry, very dependent on its employees for operational effectiveness and strategic success. The human resources function supports all the other areas of the organization in selecting and supervising the best employees for optimal performance of operational tasks. This aid is just as vital to the implementation of strategies.

As an example, imagine a hospital or MCO that has decided to expand into a new geographic market by opening a primary care clinic there within the next year. Human resources staff can advise on the types and numbers of personnel that will be required, and their availability in the job market. When the strategy is approved, they can set up a schedule for recruitment and hiring. Some strategies place great emphasis on improving the overall performance of the organization. The HR area is a good source of ideas on methodologies for managing individual employee performance, reward systems that encourage the desired employee behavior, and alternative organizational structures better suited to new strategies. When a firm decides that it must retrench, a common tactic is a workforce reduction or downsizing. Such radical steps are usually orchestrated by human resources.

Financial Management and Accounting

Money is the lifeblood of most organizations. Its careful management is necessary to fund current operations, invest in strategies for the future, and generate a return to shareholders. Because the financial management function is arguably a more essential prerequisite to strategic success, it is covered in its own chapter, Chapter 11.

Creating and Coordinating Functional Area Strategies

To be able to carry out their implementation responsibilities competently, each functional area must prepare its own strategic plan that satisfies two criteria. Its plan must support and mesh with the organization-wide plan. In addition, it must be synchronized with the equivalent plans in the other functional areas. If marketing is going to conduct a campaign designed to increase product demand, manufacturing had better be ready to achieve production volumes to meet the demand. As this may require increasing production staff, human resources must be aware of how many new hires will be needed and when. The research and development department cannot develop new product features requested by customers without some assurance that manufacturing has the equipment and expertise to fabricate them.

It normally is not feasible to draw up the functional area plans, in all their detail, simultaneously with the broader strategic plan. That is done later by the managers and employees in each functional area. To do that effectively, representatives from the functional areas should have participated in the formulation of the strategy, understood its content and context, and fully embraced it. Subsequently, communication channels should be open among the functional areas to ensure the synchronization of their efforts.

■ DECISIONS AND ACTIONS FOR IMPLEMENTATION

The action steps required to turn a strategy plan into reality are essentially the same as those employed to perform any organizational activity. The grand strategy must be broken down into manageable parts, the scope of each part must be defined, goals and deadlines must be set for its accomplishment, appropriate resources must be allocated, the right numbers and types of people must be assigned, policies and procedures must be created to direct and control their actions, a single individual must be given overall responsibility for each part, and progress must be measured and tracked.

The decisions and actions necessary for implementation come out of the strategic planning group and cascade down though the organization. The heads of the various functional areas, who are likely to have participated in the planning meetings, work with the managers of their departments, facilities, and units to formulate substrategies for each area. In turn, those managers break the work down into bundles of tasks suitable for assignment to teams, task forces, and other forms of work groups, both permanent and ad hoc. Programs and projects may be established for the specific purpose of implementing some part of the strategy. Eventually, managers and supervisors parcel tasks out to individual employees. The number of layers through which the implementation initiatives must flow depends on the size and depth of the organization.

These are generic examples of operational initiatives that may be necessary to put a strategy into effect.

- initiate new marketing campaigns, refocus existing campaigns, continue existing campaigns through different media, discontinue existing campaigns, expand or contract existing campaigns, conduct small-scale pilots of potential new campaigns.
- create new departments, offices, or teams; discontinue, refocus, expand, or split up existing units.
- open new facilities; expand, repurpose, or close existing facilities.
- raise or lower prices of various products, bundle or unbundle products/services for pricing purposes.
- reengineer operating processes, reorder the way that process tasks are performed, add new tasks, eliminate existing tasks, combine or separate the tasks performed by single individuals, perform existing tasks in different ways, perform existing tasks at lower cost, create the same value by performing different tasks.
- hire new employees, retrain/develop existing employees, transfer existing employees (including managers).
- deploy new systems for monitoring/measuring operating performance and feeding results back to the employees concerned.
- create/develop/invent new products or services, drop existing products or services, redesign or add new features to existing products or services.

Delegating Implementation to the Right People

Strategy implementation is simpler in smaller organizations. With a smaller workforce, it is possible to involve every employee in the planning phase. That involvement means that there is not much more that must be com-

Two Universal Challenges in Strategy Implementation: Coordination and Operations

The strategy implementation work of each team or task force must be coordinated and integrated with the efforts of other teams and task forces. This is to ensure that they do not interfere with each other and, preferably, interact synergistically to create the optimum result at the minimum cost. For the same reasons, the strategic activities of the several functional areas also must be synchronized with each other. The challenge is to make sure that the functional areas and the task forces talk with each other constructively.

All the activities conceived for carrying out the strategy must be interwoven with the regular day-to-day activities that maintain the firm's existing business operations. Sometimes, strategic actions are wholly separate and unconnected—as when a hospital constructs a new facility for women's health services. Quite often, however, they are enhancements of activities that are already taking place—as when that same hospital adjusts or redirects its current advertising campaign to promote the opening of that women's health center.

The work of specific team and task force members must also be reconciled with the performance of their existing operational responsibilities. It is not often that an organization can afford to assign some employees to stop what they were doing previously in order to work full time on implementing a strategy. Normally, employees will be performing strategy-related tasks while simultaneously continuing with the regular operational duties that are the business of the organization. In some cases, the "strategy" involves simply performing customary operational tasks somewhat differently. For instance, a small biotechnology research firm that is making good progress in developing its initial drug product decides to begin discovery work in a second drug class. The current lab director is asked to begin setting up another lab for the new initiative, while continuing to move the first product toward completion. The challenge is to find the appropriate balance between the individual's strategic and operational assignments.

municated about the strategy. The employees will already know what the organization is trying to accomplish strategically and will be predisposed to thinking about how to accomplish it.

Most organizations are large enough that the planning has to be conducted by a small subset of the workforce. Although the majority of employees will not be in on the planning, almost every one of them could conceivably have a role in the implementation. The planners, in effect, delegate implementation to the rest of the organization.

It is important to select the right people to carry out each step of the strategy implementation process. The nature of the assigned task must fit the area of expertise and skill set of the person. If a health plan decides to create an outreach program to communicate with its Medicare members and wishes to assign a nurse administrator to the job, it will prefer a person experienced in gerontological medicine or in diseases common to the elderly over someone who has worked primarily in an ICU. The right person for the task may not always be available. There may be an appropriate person on staff who is preoccupied with other duties. Can someone stand in for her while she shifts to work on strategic initiatives? Or can she handle both her operational and strategic assignments? Can another employee receive special training to prepare her to handle the strategy implementation responsibilities? It may even be necessary to hire someone new with the skills and experience needed. Most of these issues can be anticipated when representatives from the human resources function are involved in the strategic planning from the beginning.

Action Plans and Programs

The real implementation starts with the creation and execution of operational and action plans. Generally, operational plans are prepared annually by the overall business and by its separate functional areas. These plans describe what steps will be taken in the coming year both to maintain/improve ongoing operations and to move the organization along the path toward realizing its strategic ambitions. A strategy selected for implementation may show up in several successive operational plans before it is completed. While the strategic plans list primary objectives common to the entire organization, the operating plans list secondary objectives for each functional area and department. The operating plans are accompanied by an annual operating budget that translates them into monetary terms.

Whether at the level of the functional area or one of its departments, an action plan or program is created to describe the systematic activities that will lead to accomplishment of strategic goals and annual subgoals. The plan is prepared by the head of the functional area or department in consultation with key members of her staff. It begins with a clear understanding of the contributions their subunit must make to the organization-wide strategies. Those responsibilities are broken down into objectives for the unit and specific activities that are assigned to specific individuals. Additional resources are allocated to the process and time deadlines are set. Metrics are selected for monitoring the progress of the action plan. If the plan is well conceived and the individuals complete their activities according to schedule, the unit will meet its strategic objectives. If all the departments and functional areas in the organization complete their objectives, the overall strategies will be successsfully implemented. It may help to look at a real-life example of such an action plan.

Imagine a large physician group practice that has decided to acquire and deploy a multi-featured EMR system that will be linked to the local hospitals where the physicians have privileges and send their patients. The action plan to carry out that decision might look like Table 9.1.

In the course of designing an action plan like this and directing employees in its performance, managers will use a variety of traditional administrative tools. The above plan already includes objectives, time deadlines, and personnel assignments. The plan's creators might also rely on the following:

Policies are broad guidelines for decision-making by employees. They are written to be consistent with overall plan/program objectives, consistent with each other, and flexible enough to accommodate unanticipated circumstances. The employees affected by the policies should be thoroughly familiar with them, and consider them to be necessary and reasonable. Policies are open to regular review and change when appropriate.

Procedures direct employees in a step-by-step fashion in how to achieve the objectives within the scope of the policies. The most effective procedures are based on a detailed study of how best to realize the intent of the objectives and policies.

Table 9.1 Action Plan for Acquiring and Deploying an EMR System in a Physician Practice

Action Plan Objectives:

1. Consult with EMR system vendors about critical specifications, available options, and related costs.
2. Consult with physicians in the practice about their specific wants and needs in an EMR system.
3. Define a decision-making protocol for choosing an EMR system and vendor.
4. Establish and apply criteria for evaluating system options available from vendors.
5. Invite proposals/presentations from vendors.
6. Analyze and discuss options.
7. Select system and vendor.
8. Negotiate with vendor for purchase of system and related services.

Action Plan Metrics:

Signed system and services purchase agreement within six months.

Initial system cost not to exceed $650,000; annual service contract cost not to exceed $90,000.

Physician involvement in decision-making process—75 percent.

(*continues*)

Table 9.1 Action Plan for Acquiring and Deploying an EMR System in a Physician Practice (continued)

Specific Implementation Activities:

1. Consult vendors (weeks 1–4)
   Identify relevant vendors (IT staff) Request detailed information on products (IT staff)
2. Consult physicians (weeks 5–7)
   Initial meeting with physicians (IT manager, business manager, physician leaders, all physicians)
   Provide list of potential system capabilities (IT staff)
   Conduct written survey of physician wants and needs (IT and business staff)
   Second meeting with physicians to discuss system options and capabilities (IT manager, all physicians)
3. Define decision-making protocol (weeks 6–7)
   Draft decision-making protocol (IT and business staff)
   Discuss with physician and business leadership (IT and business staff, business and physician leaders)
   Finalize and approve decision-making protocol (business and physician leaders)
4. Establish criteria (weeks 8–9)
   Using information from vendor and physician meetings, draft criteria (IT and business staff)
   Discuss with physician and business leadership (IT and business managers, physician leaders)
   Finalize and approve decision-making protocol (business and physician leaders)
5. Vendor proposals/presentations (weeks 10–14)
   Invite vendors to make proposals/presentations (IT staff)
   Schedule presentations at the practice offices (IT staff, physician leaders)
   Debrief and critique the presentations (IT and business staff, all physicians)
6. Analyze options (weeks 15–16)
   Prepare summary sheet on the systems and vendors (IT and business staff)
   Narrow the number of systems and vendors to a few (IT and business managers)
7. Select system and vendor (week 17)
   Final meeting with physician and business leaders to make final decision (IT and business managers, physician leaders)
8. Vendor negotiations (weeks 18–22)
   Initiate negotiations with selected vendor for chosen system (IT and business managers, legal counsel)
   Complete negotiations and sign purchase and service agreements (IT and business managers, legal counsel)

Methods describe the specific actions to carry out each step of a procedure.

Rules are statements that forbid or require certain actions or inactions.

Organizations and managers may use these terms differently—for instance, viewing procedures and methods as synonyms or policies as simply sets of rules. The exact wording is not as important as the underlying concepts that organizations use to guide their employees' work behavior toward strategy implementation.

Allocation of Resources

The implementation of strategy through action plans requires a variety of resources. As mentioned above, people must be assigned to lead projects and teams and to perform tasks. In addition, a plan may require the allocation of office space, equipment, supplies, space on a company Web site, or even time on the agenda of management/staff meetings. All of those resources are in limited supply. Managers must make difficult choices about priorities not only among strategic initiatives, but also between strategic efforts and current operations.

A resource that is often overlooked because it is so intangible and amorphous is the autonomy and discretion that a manager or employee may need to carry out assigned strategic tasks. An employee involved in strategy implementation may need to be able to commandeer certain resources or give directions to other employees over whom she normally does not have authority. It may be preferable that strategy work be allowed to proceed without all the authorizations and approvals that are required. These special allowances can make sense when the strategy work calls for innovation and creativity, needs to be completed quickly, or otherwise represents a departure from typical operational work activities.

In most cases, the resource most essential to strategy implementation will be money. It is the resource that can buy all the others. It is a major concern in assessing the viability of a proposed strategy and in subsequently implementing it. There are established methods for allocating and budgeting financial resources for new strategic initiatives. Capital budget items are typically purchases of real estate, buildings, and equipment that have useful lives exceeding one year, cost over a certain substantial amount (e.g., $50,000), and are subject to depreciation. The purchase of entire businesses is also considered a capital expenditure. These items are common elements of many strategic plans, particularly the larger, more ambitious ones.

Capital expenditures are made for three broad purposes: to replace existing capital assets (buildings and equipment), to purchase entirely new, nonstrategic capital assets, and to carry out strategic plans.

Replacement Capital Expenditures

Capital assets regularly have to be replaced, for a variety of good reasons. Inevitably, everything reaches the end of its useful life, simply wearing out or ceasing to function. If the asset can still perform a useful function, even an exact-copy replacement will suffice. An asset with some remaining usefulness may become technologically obsolete. An updated version will be necessary to maintain that usefulness, which may include interconnectivity with suppliers and customers.

A new model of the asset may become available that offers greater capacity or more cost-efficient operability. A more current version might produce a higher-quality product or, in combination with the business's other processes, enable it to deliver products or services of higher quality. In some cases, a new regulatory mandate, perhaps dealing with safety, privacy, or environmental concerns, will require that a business replace an existing asset with something that is more compliant.

New Nonstrategic Capital Expenditures

Businesses regularly make investments in new capital assets that are designed primarily to improve operational effectiveness. They are sometimes misinterpreted as strategic in nature, but, in fact, lack the long-range perspective and dedication to pursuit of sustainable competitive advantage. Nonetheless, these expenditures can be worthwhile contributions to an organization's mission and keeping up with the competition.

There are numerous possible reasons for this type of capital spending. The business may wish to expand the range of services that it offers. It may see an opportunity to reduce operating expenses, promote care quality, or improve safety conditions. A desire to enhance the overall patient treatment experience also could involve a variety of capital projects.

Strategic Capital Expenditures

These are the high-cost asset purchases that are part of most strategic initiatives. They compete for funding with replacement and nonstrategic capital proposals, so it is critical that the business use a robust, objective, trusted methodology for allocating the limited supply of financial resources among the many demands for financial support. Over several decades of experience with capital spending decisions, American business corporations have developed several good tools to facilitate the process. This is one excellent approach.

1. *Identify and describe all the capital spending requests for the current budget cycle*. This includes describing the amount of the proposed expenditure, the proposed timing of the expenditure, the assets to be purchased, and the specific reasons for the purchase. Also make clear whether the purchase is a replacement of an existing asset, a new nonstrategic item, or a necessary component of a proposed new strategy.

2. *Describe the nonfinancial benefits that are expected to result from the capital expenditure.* Every effort should be made to translate these benefits into objective, preferably quantitative, terms. However, some benefits are so unavoidably subjective and amorphous that precise measurement is difficult. Even when it is possible to assign numbers to a key variable (e.g., patient satisfaction measured via a survey), it should be remembered that this does not imply the same accuracy as metrics showing an increase in the bed occupancy rate or a decrease in the hospital-acquired infection rate. Besides patient satisfaction, bed occupancy, and hospital infections, other possible examples of nonfinancial benefits of capital expenditures are lower maintenance downtime for upgraded manufacturing equipment, speedier enrollment of participants in clinical trials, and improved staff morale and lower turnover rate.
3. *Set priorities for each of the capital requests on the basis of urgency factors* like critical relevance to current operations, responsive to a legal mandate, responsive to aggressive moves by competitors, or a major contributor to the organization's strategic program. Priority assignment could be done by a simple ranking or grading the requests into a few categories (e.g., A, B, C, D). A somewhat more sophisticated method is to agree on a few generic criteria for evaluating any capital request, weight each criterion by its importance to the organization, score each request for how well it satisfies each criterion, multiply the scores by the weights, and add the results to come up with a total score for each request.
4. *Make projections of cash flows for each capital request.* This is easier for replacement purchase proposals because they have a financial track record. It is more difficult to estimate the future cash flows stemming from an entirely new strategic initiative. Some capital proposals are not designed to generate revenues. This is often true for plant and equipment purchases intended to improve operational effectiveness rather than build competitive advantage. In such cases, cash flow projections will reflect cost savings to be realized, not revenue increases.
5. *Perform financial analyses of each capital request.* There are three traditional calculations that can be used for this purpose. They are Payback Period, Net Present Value (NPV) or Discounted Cash Flow, and Internal Rate of Return (IRR). The latter two calculations (NPV and IRR) require that the business determine its "weighted cost of capital" (WCOC). Frequently, businesses add a minimum desired profit margin to the WCOC and designate that as a "hurdle rate" that every capital project must meet or exceed. The preferred and most accurate method is NPV. These analyses permit comparisons of capital requests on the basis of the financial benefits that they are projected

to deliver.

6. *Evaluate and compare the financial and nonfinancial benefits of all the capital requests and decide which ones to fund and in what amounts.* At this point, the organization should have ample information to make these decisions. If return on the capital invested is the sole standard for evaluating strategy alternatives, the proposed initiatives can be ranked by the amount of NPV that they are projected to create and funded in that order. More often, the firm will want to take other financial and nonfinancial factors into consideration. There are tools for doing this systematically. One good method is the weighted factors and scores approach described in step three above. Preliminary versions of these assessments will often have been made during the strategy formulation and selection stage.

   While assigning priorities and allocating capital, it usually is a good idea to examine the requests separately in the three groups mentioned earlier. Otherwise, using a priority system applied to all requests at once, all or most of the available capital funds might go to replacement purchases or to strategic projects at the expense of the other categories. Organizations deal with this conundrum in different ways. Some establish separate capital pools for each category; others decide in advance to approve a certain number or dollar value of requests in each category.

Objectives and Deadlines

Just as the strategy's goals guide the forward motion of the entire organization, narrower functional and departmental objectives steer day-to-day activities toward achievement of those goals. Both long- and short-term objectives will be established. It is best if those who will be asked to meet the objectives are involved in setting them. Their acceptance and commitment will be greater. The objectives serve several purposes.

- They guide and motivate employees assigned to the effort.
- They are the basis for measuring progress and evaluating the participants, particularly their manager/supervisor.
- They help establish priorities for the organizational units involved.
- Those priorities serve as the basis for allocating resources.

The objectives at each level in the strategy implementation process must contribute to achievement of the objectives at the levels above them and be supported by the objectives at levels below them, in a sort of cascading hierarchy. In addition to up-and-down consistency, objectives in one functional area or department should be synchronized with those in parallel areas or departments. For instance, if a hospital planned to repackage some of its service offerings into a women's health center and carve out a separate physical space for that purpose, the engineering department responsible for preparing the space, the human resources department responsible for properly staffing the center, and the marketing department responsible for promoting its opening would have to work together to make sure that the new facility was ready and staffed on the day scheduled for the opening.

The objectives may apply to a market segment, a geographic area, a facility, an operating department, or a particular product/service. The objectives can be stated in terms of sales, profits, market share, patient volume, employees hired/trained, or any other metric that reflects progress toward implementation of the strategy. They should be measurable, comprehensible, challenging (not too easy/not too hard), and widely broadcast throughout the organization. If the objectives are not tied directly to the compensation and other rewards for the employees involved, they at least should not conflict directly with other employee incentives.

Specific dates are set for completion of each objective. The initiation of work on one objective may be made contingent on the conclusion of work on another. Different pieces of a strategy plan have different time horizons. As an example, if the entire strategy is projected to be completed within two and a half years, its separate plans and programs may take from three to twelve months to execute. Narrower projects and tasks may take a matter of weeks or even days. Keeping all the pieces synchronized is essential to efficient and timely implementation of the strategy.

Monitoring and Control of Implementation

Strategic management does not end with the commencement of the implementation of a well-planned strategy. The process must be watched to ensure that it follows the plan and keeps to the timetable. There must also be monitoring of the assumptions on which the plan is based, and the external conditions (general environment, markets, competition) to which the strategy is responding. If implementation falters, it may be necessary to fine-tune the plan or reallocate resources. In some cases, the firm may decide to modify the plan dramatically or drop it entirely due to unanticipated changes in the outside world. This phase in the strategy-making process is so important that it is explained at length in Chapter 10.

■ IMPLEMENTATION PROBLEMS THAT NEED TO BE MONITORED AND CORRECTED

Strategy implementation can go wrong in a variety of ways. These are examples of implementation problems that need to be identified and corrected as early as possible. A strategic monitoring system does that for an organization.

- Implementation took more time than originally planned, resulting in failure to meet objectives and delays in numerous operational areas.
- Unanticipated major problems arose. The problems may be internal or external, but the best efforts could not plan for them and now they must be resolved promptly.
- Activities were ineffectively coordinated. It takes experienced, skilled managers to keep all the pieces of a strategic plan in synchronization.
- Competing activities and crises took attention away from implementation. Current operations and unexpected emergencies always seemed more urgent than long-term strategy matters.
- The involved employees have insufficient capabilities to perform their jobs. During the planning stage, insufficient thought was given to whether the organization had the human resource competencies to carry out the plan.
- Lower-level employees were inadequately trained. The training that is often necessary for employees to function effectively under new strategies was not factored into the planning.
- Uncontrollable external environmental factors created problems. Despite best efforts at forecasting, events of all sorts (legal, political, economic) can occur in the outside world to foil well-conceived plans.
- Departmental managers provided inadequate leadership and direction. If lower-level managers do not appreciate the importance of new strategic initiatives, they may be lax in guiding their subordinates to implement them.
- Key implementation tasks and activities were poorly defined. The result may be wasted resources, confusion, and delays in meeting objectives.
- The information system inadequately monitored activities. An ineffective monitoring system may reveal problems only after they have worsened and created still more problems.

Study Questions

1. Think about organizations in which you have worked. How would you describe their organizational structure, using the terminology presented in this chapter? Bear in mind that an organization's structure may not fall neatly into one category or another.
2. Imagine that you are a top executive in a biotechnology firm that has grown rapidly on the basis of its first FDA-approved drug. It now has been decided to proceed down two new drug development paths, while continuing adaptive research on the first drug. It seems appropriate to reorganize in order to accommodate these new strategic ini-

tiatives. What changes in organizational structure do you recommend and exactly how would you go about moving from the current structure to the new one?

3. Imagine that you are the head of the IT services department in a managed care organization that has made the strategic decision to expand operations into an adjacent state. Unfortunately, the functional area leaders, like you, were not invited to be part of the group that reached that decision. However, you will be partially responsible for implementing it. Prepare a list of at least ten pieces of information you want about the expansion plan in order to make sure that the IT component is carried out properly.
4. As a mid-level manager in a good-sized organization (hospital, multispecialty group practice, pharmaceutical company), you will frequently be responsible simultaneously for implementing new strategies while effectively conducting ongoing operations. How do you decide how to allocate your time, your staff, and your other resources between strategic and operational activities?
5. What is the difference between operating expenses and capital expenditures? How does a company decide how much of its available cash to allocate to operations and how much to strategic investments?

Learning Exercise 1

There are some elements missing from the action plan in Table 9.1. If the EMR system is to be integrated with similar systems at local hospitals, and the physicians fully utilize its data-sharing capabilities, representatives from the hospitals must be drawn into this implementation process. Add activities to the above list that would permit this to happen. Be sure to insert them at the appropriate points in the time line. Specify exactly which people from the hospitals and the practice will participate.

Learning Exercise 2

Do a quick search of media reports on apparent strategic failures in the health care or biotechnology industries (i.e., divestment of a business, layoff of a large proportion of the workforce, very large losses over several years). Pick one of the failure stories for which a substantial amount of information is available. Attempt to determine the cause of the failure. Was an inappropriate strategy selected in the first place? If so, exactly why was it inappropriate? Was a reasonably suitable strategy chosen, but then incompetently implemented? In exactly what ways was the implementation faulty?

References

Alexander LD. Strategy implementation: Nature of the problem. In: Hussey DE, ed. *International Review of Strategic Management*. Vol. 2, No. 1. Hoboken, NJ: John Wiley & Sons; 1991:73–113.

Chadwick C, Hunter LW, and Walston SM. The effects of downsizing practices on hospital performance. *Strategic Management Journal*. 2004;25(5):405–428.

Chandler AD. *Strategy and Structure: Chapters in the History of the American Industrial Enterprise*. Cambridge, MA: MIT Press; 1962.

Dobni B. Creating a strategy implementation environment. *Business Horizons*. 2003;46(2):43–46.

Drucker PF. *The Practice of Management*. New York, NY: HarperCollins; 1954.

Galbraith JR and Kazanjian RK. *Strategy Implementation: Structure, Systems, and Processes*. 2nd ed. St. Paul, MN: West Publishing; 1986.

Gary MS. Implementation strategy and performance outcomes in related diversification. *Strategic Management Journal*. 2005;26:643–664.

Gupta AK. SBU strategies, corporate-SBU relations, and SBU effectiveness in strategy implementation. *Academy of Management Journal*. September 1987:477–500.

Hambrick D and Cannella A. Strategy implementation as substance and selling. *Academy of Management Executive*. 1989;3(4):278–285.

Hrebiniak LG and Joyce WF. *Implementing Strategy*. New York, NY: Macmillan; 1984.

Mankins MC and Steele R. Turning great strategy into great performance. *Harvard Business Review*. 2005;83(7):65–72.

Miller S, Wilson D, and Hickson D. Beyond planning: Strategies for successfully implementing strategic decisions. *Long Range Planning*. 2004;37:201–218.

Nutt P. Selecting tactics to implement strategic plans. *Strategic Management Journal*. 1989;10:145–161.

Olson EM, Slater SF, and Hult GTM. The importance of structure and process to strategy implementation. *Business Horizons*. 2005;48(1):47–54.

Porter TW and Harper SC. Tactical implementation: The devil is in the details. *Business Horizons*. 2003;46(1):53–60.

Tetenbaum TJ. Seven key practices that improve the chance for expected integration and synergies. *Organizational Dynamics*. Autumn 1999:22–35.

CHAPTER

10

Monitoring, Fine-Tuning, and Changing the Strategy

Learning Objectives

After reading and studying this chapter, you should be able to:

- Understand why monitoring and sometimes changing strategy is essential to its eventual success.
- Recognize the ways in which unmonitored strategy implementation can go wrong.
- Define the key principles of a good strategy monitoring and adjustment program.
- Explain the steps in setting up a good strategy monitoring and adjustment program.
- Show how to choose the right metrics for monitoring a strategy's implementation, giving some examples.
- Discuss the events that might be discovered by a strategic monitoring program and the adjustments that might be made in response.

It is possible for a firm to devise thoughtful, appropriate strategies, to implement them competently, according to plan, and still fail to move closer to realizing its vision.

A complete strategic management process also includes a mechanism for monitoring both implementation of the strategy and its ongoing functioning once it is operational. The reason is that every strategy is based on best estimates of the conditions that will exist in the future. The conditions that actually occur can be, and often are, very different from the estimates.

- A physician group practice that prepared itself to operate efficiently under a capitated contract with health plans might find itself quite unprepared when those plans shift to reimbursement on the basis of pay-for-performance.
- The role of health insurers and health plans could change dramatically and unexpectedly if the nation and the Congress, out of frustration at the failure of all previous attempts at health care reform, adopted a single-payer national health insurance plan.
- A managed care organization with long-established contracts with several large employers in a major metropolitan area could find its business seriously diminished if those employers decided to form a business purchasing collective, eliminate the middleman, and contract directly with hospitals and physicians.

The purpose of the monitoring system is to notice when there has been a change in environmental conditions, in the performance of the strategy, or in the organization's strategic preferences significant enough to warrant some kind of adjustment in the strategy.

WHAT STRATEGIC MONITORING INVOLVES

A comprehensive program for monitoring the progress of an organization's strategies has several features. The foundation for the effort is a clear statement of the assumptions (about the firm's internal and external environment) upon which the strategic plans are based, and the measurable goals that the strategies are intended to achieve. A close watch is kept for significant changes in environmental circumstances and their potential effect on the continued validity of the assumptions. Similarly, the performance of the strategies is observed and compared to their original goals. Gaps between the initial assumptions and new environmental conditions, and between the initial goals and current performance, are noted and studied. When deemed appropriate, adjustments and corrections to the strategies are made.

WHY STRATEGIC MONITORING HAS BECOME MORE IMPORTANT

It used to be that an organization could review the progress of its strategic initiatives in a formal meeting once a year and perhaps make some modest adjustments. That is no longer possible, for a variety of reasons.

- There is greater variability and even instability in economic conditions, at regional, national, and international levels.

- Commercial lives of products are shorter.
- Product development times are longer and more expensive.
- New technology developments (clinical and information) occur more frequently.
- There are more competitors in the domestic market and more foreign competitors.
- There are more for-profit companies and money-driven entrepreneurs active in the health care industry.
- The resulting competition is more intense and ruthless.
- The competitive environment leads to more rapid and dramatic changes in health care business models and industry structure.
- The external environment is more complex with more variables to be considered.
- There are more laws and regulations that apply to health care and biotechnology, with new ones being issued at an accelerating pace.
- There is accelerating change in every aspect of life.
- Accurate projections are difficult to make.
- The time span for valid projections and plans is shorter, and they become outdated sooner.
- Critical success factors in the industry change more often.
- As a result of all these changes, the health care industry has become more fragmented and complex (forty-five years ago, there were no MCOs, specialty hospitals, hospitalists, physician assistants, Medicare, Medicaid).

PRICE OF FAILURE TO NOTICE AND RESPOND TO STRATEGIC CHANGE

Numerous companies, and sometimes entire industries, have failed to pay attention to changes that have occurred in the market and competitive environments around them, and they paid a high price for their negligence. Among U.S. auto manufacturers, for example, established industry-wide mental models of how to organize and compete, how to produce and deliver products, and what customers want in their cars led the U.S. companies into an ambush by foreign auto manufacturers, particularly the Japanese, from which not all may survive. Thirty years ago, private health care financing in the United States was dominated by a great many indemnity insurance companies, many of whom were unable or unwilling to adjust to the shift to managed care health plans and have since gone out of business. The health care industry is in the midst of another major swing—toward consumer-driven health care. Some provider and payer organizations will not fully recognize this move quickly enough or make the necessary adjustments in their business models in time to avoid losing market share and eventually failing.

HOW A STRATEGIC PLAN CAN GO WRONG IN ITS IMPLEMENTATION

A strategy can fail to achieve its intended aims in several generic ways. A savvy firm can anticipate, but not always prevent, these complications.

- The assumptions about the external factors (general environment, market forces, customer preferences, competitor behavior) upon which the plan is based turn out to be invalid or unfounded.
- The resources or competencies that the plan is counting upon become no longer available (e.g., key personnel leave, capital cannot be raised in the necessary amounts, legal permissions are denied).
- The plan is not implemented competently (e.g., it was implemented too slowly, or with mistakes, misjudgments, individual incompetence, or inappropriate methods).
- The plan was not a good one to begin with (e.g., it was poorly conceived, it was not responsive to identified threats and opportunities, it failed to leverage the firm's strengths and minimize its weaknesses, it paid insufficient attention to implementation, there was inadequate involvement of staff responsible for implementation, there was not enough plan detail or structure, or top management failed to inspire and mobilize the organization around the plan).

One of the primary functions of a strategic monitoring system is to catch these problems before they become so serious that the strategy is derailed.

KEY PRINCIPLES OF A STRATEGY MONITORING AND ADJUSTMENT PROGRAM

Strategy monitoring must be carried out on a continual basis—occasional, sporadic monitoring reports may reveal problems only after the strategic plan has been compromised and it is too late to make corrections. Continuous monitoring of implementation creates a record of progress, especially valuable for strategies that take years to reach fruition.

Monitoring looks at two broad areas of activity: the *context* of the strategy and the *performance* outcomes of the strategy.

The context has to do with the multitude of environmental forces that a strategy is designed to address and the resources being relied upon to put it into practice. The monitoring of the contextual forces answers questions like these:

- How have our customers' demands for products and product features changed?
- What new technologies have become available in our industry and, of these, which is essential to maintain our competitive position?
- Has the pace of economic growth in our markets increased or slowed?
- How are competitors reacting to our strategies?
- What new strategies have our competitors initiated? Have they taken actions, strategic or otherwise, that threaten the viability or success of our strategies or create opportunities for us to initiate successful new strategies?
- Have new competitors entered our industry or have existing competitors departed?
- Have new products/services been introduced to our markets or existing products dropped?
- Have new substitute products/services been introduced in our markets?
- Have new market segments emerged in our overall market?
- Have any of our competitors' strengths become weaker or weaknesses become stronger?
- Have any of our own strengths become weaker or weaknesses become stronger?
- What new opportunities have emerged in our industry or markets?
- What new threats have emerged in our industry or markets?
- Is there evidence of new demographic trends that may affect the size or preferences of our customer base, shrink or expand our markets, or create entirely new markets?
- Have new laws been enacted, court rulings been issued, or governmental administrative decisions been rendered that create legal doubts about some features of our strategies or that open up new courses of strategic action that previously seemed to be blocked?
- Do we appear to be moving closer to or farther away from our fundamental, long-term strategic objectives?
- In light of changes in external environmental conditions and in the resources and competencies that we can apply to strategic initiatives, do our current vision and mission still make sense?
- Have any key people left the organization, upon whom our strategies depended? Have new people joined our staff with competencies that make new strategies possible?

- Have conditions in the markets for financial capital (debt and equity) changed sufficiently for us to consider raising additional capital to fund new, more expansive strategies?
- As we implemented our strategies, did we discover gaps or failings in the competencies we thought we possessed?
- Due to any of these factors, has the risk level inherent in our strategies gone up or down?

The second area on which monitoring activities are focused is the performance associated with the strategy being implemented. Several categories of performance metrics deserve attention.

Performance of the strategy implementation process—time deadlines, percentage of project completion, interim objectives met, over- and under-budget expenditures.

Performance of the new operational activities created by implementation of the strategy. This depends on what the strategy was intended to achieve. Goals, objectives, and timetables should have been set during strategy formulation and incorporated into the plan.

Performance of the divisions, departments, functional areas, task forces, and project teams involved in implementing the strategy.

Performance of individuals staffing those units participating in the implementation process.

Over long periods of time, *performance of the executives* responsible for overseeing the formulation and execution of strategies across the organization.

Some form of monitoring, performance evaluation, and feedback must occur at all these levels to ensure that strategy implementation stays on track and on schedule, that all levels are in synch with each other, and to catch and correct any emerging problems.

The greatest value of (and challenge for) a monitoring system comes in accurately correlating developments in the strategic context with actual performance of the strategy. The ability to engage in true "systems thinking" is critical at this point. Changes in performance are rarely the result of a single contextual factor; normally, there are multiple forces pushing and pulling on performance. If effective corrective measures are to be taken, they must be directed at the most likely true causes.

■ MONITOR THE PAST, PRESENT, AND FUTURE

A good monitoring system will look at performance and events in the past, the present, and the future.

The easiest mechanisms to institute are those that report on the results of strategies and programs after they have been implemented. Some key variables can be assessed in no other way. For instance, the number and dollar value of reimbursement claims paid without further questioning to a hospital by a managed care organization within a certain month cannot be known until that month is over. The results of clinical trials on a new drug being developed by a biotechnology firm are apparent only after the trial has been completed. Projections, best estimates, and trend plotting can help, but events can be clearly understood only when they have become history.

More desirable is real-time reporting on performance results/outputs as they are occurring. When there are deviations from original intentions or planned objectives, corrective action can be taken before the damage spreads to other parts of the organization. In some cases, just a few hours' or days' delay can be disastrous. For instance, if a virus epidemic or environmental health crisis began spreading rapidly throughout a community, public health agencies would want to hear as quickly as possible about new cases in order optimally to deploy their resources. A health care provider organization might launch a new advertising campaign that is suddenly made irrelevant and foolish by a new product announcement from a competitor. The organization would want to learn this promptly in order to cancel or redirect its campaign. Creating a concurrent reporting system calls for highly sensitive, alert monitoring coupled with almost instantaneous communications to the appropriate decision makers.

The ideal monitoring system is one that anticipates performance problems and environmental changes before they occur—so that adjustments can be made that completely preempt/prevent damaging effects and put the strategy back on course. A good example might be tracking the progress of a new piece of legislation as it moves through the state legislature, preparing for its impact on the organization as enactment becomes more likely. Most demographic trends can be projected to endpoints many years into the future (e.g., aging baby boomers and their associated health care needs). Sophisticated prediction and extrapolation techniques are elements of a forward-looking monitoring capability, along with a degree of solid intuition.

■ STEPS IN SETTING UP A STRATEGIC MONITORING SYSTEM

In establishing a comprehensive strategic monitoring system, a business must do several things. It starts with determining which metrics best measure the factors it wants to follow. This usually requires talking in depth with the strategy decision makers and those in the organization with a profound understanding of the world in which it operates. Choosing the best metrics may be a process of trial and error, seeing which are most useful in assessing strategy effectiveness. In addition, the firm must focus on a manageable number of metrics; it can be expensive and distracting to try to gather and analyze all remotely relevant information on a strategy. As the firm proceeds with its strategy implementation, it may realize that new, additional types of information would be useful in its monitoring process.

The next step is to identify the best sources for data on the chosen metrics. Some very desirable data may not be available. The firm will have to decide whether it will use its own resources to gather the data. Other data may be available, but at considerable expense or with great difficulty. The firm will have to decide how badly it wants that data. Certain types of data may be available from multiple sources—some free, some with modest charges, and some at much higher prices. The quality of the data may vary among those sources, and the firm will have to make a tradeoff between price and quality. As time passes the firm will learn about new sources of information and data that it may wish to utilize.

Once decisions have been made about which metrics to use and the best sources for data on them, the firm must implement a system for gathering those data from those sources that is not overly complex or costly. It must be a genuine "system" that draws in, digests, analyzes, and reaches conclusions from these data.

That system must incorporate a process, perhaps with limits and trigger points, for determining when strategy changes are called for and what the changes will be. For instance, a hospital may decide in advance that when demographic trends show that the number of families with two or more children in its market area has reached a certain point, it will open a specialized pediatric clinic. A large managed-care network may condition its growth strategy of acquiring and converting small nonprofit health plans on its ability to raise debt capital at an interest rate no higher than a certain level. In most cases, however, the firm will wait to see what changes occur in its environment before analyzing their effect on its strategies and deciding if adjustments are necessary.

To optimize the value from its strategic monitoring, the firm must dedicate people with appropriate skills and sound judgment to manage these systems and processes. It is important to avoid creating a system that is too ponderous, too hard to understand, too expensive, and generally lacking in credibility. The goal is a process that is fluid and seamless, producing the right change decisions when they are needed.

Once the system has done its work, it must include procedures for passing the information on critical changes, trends, and developments on to the persons best qualified to make appropriate decisions on the basis of it. The value of a monitoring program is measured by how well it informs, and keeps informed, those executives and managers responsible for formulating new strategies and tuning existing ones.

To summarize the steps in setting up a strategic monitoring system:

1. Ascertain that appropriate, measurable goals have been set for successful implementation of the strategy.
2. Determine the metrics that will best measure progress toward achievement of those goals.
3. Identify good sources of data on those metrics.
4. Create a formal system of designated people and reporting schedules to gather the data from those sources, analyze and categorize them, and draw conclusions about their effects on strategy implementation.
5. To the extent possible, decide in advance at what points in the data trends an adjustment in the strategy will be considered necessary. At the very least, be prepared to recognize when changes in environmental variables or deviations from expected strategic progress call for a reexamination of the strategy or its implementation.
6. Communicate the data and the conclusions to those people in the best position to understand their strategic implications and with the authority to make appropriate changes.

■ STRATEGIC PARAMETERS TO BE MONITORED

The starting point or baseline for a strategic monitoring process is the few fundamental strategic objectives developed from vision and mission statements, the internal and external environmental assessments prepared at the beginning of the strategic planning process, and the specific objectives and other metrics associated with each strategy. The purpose of the process is to make sure that the strategy, as implemented, achieves what it was attended to achieve. Setting those achievement objectives should be a mandatory part of the strategy formulation process. The stage at which the strategy is being implemented is not the time to decide on the best measures of its success. If the firm does not already know what value the strategy will bring to the organization, why is it pursuing the strategy at all?

One way to track the progress in implementing a strategy is to measure how well the firm is accomplishing its grand strategic objectives—such as return on the equity invested by its owners or revenue growth. Those measurements must be made in any event. However, they are often the product of the simultaneous implementation of several strategies, and the progress and success of each, which must also be monitored. In fact one way of viewing performance evaluation within a

Table 10.1 Interrelated Strategic Objectives at Different Organizational Levels

Vision and Mission
Grand Strategic Objectives
Individual Strategy Objectives
Functional Area Objectives
Department Objectives
Team/Group/Task Force Objectives
Individual Employee Objectives

The objectives at each level feed into and support those in the level above it.

good-sized organization is in terms of a nested, interlocked cascade of objectives that looks something like the table above.

The approach to monitoring progress toward achievement of objectives is the same at all of these levels: determine metrics for each objective, identify data sources for each metric, gather the data, draw conclusions, and make decisions about strategy changes. An important question concerns the metrics to which the firm will pay attention. The following are good examples of monitoring metrics at the levels of both the corporation and the individual SBU.

Corporate-Level Monitoring Metrics

A simple global metric for a multi-SBU corporation is a set of aggregate measures for key parameters applying to all the SBUs. In a typical health care provider organization these parameters might include patient satisfaction ratings, National Committee for Quality Assurance (NCQA) scores, clinical outcomes measures, or procedure mortality rates. In a biotech research firm, the number of new drugs entering each step of the FDA approval process might be tracked. The overall corporate measure might constitute a simple average of the score for each SBU or a weighted average based on the sales revenue of each SBU.

The overall increase in the corporation's total revenues is also important, particularly in comparison with growth in the national economy or similar corporations.

A rapidly growing corporation with a large SBU portfolio might choose to monitor the number of new SBUs it has acquired or created internally, to replace existing SBUs that are moving along their life cycles toward decline.

In a corporation that is growing primarily by adding new businesses, it is often useful to measure and compare the growth in revenues derived from existing businesses and the growth that comes from simply adding new businesses. Almost ten years ago, the industry of physician practice management companies virtually collapsed overnight when it became evident that its highly publicized growth was based almost entirely on the constant acquisition of new physician practices.

Market share is always an important metric; it might be a good idea to track dynamically the market shares of all the SBUs in the portfolio.

A primary responsibility of corporate-level executives is management of the composition of its business portfolio. A helpful tool for doing this is a graphic display like a pie chart that shows the composition by geographic region, payer, or other relevant variable. An animated chart could show the shifting makeup of the portfolio.

An essential set of metrics comprises those that measure and compare the key performance variables for all SBUs, such as revenue growth rate, volume and type of assets, ROI, positive/negative cash flow, and sales and profits. As these metrics are monitored, the firm must recognize the stage at which each SBU is in its life cycle and ask itself questions like: Is it performing appropriately for that stage? Is there evidence that it is moving to the next stage?

Another useful monitoring metric would be the diversification of the corporation's portfolio and the relatedness of that diversification. Unfortunately, there are no good quantitative measures of either. However, it is possible to describe qualitatively the different industries and markets in which the SBUs compete as well as the synergies that have resulted from the relatedness among the SBUs. Examples of those synergies are the sharing of facilities, the sharing of knowledge like best practices, and the economies of scale produced by joint purchasing, manufacturing, or marketing.

No strategic monitoring process would be complete without regular examination of the traditional financial measures that are important for shareholder satisfaction, continued access to debt and equity capital, and as general indicators of SBU success. These include economic profits, market value added, market-to-book ratio, earnings per share (EPS), return on capital employed (ROCE), return on equity (ROE), and liquidity.

SBU-Level Monitoring Metrics

Strategic monitoring at the level of the individual SBU is, with a few exceptions, not very different from corporate-level monitoring. If there is only one SBU in the corporation—that is, if the corporation consists of a single business—then most of the metrics described above for corporate-level monitoring could be used. Because the corporation has no portfolio of business units, there would be no weighted averaging of SBU performance or evaluation of changes in the composition of the portfolio. In contrast, when an SBU is one of many under a corporate umbrella, it will not need to concern itself with metrics related to the raising of investment capital (debt or equity) because that function is performed by the corporate center.

A clearly unique feature of SBU-level strategies is their focus on substantive operations that are producing goods or services in competition with other similar firms for customers in defined market segments. The monitoring metrics will reflect this fact.

Traditionally, for-profit businesses in most industries have paid most attention to the measurement of financial performance variables. There is some good reason for this, to the extent that shareholders and debtors are viewed as the ultimate stakeholders of a business. However, while all organizations must be concerned with their financial resources, many nonprofit entities give greater consideration to their missions and the long-range purposes that they are trying to achieve. Health care organizations, even those that are primarily profit driven, have professed an overriding interest in patient health and quality of care. Many businesses throughout the economy have come to realize that other nonfinancial metrics must be balanced against measures of sales, profits, and other monetary criteria.

This approach to strategic assessment has been popularized in the concept of the "Balanced Scorecard" devised by Robert Kaplan and David Norton.[1] Financial metrics are just one of four dimensions along which the Balanced Scorecard looks at a business's strategic performance. The other three are customer indicators, internal operations, and innovation. Before describing specific metrics in each of these areas, it should be understood that a business can define whatever broad categories of nonfinancial measurement seem relevant to its operations. For instance, in certain organizations, supplier indicators, environmental and safety concerns, or political issues and relationships may be more important than in others. For most businesses, however, the Balanced Scorecard model works quite well.

Customer Indicators

Because customers of one sort or another, wholesalers, retailers, or end users, purchase the firm's products or services and generate its revenues and profits, it makes sense that they would be a primary focus of any strategic monitoring system. These are some examples of metrics in this category.

Sales volume (in units and dollars) and growth—by market segment, and compared to the overall economy and to competitors.

Market share of the business by product or service, geographic area, customer/market segment, or distribution channel.

Customer or patient satisfaction, not only with the products or services themselves but also with the entire purchase experience.

Brand equity of the firm's products or services, measured in terms of the price premium that they command or the increased customer loyalty that they engender.

Each of these key variables is driven by factors that also need to be watched.

Internal Operations

It is through its internal activities that an organization creates the products or services that deliver satisfaction to customers for which they are willing to pay.

Unit cost of production, where the unit may be an individual product or a definable unit of service.

Operational productivity, generally measured in terms of quantity of output per employee.

Error rate. This may refer to defects in products that are manufactured or errors committed in the delivery of the service, medication errors and outright malpractice being good examples in a health care provider setting.

Employee satisfaction. This metric, with its implications for staff morale, has effects on work productivity and the attitudes displayed during delivery of services to customers.

Quality of the products or services offered to customers. The quality of drugs or medical devices manufactured is important and relatively easy to measure; perhaps even more important and yet much more difficult to measure is the quality of medical care services provided.

Clinical outcomes. These are a metric unique to health care delivery, being a measure of how well a medical treatment or procedure achieves the desired improvement in the patient's condition.

The internal operations area. This encompasses most of the factors determining the customer-related indicators described just above.

Innovation

In an environment of even moderate competitive intensity, an organization must constantly be looking for new product ideas, new markets, and new resources and competencies.

New products or services are a leading example of the results of innovation, with good metrics being number of patents granted, number of FDA approvals received, or revenue earned from new products (or new payers, market segments, CPT codes, ancillary services).

New business models, such as the ability of a multispecialty group practice to accept a "global capitation" contract with a managed care organization.

Ability to enter new markets, as when that same group practice prepares itself to offer its own health plan to employers.

New operational processes, with examples being EMR and CPOE systems.

New distribution channels, such as the primary care clinics being installed in retail malls and stores.

New organization structures. This would be the case when a biotech firm evolves from a functional area structure to a product line structure.

Employee training and development. Firms spend money on training in order to create new competencies in their workforces.

Financial

This category encompasses the wide variety of financial metrics that businesses typically use in evaluating their performance. Some of the more common indicators are economic profit, net income, return on capital employed, return on sales, current ratio, asset turnover, and cash flow. A more detailed discussion of financial management issues appears in Chapter 11.

■ CHANGES THAT COULD BE DETECTED BY A STRATEGIC MONITORING SYSTEM

It is not hard to imagine the many kinds of changes in the strategic metrics that could be picked up by a good monitoring system. These are just a few examples:

- An announcement by the federal Center for Medicare and Medicaid Services (CMS) that Medicare reimbursement rates for physicians will be held steady for the next two years.
- A report from the state public health agency that the proportion of adults aged 25 to 64 who are either overweight or obese rose from 55 percent to 62 percent in the past two years.
- The signing into law by the president of an appropriations bill that will increase by 70 percent the available National Institutes of Health (NIH) funding for medical research in areas being investigated by a biotech firm.
- The announced merger of the two smaller hospitals in the market served by a total of three hospitals.
- The number of patient visits during the first six months of operation of a newly opened satellite clinic of a physician group practice is 45 percent below original projections.

Dashboard Graphic Displays as Monitoring Tools

Strategic monitoring systems can sometimes generate more information than strategy decision makers have time to absorb. Some simple devices are available to summarize that information and present it in a form that captures its strategic impact. One such device is the corporate "dashboard." The term refers to the instruments on the dashboard of an automobile, particularly racing cars, which with simple clarity display key variables in which the automobile driver or the corporate executive is interested. For instance, a strategic version of such a dashboard for a hospital might include five round dials representing revenues, net income, free cash flow, adverse events rates, and days' delay in receiving payment for managed care claims. Each dial would have numbers around its perimeter for the variable being measured and a needle pointing to the number of the most recent measurement. There might also be a red line on the number indicating the goal toward which the hospital was currently aiming. A quick glance at these gauges would give a hospital executive a useful, if somewhat superficial, picture of the current state of the organization. If she saw a reading that was puzzling or disturbing, she could ask for a fuller explanation.

Numerous other graphic tools can be used to display the current state of a strategic metric succinctly. To continue the automobile metaphor, "traffic light" graphics can show if an environmental variable is at an acceptable level (green), is showing some uncertainty and needs to be watched more closely (yellow), or poses a serious threat requiring immediate action (red). Animating a graph or chart is a good way of demonstrating a trend in a metric (e.g., a pie chart indicating market shares with sectors that grow and shrink to show changes over time).

- A competing biotech research firm has just begun a clinical trial for a new drug that serves the same clinical function as a drug that another firm is developing and that is at least one year away from the clinical trials stage.
- A national retail drug chain cancels its previously announced plan to build primary quick-care clinics in twenty-eight of its retail outlets in the local market.
- The lead investigator on a major biomedical research project for which a multimillion-dollar grant recently was received has been diagnosed with lung cancer and will have to cut his work schedule to half-time.
- A survey conducted by a local newspaper on patient satisfaction levels at five local area hospitals ranked your hospital third.

- A physician group practice's share of the local market for Medicare patients has increased from 8 percent to 11 percent, while the proportion of the local population that is Medicare eligible has declined from 22 percent to 18 percent.
- The firm's bond rating was raised from BB+ to BBB by Standard & Poor's.
- A hospital's plan to reduce its infection rate by 10 percent within one year has already brought the rate down by 8 percent within six months.
- The institution of new claims submission procedures in a physician practice has reduced payer claims denials by one-third.
- For the first time in twenty years, the federal government has issued a list of the nation's hospitals rated by their death rates for heart patients.
- A bill that would allow the FDA to approve generic versions of biotechnology drugs is making significant progress through Congress.
- In the past year, the company's revenues have increased 23 percent, profits have risen 14 percent, and its stock price has gone up 31 percent.

The real challenge for a business is deciding exactly what response, if any, to make to these developments.

CONCLUSIONS THAT COULD BE REACHED AND CHANGES THAT COULD BE MADE

These are some of the primary generic conclusions that may be reached and changes made on the basis of information gathered through a strategic monitoring system:

- Drop/cancel a strategy. The strategy no longer makes sense because the firm's long-term objectives have changed, the market segment to which the strategy is targeted has shrunk, the preferences of the customers in the market have changed, a competitor has launched its own strategy that preempts the firm's, or a recent court decision renders the strategy no longer viable.
- Replace an existing strategy with a new one. In response to any of the above developments, rather than cancel the strategy entirely, the firm chooses to adapt it to the new conditions. For instance, the strategy might be adjusted to accommodate the new preferences of customers, the strategy could be reconfigured in a way that preempts the competitor's strategy, or a few modest changes might permit the strategy to comply with the court's ruling.

- Initiate a new strategy, in addition to the existing ones. If the monitoring system reveals a newly emergent strategic opportunity, and the firm possesses the necessary uncommitted resources, it may decide spontaneously to launch a new strategy to take advantage of the situation.
- Reallocate existing resources, particularly financial and human, among the strategies. For a variety of reasons, usually having to do with one strategy unpredictably becoming more attractive than another, a business may choose to move money and people from the latter to the former as a reflection of its changed priorities.
- Invest additional resources in one or more strategies. Because a current strategy in progress has become more appealing or is lagging in its implementation, a firm may devote more resources, if it has them, to it in order to speed its execution.
- Stretch the objectives of a strategy (develop a drug sooner, enroll more members faster, increase revenues further). An organization may realize that it originally set its strategy goals too low or that it simply is capable of accomplishing more through the strategy, so it sets its strategic heights even higher.
- Reduce the objectives of a strategy. The firm's initial strategic expectations may have been too optimistic and it now seems appropriate to pull back on its objectives.

By responding promptly and prudently to reports from its strategic monitoring system, a firm can ensure that the strategy that finally becomes reality is the best one for the firm.

Study Questions

1. Under what conditions would it make sense to cancel or reverse the implementation of a strategy? What would be involved in canceling a strategy? It is likely that substantial funds have been invested, new people have been hired or current people retrained, new equipment purchased, new facilities constructed, supplier contracts negotiated, and marketing campaigns launched. Does the company simply forget all that effort, or does it try to redirect it in a slightly different strategic direction?
2. Imagine that you are the CEO of a managed care organization offering health plans in twenty-three states. You have made strategic decisions to expand into an additional five states over the next several years. Think about what you have been reading recently about developments that might impact those decisions (i.e., political, economic, sociocultural, demographic, technological). Pick ten of those developments and explain exactly how they might affect your plans.

Learning Exercise

You are the business manager of a fifteen-physician group practice in family medicine that at a recent strategic planning retreat agreed to open a satellite clinic on the periphery of its current market area in order to increase the number of families that it serves. The clinic will be located in an area of somewhat older, rundown homes that seems to be undergoing slow but steady gentrification. The clinic initially will be staffed by three physicians and has a maximum capacity of ten doctors. One of your responsibilities under the strategic plan to create the clinic is to establish a modest program for keeping track of the factors and variables that might affect the success of the clinic. To get started, prepare a list of ten to fifteen financial and nonfinancial metrics that you propose to monitor, including the sources you will use to gather the necessary data. For each one of the metrics, indicate the directions in which they might change and the adjustments in the plan for the new clinic that would be necessary.

Notes

[1] Kaplan RS and Norton DP. *The Balanced Scorecard: Translating Strategy into Action*. Cambridge, MA: Harvard Business School Press;1996.

References

Balkin DB and Gomez-Mejia LR. Matching compensation and organizational strategies. *Strategic Management Journal*. February 1990:153–169.

Brancato CK. *New Corporate Performance Measures*. Research Report No. 1118-95-RR, New York, NY. The Conference Board, 1995.

Drew SAW. From knowledge to action: The impact of benchmarking on organizational performance. *Long Range Planning*. June 1997:427–441.

Galbraith CS. The effect of compensation programs and structure on SBU competitive strategy: A study of technology-intensive firms. *Strategic Management Journal*. July 1991:353–370.

Goold M and Quinn JJ. The paradox of strategic controls. *Strategic Management Journal*. 1990;11:43–57.

Govindarajan V and Fisher J. Strategy, control systems, and resource sharing: Effects on business unit performance. *Academy of Management Journal*. 1990;33:259–285.

Hoskisson RE and Hitt MA. Strategic control and relative R&D investment in large multiproduct firm. *Strategic Management Journal*. 1988;6:605–622.

Kaplan RS and Norton DP. Using the Balanced Scorecard as a strategic management system. *Harvard Business Review*. January–February 1996:75–85.

Linneman R and Chandran R. Contingency planning: A key to the swift managerial action in the uncertain tomorrow. *Managerial Planning*. January–February 1981:23–27.

Lorange P, Scott Morton MF, and Goshal S. Strategic control. St. Paul: West Publishing; 1986.

Low J and Seisfeld T. Measures that matter: Wall Street considers non-financial performance more than you think. *Strategy & Leadership*. March–April 1998:24–30.

Meyer MW. Finding performance: The new discipline in management. In: Neely, A. *Business Performance Measurement*. Cambridge, MA: Cambridge University Press; 2002;51–62.

Pickton D, Starkey M, and Bradford M. Understand business variation for improved business performance. *Long Range Planning*. June 1996:412–415.

Roney CW. Planning for Strategic Contingencies. *Business Horizons*. 2003;46(2):35–42.

Schreyogg G and Steinmann H. Strategic control: A new perspective. *Academy of Management Review*. 1987;12:96.

Simons R. Strategic orientation and management attention to control systems. *Strategic Management Journal*. 1991;12:49–62.

Simons R. How new top managers use control systems as levers of strategic renewal. *Strategic Management Journal*. 1994;15:169–189.

Simons R. Control in an age of empowerment. *Harvard Business Review*. March–April 1995:80.

Stamen JP. Decision support systems help planners hit their targets. *Journal of Business Strategy*. March–April 1990:30–33.

Stivers BP and Joyce T. Building a balanced performance management system. *SAM Advanced Management Journal*. Spring 2000:22–29.

Stonich PJ. The performance measurement and reward system: Critical to strategic management. *Organizational Dynamics*. Winter 1984:45–57.

Tilles S. How to evaluate corporate strategy. *Harvard Business Review*. July–August 1963:111–121.

CHAPTER

11

Strategic Financial Management

Learning Objectives

After reading and studying this chapter, you should be able to:

- Appreciate the indispensable role of strategic financial management in the success of specific strategies as well as in the overall business.
- Describe the elements of a professional corporate finance function.
- Identify and explain the major sources of financing for capital investments in strategic initiatives.
- Distinguish the roles of debt and equity financing, and their combination in a well-crafted capital structure.
- Appreciate the role of "creditworthiness" in a firm's strategic success and the ways that it can be enhanced by competent strategic financial management.
- List the factors internal to an organization that determine its creditworthiness.
- Discuss the good and not-so-good ways that a business may allocate its limited capital funds to strategic projects.
- Understand the mistakes that often are made in the strategic management of an organization's finances.

In ensuring that the entire organization is optimally prepared to carry out strategic initiatives, every functional area must be in synch with those initiatives. This is explained in greater detail as a facet of strategy implementation in Chapter 9. One fundamental area is of disproportionately greater significance to strategic success. That one is financial planning, management, and control, and it is the subject of this chapter.

Financial terms often are the basis for measuring the performance and success of strategies. Beyond that concern, there are powerful reasons for managing the firm's finances in synchronization with its strategies. There is a symbiotic relationship between the substance and success of the strategies and the financial health of the firm. Financial resources are required to pay for all the other resources that go into implementing strategy—land, plant, equipment, salaries, contracted services. The financial achievements of the strategy determine the firm's ability to continue to obtain the capital necessary to support both future strategies and current operations.

The primary elements of strategic financial management can be summarized in this way:

- Making sure that there are sufficient capital funds to support the chosen strategies. This generally means ensuring organization-wide financial performance that satisfies the demands of equity and debt stakeholders.
- Making sure that the chosen strategies enhance the organization's creditworthiness and ensure its continued access to the capital markets.
- Making sure that the available capital is allocated among strategy initiatives according to criteria that maintain creditworthiness and maximize the value created by the organization's operations.
- Tracking performance of new strategies as they are implemented to make sure that they meet financial objectives, and to anticipate any developing problems.

The ingredients of a well-run corporate finance function are described in the sidebar on the next page.

FINANCING OF CAPITAL INVESTMENTS

If an organization had no strategic ambitions, and was satisfied continuing its current day-to-day operations for the foreseeable future, it would need to be concerned only that the revenues from those operations were enough to cover the expenses of conducting the operations. In fact, thirty years ago, most health care organizations, certainly the primarily not-for-profit (NFP) hospitals, functioned in approximately that manner. If the hospital decided that some kind of capital expenditure was necessary—to replace a failing heating plant or build a parking garage—it could factor the required funds into its charge calculations and they were accepted unquestioningly by payers.

Today, in an industry where organizations must make regular capital investments in order to survive and where payers carefully scrutinize every bill they pay, it is necessary to pay much more attention to potential sources of strategic capital financing. It is necessary to practice professional corporate financial management. This is true for large and small organizations, for-profit and not-for-profit. It does not take a large staff of financial experts, just one well-trained capital finance manager.

Ingredients of a Professional Corporate Finance Function

There is hardly a for-profit or not-for-profit corporation without a person or a department designated to manage the finances of the organization. The job description of that person or the mandate of that department typically includes the following activities:

Plays a leadership role in pushing for full integration of strategic and financial planning. It is an unfortunate fact in many organizations that financial management is conducted as a function separate from strategic planning. The result is often a disconnect between the strategies being followed and the business's finances: strategies are adopted for which there are insufficient financial resources or which have damaging effects on the business's creditworthiness. It is frequently the financial managers who best understand the importance of this integration and urge the corporate leadership to make it part of the strategy decision-making process.

Assumes responsibility for the full range of financial management activities, including performing financial feasibility analyses of strategies, processing the financial implications of proposed strategies, making financial projections on the basis of strategies proposed for adoption, determining the availability of capital resources, making decisions about the organization's capital structure, conducting negotiations with capital market institutions, shaping and overseeing the procedure for allocating capital resources among the strategies, managing the strategic and operational budgeting processes, and ensuring the effectiveness of the financial control components of the strategic planning process.

Maintains the integrity of the balance sheet and the creditworthiness of the organization. This is the one department that can be relied upon consistently to monitor and protect the financial underpinnings of the entity. It will provide input to the formulation of strategies on their financial implications. It will frequently speak up when it feels that an organizational activity threatens its creditworthiness.

Manages the capital structure of the organization to ensure maximum capital availability at the minimum cost. It will make recommendations on the various types of capital that the business might use to finance its operations and strategies. This involves

(*continues*)

Ingredients of a Professional Corporate Finance Function (continued)

choices among debt, equity, and internal cash flow; among different types of debt and equity instruments; and between long- and short-term debt.

Oversees the interplay among strategic plans, capital markets access and capital structure decisions, and capital allocation decisions. It is a difficult juggling act to ensure that there is sufficient capital to pay for strategic plans, that the available capital is allocated optimally among the proposed plans, and that the strategies have the effect of generating the capital that will be needed for future strategies and operations.

Enforces the application of a rigorous, systematic, evidence-based, unbiased assessment of capital investment opportunities. It sometimes is easy for non-financial managers to relax their scrutiny of the financial consequences of the strategies under consideration, and allow themselves to be influenced by politics, personality, or passion. A firm's finance specialists make sure that no one loses sight of the dollars involved.

Monitors and measures the financial performance of the total corporation and its individual SBUs. Money, capital, revenues, and profits are the lifeblood of every organization, for-profit and not-for-profit. It is the responsibility of financial managers, while the organization is implementing strategies designed to realize its vision, to make sure that nothing is done to compromise its existence. They are professionals at gathering all necessary data on a business's finances and drawing conclusions about the future of the organization.

The responsibility of corporate finance that deals with capital markets to ensure that there is sufficient funding for the organization's strategic initiatives is carried out at the topmost management level in a multi-SBU corporation. The corporation is the legal entity to which banks will make loans, in which investors will buy ownership shares, and by which bonds may be issued. Individual SBUs usually do not have the independent legal standing to engage in such transactions. Investors and lenders will evaluate the businesses in the portfolio, but they place their capital funds in the hands of the corporate managers and count on them to make strategically appropriate disbursements to the individual SBUs.

The sources of financing for business organizations are well established and relatively few in number, though the terms under which they may be accessed are many in number. The basic choices available to for-profit (FP) corporations are internally generated funds, bank loans, bond issues, and equity sales. Not-for-profit (NFP) organizations can turn to internally generated funds, bank loans, bond issues, and charitable donations.

Internally generated funds consist of operating surpluses and funded depreciation. Some companies generate sufficient profits and positive cash flow that they can finance a significant portion of their capital projects without going to external capital markets. This has not been the case for most health care organizations in recent years as competitive pressures and payer cost control efforts have squeezed margins to very low levels. Health care businesses with tax-exempt status are also able to solicit philanthropic gifts.

There is another source of funding that is unique to health care and scientific research organizations: grants from government agencies and charitable foundations. Government grants may go to both NFP and FP organizations; only NFP entities may receive money from foundations.

Capital financing beyond the internal sources falls into two broad categories—equity financing and debt financing.

Equity Financing

While some organizations include internal funds and charitable donations in the equity category, the term technically describes an ownership interest in the organization. NFP organizations are not "owned" by anyone, certainly not any private individual. Conceptually, they are owned by the body public, by the community, by all citizens in general. A company's equity is represented by the shares of stock owned by its shareholders. If an NFP organization can be said to have equity, it is reflected in its "net assets," the difference between its total assets and total liabilities.

Shareholders invest their money in the shares of an FP business because they want to see the value of their investment grow. This happens in two ways: the business pays them dividends on their shares or the value of those shares in the markets where they are traded goes up. The business has complete control over whether dividends are paid on its stock, though it will not have the money to do so unless the business is doing well in selling its products and services. The business has considerably less control over the price of its shares on the public stock exchanges. Superior business performance will certainly favor higher prices, but other unpredictable factors come into play. Stock prices may be influenced by the state of the national economy, by the state of the industries in which the business operates, by the opinions of financial/investment analysts, by changing expectations of investors, and by subtle, sometimes psychological trends in the market.

Equity investors have definite expectations about the monetary return they receive on their investments. That rate of return is defined by the dividends per share paid out by the company and the appreciation or increase in the market price of the shares. Through the action of the stock markets, investors demand a higher rate of return on equity shares than they would for an equivalent investment in a company's bonds. The reason is the difference in risk assumed. A corporate bond is a contract that legally compels the company to make interest and principal payments at specific times. A share of stock is evidence of ownership of a piece of the corporation, but entitles the owner to no particular return. If the business is not financially prosperous and the market price of the stock does not increase as a result, investors will be unwilling to provide equity financing to the business.

There is one feature of equity financing that severely complicates the work of corporate strategists. It is the widespread preference of investors to see returns on their investments accrue sooner rather than later. Perhaps a manifestation of a desire for instant gratification, there is a focus on short-term gains that can inhibit management efforts to pursue longer-term goals.

Access to equity financing is a unique capital financing source available only to for-profit organizations. The downside is that management is forever beholden to the whims and desires of financial market analysts and the investors that they aim to represent.

Debt Financing

The major alternative to equity financing is debt financing. Because debt is a lower-cost source of capital than equity, many businesses try to keep their overall cost of capital as low as possible by using as much debt as possible. This is true of both FP and NFP organizations. This approach works as long as the business is able to earn a return on capital that equals or exceeds the debt interest rate. In fact, any earnings over and above the interest accrue to the benefit of equity shareholders—whether paid out as dividends or reinvested in the business.

A popular form of debt financing is a bond issued directly by the organization requiring the funds. Under a bond agreement, the issuing company promises to make regular interest payments up until the bond maturity date when it will pay off the principal in one lump sum. A thirty-year bond matures thirty years from the date of issue. The bond is a negotiable instrument that can be bought and sold during its life, the price rising and falling as national interest rates change. The life of bonds traditionally extends from ten years to as much as thirty, forty, or fifty years.

Debt financing is especially appealing to NFP organizations like hospitals. It is their primary recourse for capital, in the absence of access to equity financing. Furthermore, the bonds they issue are tax-exempt bonds in which the interest payments to the bond purchasers have exempt status from the IRS. Because they do not have to pay income taxes on the interest they receive, bond purchasers are willing to accept lower rates of return or interest on those bonds. There is no backing for these bonds other than the organization's revenues, which is why they are usually referred to as "tax-exempt revenue bonds." In order to qualify for the tax-exempt status, the proceeds of the bonds may be used only for the charitable, exempt purposes of the organization that issued them.

Tax-exempt revenue bonds have for many years been the primary source of capital financing for NFP organizations. However, over the past decade, even debt financing has become less available. Increased competition and pressure from payers to reduce reimbursement levels have significantly cut operating margins and cash flow in many health care organizations. This declining fiscal performance leads prospective bond purchasers to question the ability of these organizations to support any greater debt loads.

Corporate bonds are not the only form of debt financing. The costs associated with carrying out a bond issue makes it feasible primarily for amounts in excess of about $10 million. For smaller capital projects and for smaller organizations whose capital needs are more modest, businesses typically rely on "term loans," which are the typical commercial loans made by banks. Term loan agreements require the borrower to make regular payments (monthly or quarterly) of both interest and principal until the full loan amount has been paid off in the specified number of years. The term of these loans normally does not exceed ten years and can be for as little as one year.

Term loans are frequently used for the purchase of equipment or real estate, which then serves as collateral for the loans. Conventional mortgages are a form of term loan. Sometimes the agreements for longer-term loans include language placing limits on further indebtedness and requiring that a sinking fund be set up to ensure repayment. In contrast, if the business can pass the credit checks, the cost of term loans is relatively low. The primary sources of term loans and mortgages are commercial banks, insurance companies, and savings and loan institutions.

The general rule in corporate finance is to use short-term financing (like term loans) for short-term needs (like equipment purchases) and long-term financing (like bonds) for long-term needs (like corporate acquisitions).

Because tax-exempt debt financing is a cheaper source of capital than equity financing, health care organizations try to minimize their cost of capital by utilizing more debt than equity in their financing decisions. As health care providers reach their debt limits, equity financing becomes their only source of new funds.

Capital Structure—Balancing Debt and Equity

The result of a corporation's decisions about its use of debt and equity financing is its "capital structure"—what is essentially the right-hand side of the balance sheet. The decisions cannot be made casually. They involve choices about when to seek capital, from what sources, in what amounts, in what forms, under what terms, and at what costs.

The timing of the corporation's entry into the capital markets is also important. The corporate financial managers must take into account:

The current state of the capital markets. For loans and bond issues, at what level are interest rates? Are they trending up or down? What is the mood in the markets for publicly traded stock? How welcoming would they be to a new issue of stock? What price per share could the corporation expect to receive? For smaller, younger businesses, is the venture capital community interested in a second or third round of financing?

The current capital structure of the business. What proportion of its potential debt capacity is the corporation currently utilizing? What is its credit standing with the bond rating agencies? What is the rating of any currently outstanding bonds? What interest rate should the corporation expect to pay? Does the corporation have the cash flow to cover additional debt service charges? If the corporation has taken on all the debt that the markets will allow, are there equity financing options available?

The projected demands for strategic capital. If the proposed strategies are implemented according to schedule, what amounts of new capital will be needed and by what dates? Can any of the capital requirements be postponed by a matter of months or years? What effect will the proposed strategies have on the corporation's credit rating and appeal to capital markets?

No corporation can assume that it will be able to obtain the capital it needs for its strategic initiatives at the cost and under the terms that it would like. It is critical that all strategic planning be synchronized with the realities of the capital markets and the corporation's credit standing. The best way to accomplish this is through the full participation of corporate financial management in the strategy-making process. As early as possible in the development of a new strategy proposal, rough estimates of the capital that it will require should be made. This enables the financial managers to comment on the availability and cost of those capital amounts.

In configuring a corporation's capital structure, financial management will balance these characteristics of debt and equity financing.

Equity

When it sells stock, the corporation is giving up pieces of ownership to outside stakeholders whose motives may, and usually do, differ from the strategic intentions of top management. Although a small business's initial public offering (IPO) is a celebrated moment, it is also the beginning of the erosion of the founders' and top management's unfettered discretion in running the organization. From that point on, their decisions will be influenced by statements of investment analysts and by the market prices of their stock.

The dividends that the corporation pays to its shareholders, as a form of return on their investments, are not required and are at the discretion of corporate management. When they are granted, they are not deductible as a business expense of the corporation.

The capital that shareholders invest in the business by buying shares does not ever have to be repaid. In order to realize a gain on the investments, shareholders must sell their stock to other willing investors. If the corporation's performance is so poor that it is declared bankrupt and must be liquidated, the shareholders will receive nothing unless there is something left over after all other creditors have been paid off. Conceptually, the business owes them nothing because they are the business.

Debt

When the corporation borrows money or issues bonds, it is not turning over ownership interests to the lenders or bond purchasers. To that degree, it is not yielding control or influence over management decisions. Either a loan or a bond issue involves a binding legal contract between the corporation and the person or entity putting up the money. Under that contract, the corporation is committing itself to paying a fixed amount of interest at regular intervals to the debt holders and then, when the term of the loan or bond has expired, repaying the debt principal. These commitments must be met regardless of how well the business is performing. If the corporation has a low credit rating, its debt agreements may include restrictive covenants that limit management control in certain areas.

It is a rule of thumb in capital structure decision-making that retained earnings/net assets are the preferred source of capital, followed by various forms of debt, with different types of equity being least preferred. A survey came up with the order ranking in Table 11.1 for corporate capital sources.

■ MAINTAINING OR IMPROVING ORGANIZATIONAL CREDITWORTHINESS

The term "creditworthiness" means pretty much what it says—it is an indicator of how worthy an organization is to be granted credit by banks, lenders, and other types of debt holders. A vibrant, growing organization operating in a competitive industry will seek constantly to maintain and, if possible, enhance its creditworthiness. The creditworthiness of an organization is measured by the formal credit or bond ratings given to it by the three leading credit rating entities: Standard & Poor's, Fitch Ratings, and Moody's Investors Service. The ratings take the form of somewhat arcane indicators like BBB−, BBB, BBB+, A−, A, A+, AA−, AA, AA+

Table 11.1. Preferred Sources of Corporate Capital

Ranking	Score
1. Retained earnings	5.61
2. Straight debt	4.88
3. Convertible debt	3.02
4. External common equity	2.42
5. Straight preferred stock	2.22
6. Convertible preferred	1.72

From "The Debt-Equity Trade Off: The Capital Structure Decision," in Aswath Damodaran, *Corporate Finance: Theory and Practice*, 2nd ed., (Hoboken, NJ): Wiley Series in Finance; 2001; available at http://www.stern.nyu.edu/%7Eadamodar/pdfiles/cf2E/capstru.pdf. Accessed July 1, 2007.

(in ascending order of creditworthiness, by Standard & Poor's). There are numerous benefits that flow from a higher credit or bond rating:

Greater access to debt capital. The various sources of debt financing are simply more willing to lend funds to a business with a higher rating. As that business contemplates a group of attractive, but expensive, strategy proposals, it will have access to a larger pool of debt capital to finance the proposals than would a comparable business with a lower rating.

Lower interest cost of debt capital. When a higher-rated business does borrow money, it will be able to pay a lower interest rate. Because the interest rate on debt is partially a function of the risk that the debtor will not be able to repay the debt, and because a high credit rating indicates that a business is in a stronger position to repay its debts, a low interest rate is a natural result.

Lower underwriting costs of debt capital. A variety of other costs are associated with borrowing money or issuing corporate bonds that can be lumped under "underwriting expenses." Because all the parties involved in the underwriting process have greater confidence in a debtor with a higher credit rating, those costs are usually lower.

Greater access to credit enhancement vehicles. There are also a number of instruments that an organization can use at the time that it is planning to borrow money to effectively raise its credit rating. One example is bond insurance; another is a line of credit. Ironically, a business with a higher credit rating will have easier access to these instruments, and at lower cost, than one with a lower rating. In other words, the higher the existing rating the easier it is to raise it even higher.

Fewer restrictive bond covenants. These covenants are terms of the bond issuance agreement that bind the issuing corporation to do certain things or avoid doing other things. They may be financial in nature (maintain a certain interest coverage ratio or debt-to-equity ratio) or nonfinancial (not sell additional common stock or change the makeup of the board of directors). Naturally, corporate management would prefer that its autonomy and discretion not be limited in these ways. There are likely to be fewer or no restrictive covenants for corporations with higher bond ratings.

Access to a wider range of creditors. More creditors of all sorts (e.g., commercial banks, investment banks, pension funds) will be interested in lending money to organizations with higher credit ratings. Many of these creditors, by their own rules, are permitted to lend only to entities with certain minimum credit ratings.

Access to a wider range of strategic partners. When businesses are contemplating mergers or acquisitions, the relative financial strengths are a significant factor in choosing appropriate partners. For instance, a cash-rich, technology-poor corporation might be interested in pairing up with another firm with a weak balance sheet and some valuable intellectual property. All other things being equal, the business with the higher credit rating will have more choices of partners.

Powerful communications device. Information on the firm's bond rating is publicly available. When that rating is a good one, it raises morale within the organization, gives capital markets confidence in the business, and lets rivals know that they are facing some formidable competition. Of course, if the rating is already low or has been recently downgraded, it sends a very discouraging message to all stakeholders.

The possession of a high credit rating can be a source of powerful competitive advantage, allowing the firm greater flexibility and scope in its strategic decision-making. Every business should be alert to the factors that may influence its credit rating.

External Factors Affecting Creditworthiness

There is a wide range of factors generally outside a particular business's control that credit rating firms consider in issuing their ratings.

- It is likely that Congress and the state legislatures will continue for many years in their efforts to rein in the national health care budget by limiting growth in Medicare and Medicaid spending. The result will be increasing constraints on reimbursements to provider organizations, leading in turn to revenues that grow at a slower rate than costs.

- The movement toward consumer-driven health care is intended to encourage consumer-patients to pay more attention to their health care purchase decisions. Their natural impulse will be to demand more in terms of features, quality, and service from their health care providers and simultaneously seek to pay lower prices. Many health care organizations have little experience competing for patients at the retail level. They are likely to lose out in the marketplace, with negative impacts on market share, revenues, and profits.
- Health care delivery organizations are already feeling wage and salary pressures from human resources who are increasingly in short supply. This is particularly true of nurses in general and physicians in certain subspecialties. Increasing trends in costs like these coupled with stagnant or very slowly growing revenues are not a formula for financial strength and high credit ratings.
- The current facilities and operating systems of health care organizations are aging and replacement or upgrade has not kept pace. These firms are merely postponing the day when major capital expenditures will be necessary to modernize their plant and equipment. This problem is further aggravated by the looming requirements for installation of electronic medical record and related systems. In the meantime, the current outdated assets only make operations more inefficient.
- All companies in the health care industry face increasing costs of compliance with the growing volume of laws and regulations, accreditation and certification requirements, that apply uniquely to health care organizations. Acquiring new systems and equipment, hiring new employees with compliance-related competencies, and retraining existing employees to compliance guidelines add costs that are not common to most other industries.
- The entire health care industry is experiencing heightened competition from more profit-driven, entrepreneurial, risk-taking businesses and executives that have moved into the health care sector of the economy. Old-line health care organizations have little history of operating in highly competitive markets and may suffer financially if they do not learn to adapt.
- Many health care organizations are still going through the process that began ten or twenty years ago of shifting from the historical cost-reimbursement "administration" of their institutions to modern, professional "management and leadership" of those same entities. To survive and to earn high credit ratings, they must learn and put into practice management principles and techniques, policies and procedures, and models and systems that have been developed and used for decades in almost all other industries. Credit rating firms look for evidence of these practices.

Internal Factors Affecting Creditworthiness

It should be of great interest to an organization to know steps that it can take to maintain the highest possible credit rating. The three leading credit rating firms are quite candid about the criteria they take into consideration in making their credit rating judgments. A business that relies regularly on the debt capital markets could not do better than to follow explicitly the standards laid down by these firms.

Strong strategic leaders and managers. The board members, senior executives, physician leaders, head researchers, and others with major roles in strategy-making must display a strategic mindset. Their thinking and decision making ranges across the full-time continuum, considering past performance, understanding what is going on in the present, and anticipating and shaping the future. They see the symbiotic potential of all the organization's component units, are sensitive to the dynamic interplay of environmental forces, customer desires and preferences, and competitor moves, and consistently view the business as affecting and at the effect of everything that goes on around it. More than anything, they understand that the future will be different from the present, and an organization that thrives today may go out of existence tomorrow—if the leaders and managers do not implement strategies to keep the organization alive and, preferably, growing.

The top executives also develop or hire people throughout the organization who are comfortable with constant change, and possess the competencies to carry out strategies and work in the new operational milieu that the organization is creating for itself.

The rating agencies expect the firm's leaders, including influential physicians and researchers, to be able to explain in some detail the strategies that they are in the process of pursuing.

Formal integrated strategic-financial planning process. The firm must conduct an ongoing planning process that simultaneously and integratively considers strategic and financial issues. Its output should be a plan that incorporates a mission, a vision, long-term objectives, specific strategies, financial projections, performance metrics, assigned responsibilities, and implementation plans. In addition to financial managers, the process will include managers from key functional areas and others who will play leading roles in strategy implementation.

The process will include a component that regularly monitors the strategies as they are being implemented to make sure that they are meeting their progress benchmarks. There should be a demonstrated ability and willingness to make changes in the strategies as environmental conditions and assumptions evolve.

The organization should be able to point to a history of well-chosen strategies that were successfully implemented. It is critical that a business demonstrate an ability competently to execute its strategic plans and achieve the desired results. The ratings firms may ask to see copies of earlier strategic plans and compare their objectives to what the business has actually been able to achieve. When an organization misses a target, the firms will ask its executives for an explanation and their proposed responses to the failure.

Thoughtful and comprehensive strategic plan. The firm is always carrying out a multi-year (five years or so) strategic plan whose primary aims are changed rarely but whose implementation/action plans may be adjusted regularly. The plan must consist of tangible steps with measurable goals that will move the organization toward realization of its vision. It should anticipate alternate futures, using tools like modeling, role playing, and simulations to describe several different scenarios. Its projections and assumptions are detailed, conservative, believable, explainable, objective, and based on evidence. The plan should define its capital needs and its long-term impact on the firm's finances as accurately as possible. It should be founded firmly in financial reality.

Strong competitive position. A highly rated business will fully comprehend its competitive position and it will be a strong one. Of particular interest will be the source of its customers-patients, their demographics and income levels, and their utilization (inpatient or outpatient) of the firm's products or services, the source of its revenues (employers, MCOs, IDSs, government payers), and its relationships with those sources. Ratings agencies want to know the firm's market position vis-à-vis its competitors. They prefer businesses with dominant market shares that have successfully differentiated themselves from the competition. If this is not currently the situation, top management should be able to describe the strategic path by which it will get there. It should be knowledgeable about its competitors' strategies and how its own differ from, and are superior to, them. If a health care delivery organization, it will have affiliated with the best physicians in the community; if a biotech firm, it will employ some of the top researchers in the field. It will have cultivated the referral loyalty of physicians as well as the treatment loyalty of patients.

Trends in all these data will be important, as indicators of momentum built up in the past that may carry forward into the future. The ratings analysts will not automatically accept the surface claims and explanations made by the firm's executives; they will dig deeper for more thorough and objective insights into market and industry dynamics.

Strong financial position and performance. This information goes to the heart of a firm's creditworthiness. The ratings agencies will be most interested in the current capital structure of the business (primarily the debt level), the free cash flow available to service the debt, and anything in its strategies that may alter that. In particular, they will ask to see financial projections, financial targets, capital budget requirements, current

Maintaining Creditworthiness While Pursuing Strategies

The interplay between a corporation's creditworthiness (debt levels) and its strategic ambitions presents executives with some difficult decisions. A business with low levels of debt has room comfortably to take on more debt and, therefore, is likely to earn itself a good bond rating. However, its long-term survival requires that it aggressively pursue competitive strategies, often marked by boldness and risk. Capital funds are needed to implement those strategies. Most health care organizations cannot generate sufficient strategic capital internally and must turn to debt capital markets. As soon as an organization begins to take on additional debt, with its principal and interest payment obligations, its credit rating can begin to drop. The fall will be aggravated the larger the amount of new debt assumed and the greater the risk involved in the strategies on which it is spent. For the strategies and their associated debt financing to make sense, they must result in increases in revenues, margins, and cash flow that more than cover the cost of servicing the debt. In that way, the strategies will have the effect of maintaining and perhaps improving the organization's creditworthiness.

The challenge for corporate management is to find strategies that, regardless of whatever else they accomplish, do not damage the business's credit rating.

Some firms have let their competitive position deteriorate to the point that only expensive, high-risk strategies seem capable of pulling them out of their predicament. To raise the debt capital needed to finance the strategies, they must let their credit ratings slide and accept the higher interest rates and other debt-issuance costs that come with that. If the strategies succeed, the firms will slowly begin to recover their creditworthiness. (It should be noted that, generally, it is harder for a business to earn an upgrade to its bond rating than it is to suffer a downgrade.) When the gamble fails, the business has nowhere else to turn, except the bankruptcy court.

capital structure, debt capital capacity, cash flow projections, and profit margin estimates.

In the analysis they perform leading up to the assignment of a bond rating, the rating firms survey a variety of financial metrics, falling mainly into three groups—debt capacity, cash flow, and profit margins. Note that these measures may or may not overlap with the financial goals that the strategies themselves are designed to achieve.

Debt Capacity

These are measures of how fully the business is using its ability to raise and pay for debt capital.

Debt service coverage—funds available from regular cash flow to make debt principal and interest payments.

Debt to equity/net assets—how much of the firm's capital comes from debt rather than equity (FP) or net assets (NFP).

Cash Flow

These are measures of how liquid an organization is, how much cash is easily available to meet debt service obligations.

Days cash on hand—an indication of how many days a business could continue operating if its cash inflow (revenues) stopped abruptly and operating expenses had to be paid solely out of cash on hand.

Cash-to-debt—the ratio between an organization's cash on hand and its debt outstanding, indicating how readily it could pay off that debt with nothing but its current cash.

Cushion ratio—a firm's unencumbered, free cash flow (not simply its cash on hand) balanced against debt service requirements (interest and principal payments).

Profit Margins

These are measures of the excess of a firm's revenues over the costs incurred in generating the revenues. In time, after "accounts payable" have been paid and "accounts receivable" received, this translates into cash flow that can be used to satisfy debt service obligations.

Operating margin—profits, as a percentage of revenues, whether selling pharmaceuticals or delivering patient services.

Excess margin—same as operating margin, plus profits (or losses) from non-core activities like capital investments (e.g., real estate) and charitable donations.

Earnings before interest, taxes, depreciation, and amortization—revenues left after covering operating expenses that could be used to meet debt interest and principal payments.

One other metric that is gaining growing importance among health care institutions as an indicator of their likely future need for debt capital is the age of their plant and equipment. The greater the average age, the more likely that imminent replacement will be necessary, calling for the issuance of additional debt.

Many of the sources of debt capital mention data like the following as important to their decisions on whether to lend money to a health care organization or purchase its bonds.

- *Patient origin*—proportion of the organization's business that comes from its primary and secondary service areas or particular geographic zones.

- *Demographics*—population, age, employment/unemployment rates, income (per capita and family), education, lifestyle.
- *Employers*—largest employers in the market, their growth rates and plans for expansion or contraction, health insurance plans provided.
- *Market share*—inpatient and outpatient care, by individual product or service line.
- *Competitors* (both health care and non-health care)—total business, individual product or service lines, and nontraditional competitors (for a hospital; ambulatory surgery centers, retail primary care clinics, and diagnostic facilities), competitive strategies followed by each.
- *Payer mix*—Medicare/Medicaid, commercial insurers, self-payers, relationships with these payers, terms of contracts with the payers, incentives offered (utilization management, quality assurance, pay-for-performance), proportion of bad debt and charity care.
- *Business, program, and service mix*—unique niches, overall balance, secondary/tertiary/quaternary services, performance and profitability by service line.
- *Physician staff*—age, primary care/specialty mix, proportion of revenue by specialty/physician, quality of relationships in referral base, loyalty, satisfaction, employment model, recruitment.
- *Employees*—nurse, administrative staff, and other employee retention strategies; turnover rates.
- *Utilization/case mix*—growth of good utilization/case mix (paying, high acuity) or bad utilization (nonpaying, low acuity), demand projections.
- *Competitive cost/charge position*—adjusted for outpatient volumes and case mix complexity, recent rate increases.
- *Consumer preferences/opinions*—based on formal surveys.

As an example of specific criteria used by rating firms, see the sidebar on the next page describing the factors considered by Standard & Poor's in assessing the creditworthiness of physician group practices.[1]

■ ALLOCATING CAPITAL FUNDS TO STRATEGIC INITIATIVES

There is never enough capital to fund all the strategic initiatives that an organization has in mind. Because capital resources are limited, they must be parceled out to the several strategies that are in the process of being implemented in a systematic way that optimizes the value created by those strategies—"value" measured by the new capital that they generate for future strategies, their positive impact on the organization's creditworthiness, and the progress they make toward realization of the organization's

Standard & Poor's Criteria for NFP Physician Group Practices

The ratings criteria used by Standard & Poor's for NFP physician group practices (primarily multi-specialty groups of 100 or more physicians) fall into eight categories. This is a summary of those criteria.

Physicians

Composition, qualifications, quantity, and quality of the group.

Physician leadership's philosophy and strategic vision.

Nature of the local physician market (practice patterns, availability of physicians for hire, group's competitive position).

Credentialing process.

Terms of employment contract used.

Top ten revenue-producing physicians (percentage of total revenues generated, age, and tenure), board certification rates, additions/deletions to staff in past three years.

Operations

History of the group and its organizational structure.

Likelihood that the group will remain viable for the life of the bonds.

Evidence of a competitive business position, sound balance sheet, and a history of adequate cash flow and debt service coverage.

Ongoing strategy and its appeal to physicians in the future.

Market position and breadth of patient draw.

Relationship with other medical entities.

Current physical assets and proposed future capital needs.

Debt structure including use of bond proceeds.

Competition

Physician competitors for patients (solo practitioners, groups, and hospitals).

Non-physician competitors seeking to provide medical services directly to patients (hospitals, ambulatory care, surgery, and emergency centers; HMOs and insurance companies).

Breadth and nature of managed care contracts and relationships.

Leadership (involves meetings with physician and non-physician managers)

Strategic goals of physicians and management, and their consistency with each other.

Strength of board leadership (includes community representatives in balance with group physicians).

(*continues*)

Standard & Poor's Criteria for NFP Physician Group Practices (continued)

Management's tenure, qualifications, and experience in running physician group practices.

Strategic planning issues.

Compensation, financial, and operating policies.

Institutional Relationships

Formal and informal relationships that exist with hospitals, universities, insurance companies, and other payers.

Information Systems

Plans for development of an EMR system.

Ability to measure and satisfy any quality metrics that are part of its reimbursement agreements.

Ability to generate reports from its information system on managed care member profiles, benefit plans, utilization rates, and cost per-member per-month (PMPM); encounters per FTE physician; hospital inpatient use rate and cost PMPM versus regional averages; revenue and expense by physician, payer, and service; clinical outliers and out-of-area utilization; and physician profiling reports suitable for pay-for-performance purposes.

Finances

Five years of audited financial statements.

Utilization information (patient visits, new patient growth, covered lives, encounters per physician).

Payer mix as percentage of revenues.

Overhead levels and allocation.

Physician compensation.

Sources of revenue from outside payers, and from clinical departments and research.

Trends in accounts receivable and collection rates.

Adequacy of malpractice reserves.

Strategic and routine capital needs.

Legal Covenants

Restrictive covenants and bond financing agreements (liquidity, debt-service reserve funds, physician salaries subordinated to bond repayment).

This summary is based on the publication "Public Finance Criteria: Physician Groups and Faculty Practice Plans," found at www2.standardandpoors.com/portal/site/sp/en/us/page.article/2,1,1,4,1148445424815.html (accessed June 28, 2007).

mission. An ability effectively to allocate capital for strategic purposes may be a source of some competitive advantage for a firm.

Traditional, Less-Effective Methods of Capital Allocation

A surprising number of health care organizations employ capital allocation methods that have developed without challenge over the years and do not reflect modern professional financial management. These are a few approaches to avoid.

Strategic project backed by the most influential manager or physician. In some organizations, a culture of personal power dominates. This can result in capital requests from the most influential or powerful individuals being given higher priority. It is not uncommon for patient care organizations to seek to please physicians, either employees or medical staff, who are the source of large numbers of patients.

To departments/units at the same levels as last year. One way to avoid upsetting the several departments or SBUs that may be requesting financing for their strategic initiatives and making difficult decisions about the merits of those initiatives is to spread the available capital among the units in the same proportions as in previous years. The problem is that a department or SBU that had the most attractive strategy proposals a year ago may have less interesting ideas this year.

In the order they are received. Under this approach, a single, large, all-purpose capital budget is established at the beginning of each year, and strategy proposals are simply funded in the order that they are received, until the budget runs out. No serious analysis of the proposals is performed, and those sponsors able to submit their proposals early in the funding cycle are rewarded. The earliest proposals are not necessarily the best or the best for the company.

There are other methodologies even less logical than these. Although none of them has a place in responsible strategic management, they all display a further flaw worth discussing. They do not evaluate the individual strategies, or a group of them considered as a package, for their contributions to the business's mission and other long-term objectives. They provide no assurance that the limited capital funds are being spent in ways at all beneficial to the business.

Guidelines for a Modern, Businesslike Process for Financing Strategy Proposals

There is ample experience with effective strategic capital allocation among many U.S. business corporations, including some enlightened companies in the health care and biotechnology industries, to be able to describe the basic elements of a modern allocation system.

The allocation of capital funds should be integrated with the formulation of strategic plans, not conducted independently after the plans have been proposed and approved. This feature is essential. Without it, there is a risk of approving strategies for which there are insufficient capital funds or which, taken together, do not enhance but in fact damage the firm's creditworthiness. Professional financial managers must be involved in the strategy-making process from the very beginning.

To facilitate its financial analysis, a formal business plan should be prepared for each strategy being proposed. The plan may not be especially elaborate for strategies seeking more modest levels of financing, a few hundreds of thousands of dollars, for instance. When the strategy costs run into the millions of dollars, the business plan should resemble what an entrepreneur might present to a venture capital firm from which he was seeking startup capital. This means including the standard financial components—multiyear projections of revenues, profits, and cash flow, stated on a monthly basis for the first year or two.

There should be agreement within the organization that strategy decisions will be based on objective evidence of each strategy's contribution to the firm's long-term financial and nonfinancial objectives. Deviations from the systematic strategy formulation process and the criteria should not be allowed. In particular, the influence of the individuals backing a strategy or the sheer volume of capital funds that a strategy sponsor may have received in the past should not be considered. If a strategy must be selected for subjective, qualitative reasons, at the sacrifice of financial metrics, the decision should be made explicitly, acknowledging the compromises being made.

Every strategy proposal should be subjected to rigorous scientific analysis using modern corporate financial management techniques that take into account the time value of money, the cost of capital, and the risk inherent in each strategy. The same methodology is applied to all strategy proposals to ensure that the calculations made and the conclusions reached can be compared across all proposals.

The allocation approach that best meets these requirements relies on net present value (NPV) analysis. NPV measures the cash inflows and outflows associated with the strategy then uses a "discount rate" (composed of the cost of capital plus an allowance for the risk involved in the strategy) to calculate the present value of all the cash flows that occur beyond the first year.

A business can rank several strategy proposals by the NPV that they generate and allocate capital to them in that order until none is left. It may also take into account other factors (financial and nonfinancial) by assigning weights to each factor, scoring each strategy for how well it satisfies each factor, multiplying the weights by the scores, and adding the results to get a grand total score for the strategy. Those overall scores are then compared among all proposed strategies. Those receiving the highest grand scores receive capital funding.

A challenge of strategic resource allocation is deciding how many proposals to review at one time. Consider these two extremes.

One at a time, at various times throughout the year. Each strategy is evaluated and funded or not whenever the proposal documents are complete. Much of the time, this will result in strategies being reviewed one at a time, without an opportunity for simultaneous comparison with other strategies. The advantage and disadvantage of this approach lies in the fact that strategy proposals are not always ripe for review at the same times. Conditions warranting the implementation of a new strategy arise at unpredictable intervals. Some strategy proposals take longer to prepare.

An allocation system that can accommodate strategy proposals at any time allows a business to take advantage of opportunities, or react to threats, spontaneously. Such organizations are more strategically nimble, more likely to catch their competitors off guard. The problems with one-at-a-time, whenever-the-proposal-is-ready systems are that the proposals that come in first may not be the best strategies that will be proposed that year. Even if the early proposals are pretty good, they will consume all the available capital, leaving none for much better ones that come along later. That is why most strategic management scholars recommend looking at batches of strategy proposals.

Once a year, in a single large bundle of proposals. In order to review a large batch of strategy proposals at one time, it usually is necessary to put on hold some proposals that have been completed, speed up the preparation of others, and generally wait until a large-enough number of finished proposals has been accumulated. The question is how many proposals must be in a batch for a balanced review of a firm's strategic options, how long a completed proposal should be kept waiting while a minimum batch is assembled, and how often will such batch reviews and allocation of resources take place? The major handicap of this approach is that spontaneity is lost—much of the force of a strategy may be weakened by delaying its implementation.

There are ways to moderate the disadvantages of these two extremes. Most companies settle on something in the middle, requiring batches, but smaller batches reviewed at more frequent intervals, perhaps with some room for evaluating and funding on short notice strategy proposals that are especially attractive.

It is important that the organization and its key managers commit themselves to following the allocation system adopted whenever capital funds must be devoted to strategic purposes. Implicit in this pledge is that the strategic decision makers and implementers are well tutored in the principles of modern, systematic resource allocation, and that the functioning of the system and the resulting decisions are fully communicated to those affected by them.

■ TRACKING THE FINANCIAL PERFORMANCE OF NEW STRATEGIES

The integrity of proficient financial management requires that capital resource allocation be followed by a mechanism for monitoring the implementation and performance of the chosen strategies, and making adjustments when necessary. The full scope of this function is explained in Chapter 10. As that chapter makes clear, effective strategic management requires more than periodic spasms of effort that produce elaborate plans that are then set on a course to implementation without much further attention. The true "management" of strategy requires watching it closely and constantly, making sure it is on course or deciding to plot a new course, and being willing to make appropriate changes at any time.

There are good reasons for a firm's financial managers to monitor financial metrics in three slightly different areas: the very long-term financial goals that the firm is pursuing to meet the needs of its major stakeholders (shareholders, insurance company regulators), the financial criteria important to maintain the firm's creditworthiness, and specific financial targets associated with the individual strategies being implemented. For instance, shareholders may be looking for general increases in revenues and profits that drive up market prices of their shares, or sufficient free cash flow to allow the business to pay out dividends. The state agency regulating the operation of insurance-type companies (health insurers, HMOs, managed care organizations) will focus on the maintenance of reserves against unanticipated losses or payouts to beneficiaries or members. As mentioned earlier, creditors and rating agencies pay particular attention to cash flow, debt capacity, and profit metrics. The financial objectives of a specific strategy might include increasing sales in selected market segments, reducing manufacturing costs to a level that would permit pursuit of a low-cost leadership competitive strategy, or aiming for higher cash flow levels in certain more mature SBUs of a corporate portfolio in order to subsidize the lower cash flows in other SBUs that are at earlier stages in their life cycles.

With this information in hand, the financial managers are in a position to draw conclusions about the effects of the strategies-in-progress on the future fiscal viability of the business. This leads to concrete recommendations for adjustments to the strategies to increase the chances that all of these financial objectives will be achieved.

COMMON MISTAKES IN STRATEGIC FINANCIAL MANAGEMENT

As an indication of practices to avoid, these are some of the ways that businesses, particularly in the health care industry, mismanage the financial component of strategic planning and management.

Failing to integrate the strategic planning and capital allocation process. Strategic plans without a foundation in the firm's financial strength and potential can lead to overspending, wasting available capital, damaging creditworthiness, and failing to meet strategic targets. Financial plans without an awareness of strategic initiatives may miss both competitive opportunities and threats and fail thereby to protect the firm's long-term financial strength.

Defaulting from a strategic financial planning process to a budgeting process. This occurs when the strategic planning process lacks a capital allocation component. Because annual budgets have a shorter time perspective than three- to five-year strategic plans, their allocation of capital funds does not adequately optimize the long-term well-being of the organization.

Spending more on strategic initiatives than is justified by the strategies' financial prospects and the organization's credit rating. When a business persistently borrows money to spend on strategic projects that do not generate acceptable, preferably above-average, returns, it eventually will use up its capital reserves, suffer bond rating downgrades, and fall into financial crisis.

Failing to thoughtfully manage the organization's capital structure. An organization that does not consciously and intelligently manage the proportions of different types of debt and equity in its capital structure is quite likely to pay higher costs for the capital it consumes and have less access to the amounts that its strategies require.

Inadequately monitoring strategic financial performance. Without an effective mechanism for monitoring strategic financial performance, there is a good chance that the invested capital will be wasted, the strategies will fail to achieve their objectives, revenues and profits will suffer, cash flow will prove inadequate, and financial weakness will develop.

Study Questions

1. Money is the lifeblood of any organization—for-profit, not-for-profit, or public. In most for-profit corporations, maximizing sales and profits, and returns to shareholders, is the primary objective. Many have criticized the health care industry for its growing fixation on profit maximization, claiming that health care should be treated as a "social good" rather than a "commercial good." How can the

leaders of health care organizations reconcile these two positions? How do high-level executives manage the tradeoffs between maintaining the fiscal solvency of their organizations and providing health care services to all who seek them?

2. Explain the different preferences that an organization might have for debt versus equity financing. Should all its financing come from one source or the other? If it is going to rely on both debt and equity, what criteria should determine the proportions of each capital source that it uses? Are the answers to these questions different if the organization is NFP rather than FP?
3. Imagine that you are the founder and CEO of a one-year-old biotech research firm that is making significant progress toward development of a new drug with high commercial potential. You have run through the initial capital with which you started the business and have begun negotiating with private investors and venture capital firms for the additional financing that you need to continue operations. All of them are insisting upon majority ownership positions in the business in return for investing the money that you need. It pains you to think about surrendering control of the business that you have built from almost nothing. How do you decide how much control you are willing to trade for investment capital? What are some of the factors that enter into an entrepreneur's decision-making at this critical point in a new venture's history?
4. During the strategy formulation process, what benefits result from the participation of a business's financial managers? What detriments may occur if they do not participate?

Learning Exercise 1

The three primary credit rating agencies, Standard & Poor's, Fitch, and Moody's, regularly announce when they are upgrading or downgrading an organization's credit rating. Identify one of those organizations whose rating has gone down, preferably one that you are already familiar with. Do some extended research to discover the reasons for that downgrade. Read the explanation given by the rating agency. Collect data on the organization's financial performance over the past few years—from annual reports and SEC 10-K filings. What changes in the financial metrics led to the downgrade? What were the apparent causes of those changes? Were those causes within the control of the organization or not? If the organization did have control, what could or should it have done differently? Which of the causes were related to the organization's strategies?

Learning Exercise 2

Identify a venture capital firm in your local area that invests in new health care or biotech ventures. If there are none that specialize in that way, choose any venture capital firm. Interview one of the firm's partners who makes decisions about which ventures the firm will invest in and on what terms. Use the interview to learn what criteria the firm looks for in a new venture, at what point in the venture's history it prefers to make investments, how it decides how much money to invest, and what terms it demands in return from the venture's owners. How closely does the firm monitor the performance of the ventures in its investment portfolio? What steps is it willing to take when that performance does not measure up to its expectations?

Notes

[1] For comparison purposes, look also at Standard & Poor's points of inquiry for not-for-profit freestanding hospitals and multi-hospital systems at www2.standardandpoors.com/portal/site/sp/en/us/page.article/2,1,1,4,1148445424815.htm l (accessed June 28, 2007) and the U.S. Health Insurance and Managed Care Rating Criteria used by Fitch Ratings at www.fitchratings.com/corporate/reports/report_frame.cfm?rpt_id=317228§or_flag=4&marketsector=1&detail= (accessed June 28, 2007).

References

Baker JJ and Baker RW. *Health Care Finance, Basic Tools for Nonfinancial Managers*. 2nd ed. Sudbury, MA: Jones and Bartlett; 2006.

Berger S. *The Power of Clinical and Financial Metrics, Achieving Success in Your Hospital*. Chicago, IL: Health Administration Press; 2005.

Gapenski LC. *Healthcare Finance for the Non-Financial Manager*. Chicago, IL: Irwin Professional Publishing; 1994.

Kaufman K. *Best Practice Financial Management: Six Key Concepts for Healthcare Leaders*. 3rd ed. Chicago, IL: Health Administration Press; 2006.

Narayanan MP and Nanda VK. *Finance for Strategic Decision Making*. San Francisco, CA: Jossey-Bass; 2004.

Nowicki ML. *The Financial Management of Hospitals and Healthcare Organizations*. 3rd ed. Chicago, IL: Health Administration Press; 2004.

O'Brien JP. The capital structure implications of pursuing a strategy of innovation. *Strategic Management Journal*. 2003;24(5):415–422.

Sussman JH. *The Healthcare Executive's Guide to Allocating Capital*. Chicago, IL: Health Administration Press; 2007.

Wrightson CW Jr. *Financial Strategy for Managed Care Organizations, Rate Setting, Risk Adjustment, and Competitive Advantage*. Chicago, IL: Health Administration Press; 2002.

Zelman WN, McCue MJ, Milliken AR, and Glick ND. Financial management of health care organizations: An introduction to fundamental tools, concepts, and applications. 2nd ed. Boston, MA: Blackwell; 2005.

CHAPTER

12

Strategy in Other Types of Organizations

Twenty years ago, management was a dirty word for those involved in nonprofit organizations. It meant business, and nonprofits prided themselves on being free of the taint of commercialism and above such sordid considerations as the bottom line. Now most of them have learned that nonprofits need management even more than business does, precisely because they lack the discipline of the bottom line.

—P. F. Drucker[1]

Learning Objectives

After reading and studying this chapter, you should be able to:

- Comprehend the diverse types of organizations that make up the health care and biotechnology industries, with specific examples of the dominant types—NFP organizations, public government agencies, and entrepreneurial new ventures and startups, in addition to FP corporations.
- Explain the benefits of formal strategic planning and management to each of the three dominant organizational types.
- Describe the features that distinguish each of the three types from the traditional FP corporate model.
- Give the reasons why and how the basic strategy management principles must be adapted for each different organizational type.
- Lay out a model strategic planning and management process for each organizational type.
- Provide examples of actual strategies that might be pursued by each type of organization.

The bulk of this book's recommended strategic management practices and principles is aimed at good-sized FP corporations, many of them composed of multiple SBUs. However, there is a variety of other organizational types, quite prevalent in the health care industry, that call for different approaches to strategic planning and management.

Beyond health care, there is no other industry composed of such a diverse mixture of large for-profit corporations, small "mom-and-pop" businesses, entrepreneurial new ventures, large not-for-profit organizations, small not-for-profit organizations, partnerships and professional corporations, and federal, state, and municipal government agencies. These are some of the examples in each category.

- *Large for-profit corporations*—health insurance companies, managed care organizations, multi-hospital networks, and pharmaceutical companies.
- *Small "mom-and-pop" businesses*—medical transcription businesses, IT vendors and technical support, home health providers.
- *Entrepreneurial new ventures*—biotech research startups, innovative medical device ventures, health-related IT ventures.
- *Large not-for-profit organizations*—major teaching hospitals, Blue Cross/Blue Shield insurance companies, national disease-focused associations, health care-oriented charitable foundations, think tanks, and clinical research institutes.
- *Small not-for-profit organizations*—patient advocacy groups, neighborhood health clinics.
- *Partnerships and professional corporations*—physician solo and group practices.
- *Federal government agencies*—provider reimbursement for health care delivery, legal regulation of health care industry structure and operations, sponsorship and conduct of bioscience/biomedical research.
- *State government agencies*—provider reimbursement, regulation of health care organizations, monitoring and management of public health, and sponsorship of public health programs.
- *Municipal government agencies*—ownership and operation of provider facilities (city hospitals and neighborhood health centers), regulation of public health practices in the private sector.

Three of these categories play especially prominent roles in health care: NFP organizations, public/government agencies, and entrepreneurial startups/new ventures. Many of the strategic management principles throughout the book can be applied to all three of these organizational types. What follows are exceptions and adjustments that must be made to accommodate their unique features.

Not-for-profit (NFP) organizations. These entities are established under state nonprofit incorporation laws. Invariably, they apply for and receive some form of tax-exempt status from the federal Internal Revenue Service (IRS), most often under section 501(c)(3) of the U.S. tax code. In return for focusing its activities on certain charitable purposes, the organization is exempted from paying most forms of tax, including income, sales, and property taxes. In addition, individuals and organizations that donate money to these entities may deduct the donations from their own income taxes. The tax exemption saves the organization the money that it would otherwise have paid in taxes. The tax deductibility encourages charitable contributions to the organization.

Among the purposes to which exempt organizations must be dedicated are charitable, educational, and scientific. The term "charitable" is defined to include relief of the poor, the distressed, or the underprivileged; advancement of education or science; and lessening the burdens of government.

Not-for-profit organizations are a major presence in the health care industry. Though their percentages are declining, they are found among acute care hospitals (60 percent),[2] health maintenance organizations (26 percent), nursing homes (34 percent), home health agencies (51 percent), and substance abuse treatment center facilities (76 percent).[3] There is also a variety of other "human service" organizations, virtually all nonprofit, whose activities border at many points on the health care field.

Some of these not-for-profits look and function like for-profits. The vast majority of teaching hospitals in the country, many of them large, well-managed enterprises, are nonprofits. Kaiser Permanente, one of the oldest, largest HMOs in the country, is a nonprofit. Yet, when observing its operating methods and style, and its behavior in the marketplace, it is almost impossible to distinguish it from profit-driven entities. One reason is that any organization of the size and complexity of a major teaching hospital or an HMO with more than eight million members must operate at the highest levels of management proficiency. Many of these organizations are also in highly competitive markets. The most altruistic, mission-driven nonprofit must adopt more aggressive practices if just one for-profit business enters its market. When several substantial nonprofits share a market, as teaching hospitals do in Boston, they usually compete with each other like for-profits. All these organizations need to plan and manage their long-term strategies like a Fortune 500 corporation.

Things are different for smaller NFP health care/human service organizations that do not face obvious competition. This category may include provider organizations like small community health centers or clinics operating in low-income or rural areas. It also encompasses a variety of organizations engaged in representing the interests of certain constituencies (American Medical Association, American Hospital Association, American Association of Health Plans), rating and certifying the performance of provider organizations (Joint Commission on Accreditation of Healthcare Organizations, National Committee for Quality Assurance), working for the elimination of specific diseases (American Lung Association, National Multiple Sclerosis Society, National Alliance for the Mentally Ill), advocating for system reform (Health Care for All, National Coalition on Health Care, Center for Studying Health System Change), and funding or conducting health care research (Robert Wood Johnson Foundation, Center for Science in the Public Interest).

Public/government agencies. These organizations are in a different legal class from FP and NFP corporations. These are units of the political establishment that maintains order and provides for the welfare of all the residents of its jurisdiction. They exist at several different levels throughout the country, including federal/national, state, county, and municipal. The sizes of their workforces range from two million people in the federal government to just a handful in the smallest rural towns. The annual federal budget is more than $2 trillion while some towns and villages have no more than a few tens of thousands of dollars to spend each year.

Public agencies do not rely on shareholders to buy their stock or charitable givers voluntarily to make contributions. The bulk of their revenues are the product of taxes imposed involuntarily on individuals and businesses within the government's jurisdiction. Taxpayers may influence their tax rates by voting for or against members of the legislative branch of the government. They may also communicate to those legislators their preferences for the types of agencies and programs to be funded from the tax revenues.

In the health care field, public agencies have taken on several major roles. The federal Center for Medicare and Medicaid Services and the fifty state-level agencies that manage the state Medicaid component directly reimburse providers for the delivery of services to Medicare and Medicaid beneficiaries. The National Institutes of Health is a major source of funding for medical and biomedical research, in addition to the research it conducts on its own. Several federal government agencies are responsible for enforcing laws that apply to different aspects of health care organization operations: the IRS watches over tax matters, particularly as they apply to tax-exempt entities; the Antitrust Division of the Department of Justice monitors anti-competitive behavior within the health care industry; and the Office of the Inspector General in the Department of Health and Human Services works to prevent fraud, waste, and abuse in the industry. Many states have similar agencies performing comparable enforcement functions.

Entrepreneurial startups/new ventures. These are FP corporations at their moment of birth. They are created by men and women who intend to grow them to considerable size as rapidly as possible, with the expectation that they personally will be able to earn a great deal of money either through appreciation of their ownership interest in the business or sale of the business to another corporation. They are willing to assume great risks in the pursuit of their vision—risk of the loss of their financial investments in the venture, risk of failure and collapse of the business itself, and risk of personal failure.

The venture may be based on a product or service concept that exists only in the founders' imagination, or on an idea or technology that has been tested in the early stages of research or development in a laboratory. The initial financial capital for the business may come entirely from the founders and their friends; if the initial concept shows promise, angel investors may be found to provide seed capital. Either way, ventures like these typically consume money at a rapid rate and require several successive rounds of additional investment before stable growth is achieved.

The founders of new ventures frequently have minimal prior managerial experience. A strong strategic mindset may be completely lacking. With luck and determination, and by accepting advice from more business-savvy mentors, however, the business can be built to a state of relative stability. Bill Gates and Steve Jobs aside, the point eventually is reached where the company requires the skills of more sophisticated and experienced leaders if it is to continue growing. The founders must step aside.

Rivaled only by the broader high-technology industry, the health care industry is one of the most fertile grounds for entrepreneurial startups and new ventures—in its biomedical, bioscience, and biotechnology subsectors.[4] The classic model is a researcher at a university, teaching hospital, or medical center who makes what he considers to be a scientific breakthrough with commercial product potential. Alone or with a few partners, after securing the intellectual property rights to the breakthrough and gathering sufficient initial capital, he creates an independent FP corporation for the purpose of developing the potential. The projected output of the venture may be a completed product ready for the end-user market or a concept or component that will be used by another business in developing its own finished products. An example of this is biotech research companies that do early-stage drug development that is then passed on to larger pharmaceutical companies for commercialization. One of the distinguishing features of this category of organizations is their emphasis on innovative science and technologies, leading to innovative products, and employing innovative business practices when necessary.

Two other types of organization are worth mentioning in passing—small businesses of a less-than-entrepreneurial nature, and partnerships/professional corporations frequently employed by physician groups. The general model of "small business" is a significant factor throughout the U.S. economy, and no less so in the health care sector. Both small businesses and entrepreneurial startups may look similar at the outset; their differences have to do with the long-term ambitions of their founders. In contrast with entrepreneurs who have a passionate desire to introduce bold new products to the marketplace, a willingness to take great risks in the process, and the hope of earning great financial rewards in the end, *small business* owners usually wish only to establish their firms and grow them to a size that will support them and their families. Rather than offering innovative new products, they are likely to enter well-established market niches with room for additional small competitors. Because of their modest size and ambitions, they are not seen as a threat to existing businesses in the market. A good example of this organizational type might be a medical transcription business serving a handful of physician practices.

While a growing number of physicians are directly employed by hospitals or health plans, most of them are still gathered into solo or group practices using the legal form of a *partnership or professional corporation*. Many are relatively small entities, comprising less than ten physicians and twice that number of clerical and clinical staff. In many ways, they function like the small businesses mentioned above. The physician-owners have not set ambitious growth objectives for their practices; they often are quite happy if their operations generate revenues and income that meet their personal needs. There is also a subgroup of large multispecialty group practices that may include several hundred physicians. They tend to have a substantial administrative infrastructure and a professional, experienced team of managers. These organizations usually take a strategic attitude about their position in the market for physician services. The strategic planning and management principles of medium-sized FP corporations can be applied to them.

BENEFITS OF STRATEGIC PLANNING FOR NFP ORGANIZATIONS, GOVERNMENT AGENCIES, AND NEW VENTURES

The basic argument for carrying out some kind of strategic planning, no matter how constrained, is just as relevant to all these other organizational types as it is to large for-profit corporations. If they do not have some sense of the long-term direction in which the organization is headed, they are likely to wander all over the competitive landscape, wasting their resources along the way. When those resources are more limited to begin with, anything that might preserve and extend them is worth considering.

An organization's performance, measured by whatever metrics it chooses, financial or nonfinancial, will be significantly improved by a strategic outlook. It would be a mistake to believe that strategic management has meaning only for organizations that measure their success in dollars. It is just as useful for a disease-focused advocacy group whose mission is to reduce the incidence of the disease, or a municipal public health agency that is aiming to improve the level of neonatal care to teenage mothers.

Many of these organizations devote most of their energies to serving their clients. Performing a strategic planning function helps them think about how well they are satisfying their other constituencies, particularly their revenue sources. The net effect is to increase their chances of long-run success and outright survival.

After completing such a process, the organization will be left with a much more complete understanding of the strategic issues that it faces, even if it does not use the term "strategic" to describe them.

Participation in strategic planning compels the organization's managers to recognize and evaluate a variety of factors, both within and without the organization, that determine how well it will be able to carry out its mission. Over time, the managers develop a form of "systems thinking" enabling them to see how intertwined their success is with that of numerous other stakeholders.

Completion of even a modest strategic planning process will give the organization a wealth of new strategic knowledge. With this new awareness, it will instinctively become more innovative in its operating practices.

In the competition for capital from various funding sources, whether a legislative body, a charitable foundation, or a venture capital firm, an organization's practice of professional strategic management principles will carry great weight. Such an organization is more likely to obtain the funding it needs to pay for its operations and strategic initiatives.

NFP ORGANIZATIONS

Organizations in the NFP category typically are founded for passionate ideological/charitable purposes that have little to do with maximizing revenues and income. In fact, it sometimes is a challenge to persuade NFP staff to pay attention to the business aspects of their organizations, not to mention the strategic dimensions of what they are trying to accomplish.

In many cases, the funding for NFP organizations comes from sources that are not the direct beneficiaries of their services. Such sources may include individual donors, charitable foundations, and government grants. The interests and demands of those various revenue sources can change unpredictably from one year to the next. The organization must keep one eye on the needs of these important stakeholders while simultaneously fulfilling its own altruistic vision. There is vigorous competition among like-minded NFP organizations for the limited funds that these sources have to give. It is not uncommon for an organization to become dependent on the charity of one particular donor only to suffer a financial calamity when the donor changes the focus of its giving. Most modest-sized NFP organizations lack sufficient creditworthiness to be able to borrow significant amounts of capital.

Occasionally funding is provided on a somewhat more reliable multiyear basis. Quite often, however, the funding must be renewed annually and simply cannot be counted upon. This can make it difficult to embark upon any capital-intensive long-range projects. Furthermore, it places a premium upon the organization's leaders' ability to cultivate and maintain positive relationships with its funders.

The one key exception to this limited mix of funding sources are major teaching hospitals and some health plans. These important components of the U.S. health care system are able to rely extensively on revenues from the patients they treat, although most of them come through third-party payers, and on significant amounts of debt. Nonetheless, due to the "public interest" altruistic nature of NFP organizations, they cannot be privately owned and therefore have no access to the equity capital that is a major source of financing for FP corporations. Apart from that capital financing limitation, these entities normally should be following the general strategic management principles of FP corporations.

If NFP organizations can maintain a fairly steady stream of revenue from their funders, they have an advantage over FP organizations that are beholden to shareholders demanding dividend payments or capital gains. Charitable donors have performance expectations of the recipients of their money, but they are usually more forgiving than investors in FP corporations.

In addition to competing with other NFP corporations for funding, a charitable organization may also be vying with them for clients and volunteers. It may seem anomalous and wasteful for such well-meaning entities to fight with each other for customers, but that is exactly what happens with some social service agencies and certainly with NFP hospitals operating in the same market area. In addition, some of these organizations are very reliant on the work of volunteers—common citizens who have a choice of organizations to which they will contribute their services.

In trying to demonstrate performance and progress to their clients and revenue sources, public agencies and NFP organizations will often try to identify objective criteria. This can be rather difficult. For instance, a lot of research is being conducted in the search for metrics of health care quality. How to measure the effectiveness of a hospice program for dying AIDS patients? How to evaluate the success of an organization whose mission is to create universal access to the health care system? Is it possible, is it acceptable, in some cases to pursue long-term goals that cannot be quantified or even measured with much precision?

Measures of success are important both for internal performance management purposes and for satisfying an organization's funders. There are relatively few appropriate financial metrics. Two that stand out are the shares of total revenues devoted to substantive program purposes and to fund-raising purposes, and the salaries of top executives. Otherwise, the standards of performance are nonfinancial and often unquantifiable. The best recommendation probably is to use quantitative measures when they are available and make sense. When the goals that are being pursued are truly subjective and amorphous, it may be possible to communicate success through anecdotes and case studies. Funding sources that share the same concerns as the organization usually understand the difficulties in measurement.

One of the hurdles to vigorous strategic management in NFP organizations is the tradition of large governing boards composed of diverse community representatives relatively inexperienced in business or strategic thinking. Sometimes, state NFP law requires such board composition. Efforts to reach a consensus on mission, vision, and specific strategies can take a long time and result in "lowest common denominator" decisions.

The external environments in which NFP organizations and public agencies operate are changing just as rapidly as they are for FP corporations, though perhaps not quite as dramatically. The interests of citizens in various causes and their willingness to donate to them can change unpredictably. It sometimes is possible to establish more reliable giving relationships with charitable foundations, though their priorities and available funds can also vary from year to year. Not-for-profit organizations not engaged in health care delivery or financing are subject to fewer legal constraints, but the IRS always shows a keen interest in the organization's adherence to the charitable purposes upon which its tax-exempt status is based. More recently, legislative and administrative officials at federal, state, and county levels have become concerned that NFP hospitals are showing less regard for their charitable purposes as demonstrated by aggressive debt collection practices, extensive sharing of hospital assets with private physician groups and other FP entities, and inadequate free or discounted medical care for uninsured patients.

Adjustments/Adaptations to Basic Strategic Management Principles

There is little doubt that few NFP organizations have an existing pool of resources and competencies as large as that possessed by a good-sized FP corporation. Nor are they in a strong position to expand the pool. They do not have access to equity capital markets. They frequently lack the collateral or creditworthiness needed to borrow money. While they can become more competent and aggressive at fund-raising, they are still reliant on the discretionary generosity of others. Staff members of NFP organizations can be quite adept at the tasks they perform, but they rarely have the sophisticated training and experience of managers in FP corporations. It is not surprising if they do not have an appreciation for the value of strategic planning and management.

For organizations that do not face anything like the ferocity of competition encountered in profit-driven industries, NFP entities are particularly fragile. If a customer needs the product or service offered by an FP corporation and likes the value that it offers, he or she will purchase the item, adding to its revenues. The sources of funding for most NFP organizations, individuals and charitable foundations, do not "need" the activities of those organizations. They may care about the mission of the organization and they may be impressed with its efficiency in pursuing that mission, but their continued financial support is ephemeral. When an individual's income declines or expenses rise, charitable giving is usually one of the first budget items to be sacrificed.

If an NFP organization's mission is cause-based, what happens when it accomplishes its strategic goals? As an example, the American Lung Association has struggled somewhat in its fund-raising as a result of its past effectiveness in combating smoking and its contribution to lung disease. Perhaps there's nothing wrong with acknowledging that an organization has accomplished what it set out to do and cheerfully discontinuing its operations. More likely, the organization subtly adjusts its mission to focus on a different but related cause.

The board of trustees of the NFP organization represents the interests of the general public in the types of altruistic work that it is doing. These interests are often hard to define and to measure. They are not selfish interests, in the sense that citizens are looking for capital appreciation or dividend payments. In fact, because NFP board members frequently come from disparate backgrounds in an effort to reflect a cross-section of the general public, the views of each of them about the mission of the organization will differ. This not only makes it hard to satisfy all of them, it also complicates the efforts to reach consensus on strategic proposals.

Because NFP organizations are so dependent on often unpredictable flows of revenue, because their clients may be receiving services for free and are not in a position to complain, and because the beneficial effects of their operations are often difficult to measure, there is a tendency to focus on the needs of the funders over the needs of the clients. In other words, these organizations pay more attention to their inputs than to their outputs. This may be inevitable in the nature of NFP organizations, but the imbalance is worth acknowledging.

Complex and passionate values typically drive the mission and activities of NFP organizations—to a much greater extent than is true for FP corporations. The effect of this pattern is that stakeholders of NFP organizations, including staff, clients, and funders, can develop somewhat irrational attitudes about the running of the organizations. This can make it hard to introduce objective, businesslike principles and practices to such organizations.

Model Strategic Planning and Management Process

The guidelines recommended for strategic planning and management in an NFP organization are somewhat different from those followed in an FP corporation.

1. Be clear on the one or more good reasons why the organization is going to embark upon strategic planning. See the list of good reasons for NFP strategic planning above.
2. Establish that the executive director of the organization is firmly behind the strategic planning effort, and will use his authority and influence to see it through to implementation. If that person's unequivocal commitment is not present, do not even begin the process.
3. Designate a leader for the strategic planning initiative, if that person is not already obvious. The leader will guide the effort and keep it moving forward, not make independent strategic decisions outside the planning group. He may or may not be the one who actually facilitates the strategic planning meetings.
4. Define and agree upon a planning process, in all its steps, that is suited to the organization and its circumstances. Do not copy another organization's planning process or use one taken from a book. Those may be starting points that are then adapted and tailored to the organization.
5. Acknowledge from the beginning that the primary benefit from this process is likely to be in the process itself (information gathered, issues identified, dialogue among managers and staff) rather than whatever plan emerges. If the process can be followed to completion, the participants will come to realize that.
6. Because of the more modest size of many NFP organizations, there is an opportunity to involve literally the entire staff in the strategic planning process. The payoffs from this can be tremendous, in terms of loyalty to the organization and commitment to the plan. This is an option not available to large FP corporations.
7. The broad public charitable mission of most NFP organizations also suggests the possibility of using the strategic planning process as an opportunity to at least consult with, if not actually involve, a wide range of stakeholders in charting the organization's future. While retaining in the board of trustees and top managers the authority to make the final strategic decisions, representatives of the organization's various constituencies may be asked to contribute to the plan's formulation.

8. Bring in a facilitator experienced in working with not-for-profit groups in conducting strategic planning. This is particularly true if none of the group's leaders themselves have gone through a strategic planning process. It may even be a good idea if they have, because it allows the facilitator to take responsibility for overseeing the process while the leaders, managers, and other staff concentrate on their substantive participation.
9. Have a staff member knowledgeable about the organization and its internal workings and external environment prepare a roughly ten-page draft of a SWOT (strengths, weaknesses, opportunities, threats) analysis. Circulate the draft among managers and staff and encourage them to freely add their comments and insights. This is a much abbreviated version of what larger corporations are able to do in a far more expanded form, as described in Chapters 2–5.
10. Schedule a formal meeting of several hours for the purpose of carrying out the strategic planning process. The traditional practice of conducting the meeting at a comfortable off-site location separate from the workplace, where interruptions can be minimized, is a good idea if the organization can afford it.

Examples of Strategies

For those health care NFP organizations that compete in industries and markets against FP corporations, such as hospitals in major metropolitan areas and managed care organizations, the most plausible and unavoidable strategies are likely to be those described throughout this book for profit-driven entities. Indeed, those organizations may face the most daunting strategic challenges of any businesses anywhere in the health care industry. They must compete with the same intensity as their for-profit rivals without access to the same amounts of investment capital.

To augment their revenues, a variety of NFP health care organizations have two other popular strategic options. One is to expand into new business areas that are related to their primary health care mission and are selected mainly for their revenue-generating potential. Hospitals offer some good examples. There is the traditional gift shop, typically used by visitors to acquire items that they give to their relatives or friends or patients in the hospital. Other hospital-based related business ventures are on-site dining facilities for visitors (often fast-food chain outlets), parking garages for visitors, and luxury floors of single occupancy rooms for patients willing to pay for added amenities during their hospital stays.

The second option available to certain types of NFP health care organizations is to rent the organization's name and good reputation to a commercial product and a separate for-profit industry. The classic example is the endorsement in 1960 of Crest toothpaste by the American Dental

Association (ADA).[5] Toothpaste consumers had respect for what they considered to be the objective opinions of the ADA on dental health issues. When they saw the ADA name associated with Crest toothpaste, they were more inclined to purchase the product.

There is a legal restriction on the freedom of NFP organizations to take advantage of this "related business" revenue-generation strategy. In return for granting these organizations tax-exempt status, the Internal Revenue Service (IRS) insists that there be some close relation between the purpose of the new business activity and the charitable purpose of the organization that is the basis of that status. An NFP organization risks losing that status and the benefits that come with it if its new business ventures stray too far from its primary mission. The IRS also is likely to become more concerned when the proportion of organization revenues from those ventures gets too high, certainly when they exceed one-fifth of the total.

If an NFP health care organization engages in a significant amount of medical research, as do many medical school-related teaching hospitals, it is possible to enter into agreements with FP corporations that are in the business of commercializing biomedical discoveries. The corporations pay for the research conducted at the hospitals in return for a right to acquire or license the outcomes of the research.

When health care organizations share common missions or operate in overlapping markets, strategies of merger or partnership may be attractive. Through this process, the organizations can enjoy reduced costs (from economies of scope) and enhanced power in carrying out their missions (as a result of greater combined size). For instance, two NFP entities engaged in health promotion, education, or advocacy might find that they carry greater weight in advancing their related causes and sponsor more-ambitious related programs by pooling their resources. Sometimes, a merger/acquisition strategy is necessary for outright survival. Many hospitals discovered this during the shakeout of the hospital industry in the late 1980s and early 1990s. In any of these situations, a challenge for the leaders of the NFP organizations is to find ways to hang on to the visions that have motivated them for years. In some organizations, the allegiance to the founding purposes and current organizational culture are so strong that the managers prefer to go out of existence rather than compromise with a potential partner.

A last strategic resort for an NFP entity is to surrender its tax-exempt status and convert to FP corporate status. This is rather difficult for the organization to do entirely on its own, because tax law requires that its assets, acquired over many years of tax-exempt operation, be turned over to another tax-exempt entity with similar charitable purposes. The original entity is then left with virtually no resources to carry on business in FP or any other form. Normally, this strategy is carried out by an existing

FP corporation that pays money for an NFP organization, transfers a significant portion of its assets to another comparable NFP entity, but retains its name, brand image, goodwill, and customer base and continues operations on a profit-driven basis. This is a strategy that has been followed by Wellpoint Health Networks in acquiring and converting Blue Cross/Blue Shield plans in fourteen states.

■ PUBLIC/GOVERNMENT AGENCIES

In a few cases, public agencies may provide services to paying customers in competition with FP and NFP entities. Imagine a large metropolitan area with two or three FP hospitals, five or six NFP hospitals, and a single public city-owned hospital. Quite often the public hospital actively fights its image as a source of medical care primarily for low-income patients and markets itself to the same insured or self-pay customers sought by the other hospitals in town.

The role of politics and ideology in operational and strategic decision-making is usually greater in a public organization. The chief executive officer of the overall governmental structure, whether president, governor, or mayor, pretty much dictates to his or her subordinate secretaries and commissioners the strategic directions in which they will be allowed to steer their agencies. The rationale behind those directions is based to varying degrees on the political ideologies of those people in authority. Consider the different public sector versus private sector approaches to resolving the problems with the U.S. health care system.

The strong influence of political considerations, as manifested by politicians who may be in and out of office within a short period of years, makes long-term planning difficult. It is not uncommon for a new state governor to replace all existing cabinet secretaries, who in turn replace all their agency commissioners, who then cancel or redirect the strategic initiatives currently in process.

A public agency, whether a county hospital, municipal department of public health, or state Medicaid agency, can almost never enjoy the managerial freedom of an FP or even an NFP corporation. It is subject to the control of a larger political unit of which it is a part (state department of medical assistance within an executive office of human services), of the current governor of the executive branch of state government, of the current legislators whose laws authorize and constrain the agency while also providing all of its funding, and of the citizens who elect the legislators and governor and pay the taxes that are the ultimate source of its funding.

Like their FP counterparts, NFP organizations and public agencies are very much concerned with maintaining steady sources of revenue to ensure their survival. Because their sources are different, the strategies they adopt must have a different focus. To begin with, the beneficiaries or clients of their operations are frequently not the major source of their revenues.

Consider a municipal public agency that operates community health centers that provide basic health care services to low-income residents. As patients, the residents pay little or no money for the services they receive. The funding of the health centers comes from the city's general budget, as allocated by the city council. The city council also sets the tax rates that determine the amount of revenues flowing into the budget. The ultimate payers for the services delivered to the low-income patients are the tax-paying citizens and businesses of the city. The managers of the health centers will want to formulate strategies that both maximize the value provided to those patients and satisfy the interests of the city council members and the general public. Only if those external stakeholders are happy with the operations of the health center will they continue to fund them. It is not surprising that occasionally the interests of the recipients of the services do not coincide with the interests of the payers for the services. The strategies must take that into account.

An NFP organization that advocates for the rights of the mentally ill faces a different set of funding concerns. For its funding, it is likely to rely on donations from individuals, frequently relatives or friends of those suffering from mental illness, and grants from charitable foundations with a focus on such diseases. The immediate beneficiaries of the organization's efforts, mentally ill patients, are rarely a significant source of revenues.

A public agency's sources of revenue are probably more constrained than for any other type of organization. The funding of its operations and any strategic initiatives comes exclusively from tax revenues as determined and allocated by the relevant legislative body. It is given an annual budget that it must live within. If it charges fees to its clients for the services it provides, those revenues go into the general government fund, not to the agency itself. If a unique strategic opportunity or threat arises during the year to which the agency would like to respond, it will have no flexibility to obtain the additional funding that it might require.

The agency's service mandate will be defined by the law that authorizes it. It is normally required to provide its services to any member of the general population; there is no freedom to concentrate on a market niche.

It is important to distinguish between public agencies that are headed by elected officials or political appointees, and those with directors who are career civil servants. There is often turnover among the former at every election, making it difficult to maintain any sort of strategic continuity. In the latter situation, the top agency official is likely to be around for several years and, within certain political limits, able to formulate and carry out the completion of strategic plans.

Both public and NFP organizations benefit from a lack of scrutiny by shareholders expecting certain levels of return on their investments in the form of capital appreciation or dividend payouts. However, public agencies must anticipate complaints from citizens who feel that their tax dollars are not being well spent and from legislators who feel that their campaign promises are not being fulfilled. Not-for-profit organizations experience the least stakeholder pressure. However, donors and grantors dissatisfied with the organization's pursuit of its mission may, without a lot of fanfare, simply stop giving.

There is an interesting dynamic among agencies, particularly those in the health care field. On one hand, they clearly do compete with each other for shares of the total government budget. It is a painful zero-sum game that even well-intentioned politicians must play. To increase or even maintain the budget of one agency may require a decrease in another agency's budget. On the other hand, there is a trend toward cooperation among agencies in meeting the multifaceted needs of their clients. For instance, a Medicaid patient with recurrent health care problems may also require the services of agencies dealing with housing, job training, and developmental disabilities.

Adjustments/Adaptations to Basic Strategic Management Principles

Whereas the time horizon for strategic plans in the private sector (FP and NFP organizations) can stretch for five or ten years, the strategy decision makers in governmental agencies cannot plan with confidence beyond the term of the current administration. This does not mean that changes and initiatives of a strategic nature are impossible. It simply requires emphasizing efforts of somewhat narrower scope that can be accomplished within a shorter time frame.

Politics play a role in the strategic planning and management process in any organization, whether FP, NFP, or public sector. However, they are a much more dominant force in government agencies and must be given serious attention in any strategic thinking. In fact, developing or taking advantage of political forces favoring the agency may be the purpose of a strategic initiative.

In addition to the politicians concerned with an agency's operations, numerous other stakeholders must be attended to—more than most FP or NFP corporations have to worry about. The media and special-interest groups, for instance, watch the agency constantly, and are quick to notice and broadcast any failures or shortcomings. Staying on good terms with these entities is an essential strategic duty.

Most of the strategic options available to FP corporations are not feasible for government agencies. For one thing, there are so many constituencies and stakeholders to be satisfied that any genuine strategic decisions are reduced to the lowest common denominator, the least innovative and the least transformational.

Although there will not be much opportunity radically to redefine an agency's mission or mandate, it may be possible to expand its activities incrementally at the fringes of its current domain. Occasionally, a wave of revolutionary fervor sweeps through the executive and legislative branches of a particular governmental unit, most likely at the state or municipal levels. A consensus develops for reorganizing many parts of the governmental infrastructure, combining or eliminating existing agencies and creating new ones. Agency mandates are expanded or reduced. Through prior reflection on its optimal strategic role, an agency may be well positioned to influence such reorganization debates when they occur.

For strategic planning purposes, public sector agencies vary in two significant ways. Many of them have an effective monopoly on the kinds of work that they do. This is because they are engaged in functions that are reserved for government—regulation of private health care organizations and management of health issues that impact the general public, for example. Other government agencies do face competition from private-sector counterparts. This is true for most agencies engaged directly in the delivery of health care services. They are doing work performed by some private entities like health clinics or even hospitals; their clients often have a choice of visiting the public or private provider organization.

The second organizational variable is the agency's degree of managerial autonomy. In a common model, the agency is an element in a large government bureaucracy. Its leaders report to other leaders above them who eventually report to a governor or a mayor, all of whom are concerned with the political expediency of what their subordinate agencies are doing. However, a number of public-sector health care organizations are not as strongly influenced by political whim. Several large city governments own and operate their own tertiary care hospitals or hospital systems. The complexity of managing institutions like these places great value on continuity in their top management. Newly elected mayors of cities are wise enough to leave in place the CEOs of well-run hospitals. Executives in such public sector positions have greater freedom in their strategic decision-making.

Model Strategic Planning and Management Process

Because of their unique public nature, government agencies must employ a variant of the traditional strategic planning and management process.

1. Determine that the commissioner or director of the agency actively supports some form of strategic thinking and planning. Through that person, try to find out if his or her superior will at least tolerate a strategic planning effort by the agency and perhaps lend some influence to it.

2. Make a realistic assessment of the viable time horizon for any strategic decisions, as well as the range of activities that might be covered by those decisions. It also is a good idea at this point to establish what financial resources are available for dedication to strategic initiatives. In other words, are there any somewhat discretionary funds, above and beyond what is required for ongoing operations, that could be applied to special projects?
3. Perform an analysis of the receptivity of key external stakeholders to strategic initiatives by the agency. Look particularly at the likelihood of shifts in political mood in the local jurisdiction, as reflected in changes in the top leader (e.g., governor or mayor), the head of the agency itself, and legislators or council members who have shown an interest in the agency's mission. Notice also any trends in the policy concerns of special-interest groups and the general public. Describe several alternative scenarios for the future direction of support for the agency's programs.
4. Conduct a quick audit of the agency's core competencies, those tasks at which it is especially proficient and that could be exploited to build new programs. It may be worth also identifying critical areas in which the agency is weak if there are prospects for correcting those weaknesses.
5. Carry out an analysis of the agency's existing programs and activities, to see where improvements are possible and where there are gaps that could be filled by new programs. Some possibilities are offering new services to existing clients, offering existing services to new clients, serving clients in new geographic areas, and generally increasing the total number of clients served.
6. Any private sector competitors must be watched closely. The public agency will pay special attention to the strengths and weaknesses of each, their market positioning, and their apparent strategic initiatives. The agency must be prepared to respond to its rivals' strategies and expect them to respond to its own strategies.
7. Whether or not the agency has competition, it is a good idea to benchmark its activities against those of other organizations, in both the public and private sectors, that are providing similar products and services to similar markets. The goal is to identify and borrow the best practices of other comparable organizations.
8. These analytical tasks would benefit from the involvement of virtually the entire agency staff, plus clients, interested legislators, and special-interest groups as well. It is especially befitting an agency with a broad public mandate to include a wide range of constituencies in its decision-making.
9. On the basis of these audits and analyses, draw up a list of proposals for new and improved programs, as well as upgrades in the agency's

current competencies and organizational infrastructure. Fill out the proposals with information on their projected costs, their added benefits to various constituencies, their likely appeal to significant stakeholder groups, and their general political acceptability.

10. Choose for implementation one or two proposals that are a) most likely to win the support of political leaders above the agency's level as well as relevant legislators, and b) that when successful will reflect well on the leadership of those politicians and legislators. Give high priority to proposals that are likely to impress taxpayers with the foresight and efficiency of the agency.
11. Work diligently to implement the proposals and meet their objectives, demonstrating the agency's ability to perform at high levels and consistently improve its operations.

Examples of Strategies

The mandate of a government agency may be to meet certain health care needs of a defined population but, because of budgetary constraints, it has not had the resources to serve all the people who seek its services. One strategic decision might be to reengineer its operations in such a way that it can deliver services more efficiently, serving more people within its existing budget.

As it has served its existing client population, the agency may have discovered other related unmet needs in the same people. If those needs could be satisfied, the quality of life of the clients would be improved and their demand for the agency's existing services might actually decline. The agency could set out to expand the range of services that it offers, either by improving the skill sets of its existing employees or by seeking budget increases to support the hiring of new employees with new competencies.

As a matter of strategic choice, the agency may dedicate itself to currying the favor of influential politicians and legislators with a view toward seeking enactment of laws that would expand its mandate, increase its flexibility in structuring activities and managing resources, and augment its budget.

Develop and grow the competencies of the agency staff to meet the needs of its clients better. This strategy is part of a broader plan that involves selecting new services to offer or new clients to serve in ways that do not require significantly more staff or additional funding, but rather emphasizes expanding the skills of the current staff through training and selective hiring.

Negotiate strategic partnerships with other government agencies or NFP organizations for the purpose of taking an integrated, multidisciplinary approach to carrying out their respective missions and meeting the needs of their clients. There is a growing awareness that the health care problems people face often have multiple causes, which are being addressed by several different agencies. For instance, a program delivering health care services to low-income clients may find it useful to work closely with agencies responsible for public welfare, public housing, and juvenile justice.

Work to develop more amorphous strategic qualities of the agency, such as its dominant culture or its reputation with its clients or the general public. Efforts like these are less likely to be criticized, restricted, or prohibited by higher-level political leaders or legislators. They can usually be carried out without significant additional expenditure.

ENTREPRENEURIAL STARTUPS/NEW VENTURES

The organizational structure of new ventures tends to be simple—minimal overworked staff, shallow flat managerial hierarchy, cross-discipline sharing of tasks, informal communication of information, and few policies, procedures, or rules. Decision-making authority is concentrated in the founder/owner/CEO and everyone reports to that person.

In the early stages of a new venture, strategy formulation is conducted almost entirely by the founder/owner/CEO. It is not based on a lot of deep analysis, but rather is intuitive, reflecting the founder's personal experiences, values, and preferences. Although strategies in these kinds of organizations are intentional and explicit, they often take shape by fits and starts. The entrepreneur may start with a germ of an idea, talk to a few people about its market potential, discover one or two immediate problems or barriers, explore those further and find ways to resolve them, move to the next step of a strategy development, find and overcome additional complications, and proceed in this cumulative step-wise fashion until a distinct strategy emerges or the original idea is thoroughly discredited.

Entrepreneurial new ventures are aggressive and reckless. They engage in a constant search for new opportunities that will keep the firm alive. They try to avoid markets that would pit them in head-to-head competition with much larger established corporations. Their preference is for narrower market niches that are less populated by rivals but offer a less-certain flow of revenues and profits.

Conduct of the full and comprehensive strategic planning process described throughout this book would not make sense for a small entrepreneurial new venture or startup. The founder of such a venture rarely has the resources (including money and time) or expertise. In fact, to follow such an extended process at this stage could inhibit the spontaneity and adaptability to new circumstances that are a hallmark of successful new ventures. That does not mean that any form of strategic planning is inappropriate for a startup. The venture's choice of strategic direction must be the result of more than sheer guesswork.

New ventures are clearly more fragile than their larger, more established counterparts. They are highly sensitive to changes in their external environment. Because of their more limited resources, they have little room for error. Ironically, at a time when it may be hardest for them to practice rigorous strategic planning, new ventures need the insights that come from that planning simply to survive.

Smaller, newer businesses have less physical and psychological investment in their current products and practices, with the result that they may be more willing to give them up for something new and better and more competitive.

Adjustments/Adaptations to Basic Strategic Management Principles

When established FP corporations engage in strategic planning, their intention is to find new ways to leverage their existing internal strengths and weaknesses to respond to new opportunities and threats in the external environment. In contrast, a new venture is brought into existence by its very first strategic decision—the new product or service that it will offer, the unique market niche that it will target, or the new channels of distribution that it will employ. So, strategic planning of a very different sort occurs at three points in a startup's early life. There is the strategic planning, if it can be called that, that the founder does as he or she contemplates creating a new business. Then, there is the planning that is carried out after the venture has been established, with the purpose of propelling it into the future, ensuring its continued existence, and growing its revenues and profits. The defining strategic moment in a new venture's history is when it first seeks outside financing, whether from a bank, an angel investor, or a venture capital firm. As long as the founder is using his or her own money, the strategic plans can be sketchy or nonexistent. Outside capital sources want much more detailed information about the prospective risks and rewards that the venture offers. This will usually take the form of a document like a formal business plan. Much of the preparation, analysis, and projections that are part of a good business plan closely resemble the steps in a strategic planning process.

Until a business plan is requested or the venture otherwise grows to a size in which more rigorous strategic thinking makes sense, its strategic thought processes will be much less formal. Rather than go through all the strategic planning steps in the detail described throughout this book, it is more important that a venture's leaders give some serious attention to the issues raised at each of those steps. The rewards will come from the heightened awareness of the business's resources and competencies, the markets in which it is trying to compete, the rivals it is facing there, and the strategic direction it is pursuing. If that consciousness-raising occurs, it is much more likely that productive strategies will emerge. Indeed, this may be the first time that those leaders have acknowledged the strategic dimension of what they are trying to accomplish.

In the quick pass that a startup takes at strategic planning, it should not forget the role of functional area strategies. The various functional areas may not yet have taken clear shape. The managers of those areas may not understand instinctively the contribution they must make to the implementation of strategy.

The much smaller size and resource base of these organizations narrows the range of generic strategic options available to them. At the outset, and often for many years to come, the best choice will be a concentration growth strategy in a focused market segment. It would be extremely difficult for a business with 100 to 200 employees and modest revenues to pursue a low-cost leadership growth strategy across the full breadth of its market, going head-to-head with much larger competitors. A full market differentiation strategy would be only a little less challenging. Until its resources have expanded, the small organization is limited to a strategy that focuses on a smaller segment of the overall market. Within that narrower domain, after accumulating resources and experience in a concentration strategy, it might be able to move on to low-cost leadership, differentiation, or hybrid strategies.

The acquisition of other businesses, when it involves the expenditure of large amounts of capital, is out of the question for quite a few years. That includes vertical and horizontal integration strategies, as well as any attempts to diversify into unrelated markets or industries. However, a friendly legal merger of two corporations, without the exchange of funds, is quite possible. Even smaller organizations may overextend themselves, in which case some form of retrenchment (cost cutting, staff reductions, modest reorganization) is possible and may be necessary.

Model Strategic Planning and Management Process

Due to their more limited resources, entrepreneurial new ventures usually follow a more abbreviated form of the standard strategic planning and management process. This is a model process for a new venture that has been established for a year or two. It does not address whatever rudimentary strategic thinking the founders may have gone through when they first created the venture. In a biotech startup, for example, the creation may have been based upon a research breakthrough by the founder in his laboratory at a local medical school. Because of the founder's familiarity with the level of progress and interest in the biotechnology field in which he works, he had a strong intuitive sense that there was commercial potential in the breakthrough. Without a lot of further investigation or study, he formed a new venture. This model process also does not go as far as the level of strategic analysis and planning that will be required eventually by venture capitalists or other sources of investment capital.

1. The creation of an entrepreneurial new venture can take several routes, each with different requirements for strategic planning. As just mentioned, the founder may get started with an interesting new idea, capital drawn from his own savings and personal assets, and a lot of intuition. On the other hand, he may choose to prepare a business plan with strong strategic elements, either to attract other investors or because it makes good business sense. One of the ultimate goals of many entrepreneurs is an "initial public offering" (IPO), and a business cannot be brought to that point without some serious strategic thinking.
2. Conduct a good, solid SWOT analysis, with particular emphasis on the strengths and weaknesses in the business's resources and competencies. This analysis will be the guide for the product and market areas into which the business should move next. It almost certainly has demonstrated some specific, valuable research capabilities that can be employed to discover and develop new products. Perhaps the organization has found that it is quite effective in applied research but needs help to develop its discoveries into marketable products.

   Pay some attention to the opportunities and threats that face the organization. Again, the founder should have a general understanding of market and competitive developments in the business's field of concentration. It now is supplemented by knowledge and inputs from its employees and other stakeholders. Do some systematic data gathering on that field. Collect competitive intelligence on other firms that are developing similar or substitutable products.
3. A couple of basic decisions about overall strategic direction should be made at this point. One concerns the rate at which the business desires to grow. If it is an entrepreneur-driven organization, a commitment to aggressive growth is assumed. A decision to stabilize the growth of the business, its revenues and profits, around its initial product or service consigns it to the category of "small businesses." Placing it on a growth curve still leaves open the question of how steep the curve will be, how rapidly the venture will attempt to grow, and what risks it will take in the effort.
4. As it proceeds through the SWOT analysis, the business should rapidly generate a large number of potential strategic opportunities. They may not be well fleshed out or their potential validated. All that is required is some plausible basis for interest and further study.
5. The competitive strategies worthy of even preliminary consideration should be limited to concentration strategies or market-segment focus

strategies, either low-cost leadership, differentiation, or a hybrid of the two. Only these types of generic strategies are within the scope of a small new venture's resources and competencies.

6. A process of progressive screening and winnowing is performed on the list of opportunities. The most critical acceptance hurdles are dealt with first. For instance, because a biotech company is likely to be looking at new products to research, an initial question might be whether it has scientists with the requisite expertise to carry out such research. As each hurdle is addressed, the screening moves on to the next one (e.g., market size, compatibility with the company's current large pharmaceutical company partner). The process continues until the company satisfies itself that the proposed strategy meets all its strategic criteria and can be seriously considered for implementation, or it fails to pass a hurdle and is dropped from the list.
7. As the list is narrowed to a handful of more attractive strategy candidates, a fairly rigorous effort should be made to project the cash flows of each proposal and compare them to the capital that the business expects to have available. Launching a new strategy with insufficient working capital is one of the leading causes of ultimate failure.
8. In a process guided substantially by intuition and fragments of information about markets and competitors, one or more of the proposed strategies will be selected for implementation. If this is the first strategic initiative after the founding of the venture, its leaders should probably restrict themselves to pursuit of a single new strategy. It is unlikely that they have the managerial capacity to oversee the implementation of two or more strategies.
9. To guide implementation of the strategy toward success, the firm should set a modest number of measurable, time-based benchmarks or objectives. The point is to have some way of determining if the strategy is on course and ultimately fulfills the firm's long-range aspirations.
10. It would be nice if a moderately detailed implementation plan could be prepared. However, there may not be the time and resources for that. At the very least, ultimate responsibility and accountability for implementation, according to the previously set benchmarks, should be delegated to an authoritative individual in the organization. If that person is not the founder/owner, he should give his unequivocal support to the person chosen.
11. At some stage during the implementation, it may appear that the strategy is no longer viable—at least in its original configuration. Some kind of change or adjustment may seem called for. One of the advantages of being a small, risk-taking organization is the ability to make sudden shifts in direction, in response to either changing market

conditions or unanticipated moves by competitors. Such spontaneous action is constrained by the commitments of limited resources that the firm has made to the new strategy. It may be painful, perhaps even impossible, to drop one strategy and launch an entirely new one.

Examples of Strategies

Every entrepreneurial new venture worthy of the name is committed to growth, and to revenues and profits. A fundamental strategic decision is how rapidly it will attempt to grow. One choice is to take modest risks in order to grow at a relatively conservative rate. This might seem like a safe, if unambitious, course. In a market that is rapidly expanding or filled with aggressive competitors, however, a slow growth strategy will mean falling behind and losing out to rivals. It also may disappoint the firm's financial backers who are counting on rapid expansion to enable them to cash out their investments. At the other extreme, the managers of a new venture can accept much greater risks in the pursuit of much more dramatic growth. If the risks are mishandled, the business may fail. It is a frequent occurrence that ambitious new ventures overextend themselves and disappear. When the risks are judged correctly, the payoffs can be tremendous.

In a no- or slow-growth strategy, a business carries out no development of new products or entry into new markets. It concentrates on protecting its current share of the markets in which it operates primarily by reacting to initiatives by competitors. A biotech firm might try to increase the number of customers using its products in those markets or increase the rate of consumption by existing customers.

In a slightly more ambitious strategy, a business would continue to defend its existing market shares and simultaneously seek growth at the fringes of those markets. This might involve moving into adjacent geographic markets, employing new distribution channels in existing markets, and selling to market segments closely related to the ones currently served. For instance, a vendor of medical devices that is currently using a wholesale distributor to market its products to large physician group practices could decide to employ in-house salespeople to sell directly to smaller physician practices.

The first growth strategy likely to be considered by a new venture with an established product is expansion of sales of that product within current market segments. The most common tactics for achieving this will be advertising and promotion, sales and distribution, increased production capacity, and some tentative attempts at differentiation of the product.

Growing within an existing market can be a slow process, and the core competencies of a biotech research firm are likely to lie more in the areas of new product development than in marketing and sales. Its innovation abilities could be employed to create variations of the existing product that will appeal to new market segments. Further research on a pharmaceutical product could discover new disease treatment applications.

Eventually, an ambitious firm will want to deploy its innovation resources and competencies to the generation of entirely new products. Because those assets will be concentrated in narrow scientific research disciplines, any new work will take place on product concepts somewhat related to the products already developed. Efforts to discover new drugs will be in the same "family" as existing drugs and take advantage of the research knowledge already acquired.

A small research firm may find that it lacks the resources and competencies to move into desirable new markets and offer compelling new products. Entering into a joint venture with another firm possessing complementary resources and competencies is a good strategy for rapidly acquiring the necessary assets. A good example was the announcement in the summer of 2007 of the formation of a joint venture, to be located in India, between a German firm, Evotec AG, and an Indian firm, Research Support International Ltd. (RSIL), to design, synthesize, and manage drug compound libraries for other drug companies. The joint venture was felt to make sense because it would "combine Evotec's expertise in library design, synthesis, analysis, purification and project management with RSIL's first-class scientists coupled with a low cost structure in India to provide a high quality, cost-efficient solution for the provision and management of compound libraries to the pharmaceutical industry."[6]

Study Questions

1. What benefits do the presence of for-profit corporations bring to the health care industry? Would the industry be better off if it was composed primarily of not-for-profit and public entities, as it was thirty years ago?
2. During the first year or two of its existence, what reasons are there for a biotech startup to engage in any sort of strategic planning? This is a time when the venture's resources are stretched to the limit and all its attention is focused on bringing its first product to market. Are there any disadvantages for the firm if it fails to think about long-term strategy?
3. Review the reasons why it is hard for public agencies to practice strategic planning. As a citizen whose interests those agencies are meant to represent, what changes in government principles and practices would you be willing to accept so that they could take a longer-range perspective?

Learning Exercise 1

You are the CEO of a biotech research company. Since startup three years ago, you and a staff of five highly qualified researchers have developed a new drug that shows great promise in combating resistant strains of malaria. The intellectual property rights to the drug have been licensed to a large pharmaceutical company. Under the licensing agreement, your firm will receive an upfront payment of $5 million plus a minimum of $1 million a year for the next ten years or a share of the pharmaceutical company's revenues from the drug, whichever is greater.

Since starting this company you have discovered that you have rather good managerial skills and a hunger for building and growing new businesses. Bearing in mind the resources that are currently available to your company, what are your strategic options at this point? What are the strengths and weaknesses of your organization? Think in terms of new products, new markets, and potential strategic partners. Consider also what new resources and competencies you might wish to develop.

Learning Exercise 2

Contact and arrange an interview (in person or by phone) with one of the following people: the head of a local state or municipal health-related government agency, a state legislator or city counselor with a special interest in health-related issues, or the head of a local NFP organization that provides health-related services to its clients. Use the interview to obtain answers to the following questions:

1. Do you or does your organization carry out any sort of long-range/strategic thinking or planning about the health care issues that you deal with? (Be prepared to explain to the interviewee the meaning of "strategic thinking" and "strategic planning.")
2. Would you be willing to tolerate or actively support a strategic planning process, as well as specific strategic plans that might result, in your government agency or NFP organization?
3. To what extent does such strategic planning take place now? What are the specific reasons that your government agency or NFP organization does not do more strategic thinking and planning?
4. To what extent are there funds available in the budget of your agency or organization to pay for strategic projects, in contrast with ongoing operations?
5. Can you briefly describe the strengths and weaknesses of your agency or organization? Think in terms of resources that you

possess or competencies that your people are able to apply to their work.

6. Does your agency or organization have competitors? Do you face any sort of competition for the financial or other resources, employees or volunteers, and customers or clients that are essential to your operations?
7. Do you ever worry about the long-term survival of your agency or organization? What threats does it face to its continued operation and existence? What steps could you take to reduce the effect of those threats?

During the interview, ask any other questions that will help you get a sense of whether the organization engages in any sort of strategic decision-making, and if it does not, why not and what would it take in order for even rudimentary strategic planning to occur?

Learning Exercise 3

Select an NFP organization or government agency that deals with a relatively narrow and specific set of health care issues, whether through service delivery, consumer advocacy, education/promotion, financing, or regulation. Look for an entity for which there is abundant information about the nature of its operations. Define a set of strategic performance measures for the entity. These should be metrics that are as objective and measurable as possible. It is preferable that they be quantitative, but do not try to quantify something that is truly subjective. By tracking these measures, the organization or agency should be able to determine whether it is making progress toward achievement of its strategic mission. If it helps, imagine that you are the head of the entity and will be using these metrics to determine how well you are doing and to persuade your funding sources to continue supporting your work.

Notes

[1] P.F. Drucker, "What Business Can Learn from Nonprofits," Harvard Business Review (July–August 1989), p. 89.

[2] "Health, United States, 2006," Table 112, National Center for Health Statistics.

[3] From Gray BH and M Schlesinger. Health. In: Salamon L, ed. *The State of the Nonprofit Sector*. Washington, D.C.: Brookings Institution Press; 2002;65–106.

[4] For the purposes of this book, these terms have the following meanings. "Bioscience" includes branches of the natural sciences dealing with the structure and behavior of living organisms. "Biomedical science" is that area of general medical science that studies the biological and physiological principles inherent in the clinical practice of medicine. The concept of "biotechnology" encompasses the use of cell and tissue culture, cell fusion, molecular

biology, and recombinant DNA to develop unique organisms on which clinical medical products can be based. Some of the specific fields included within biotechnology are bacteriology, biochemical engineering, bioinformatics, bioprocessing, cell biology, developmental and molecular genetics, embryology, immunology, microbiology, protein engineering, and virology.

[5] "How Crest Made Business History," HBS Working Knowledge, January 17, 2005, http://hbswk.hbs.edu/archive/4574.html. Accessed July 31, 2007.

[6] Bio Screening Industry News, July 16, 2007, reporting a press release by these two companies on July 11, 2007 simultaneously in Hamburg, Germany and Oxford, England, found at http://www.bioscreening.net/2007/07/16/evotec-and-research-support-international-limited-announce-the-formation-of-evotec-rsil-ltd-a-joint-venture-for-the-design-synthesis-management-and-commercialisation-of-compound-libraries/

References

Allison M and Kaye J. *Strategic Planning for Nonprofit Organizations.* 2nd ed. NewYork, NY: John Wiley & Sons; 2005.

Brouthers KD, Andriessen F, and Nicolaes I. Driving blind: Strategic decision-making in small companies. *Long Range Planning.* 1998(31):130–138.

Bryce HJ. *Financial and Strategic Management for Nonprofit Organizations.* Upper Saddle River, NJ: Prentice Hall; 1987.

Bryson JM. *Strategic Planning for Public and Nonprofit Organizations.* 3rd ed. San Francisco, CA: Jossey-Bass; 2004.

Chen M and Hambrick DC. Speed, stealth, and selective attack: How small firms differ from large firms and competitive behavior. *Academy of Management Journal.* 1995(38):453–482.

Deber RB. 2002. Delivering health care services: Public, not-for-profit, or private? Commission on the Future of Health Care in Canada, Discussion Paper No. 17, August.

Horowitz JR. MARKETWATCH: Making profits and providing care: Comparing nonprofit, for-profit, and government hospitals. *Health Affairs*; May/June 2005:790–801.

Ireland RD, Hitt MA, Camp SM, and Sexton DL. Integrating entrepreneurship and strategic management actions to create firm wealth. *Academy of Management Executive.* 2001;15(1):49–63.

Reeves TC and Ford EW. Strategic management and performance differences: Nonprofit versus for-profit health organizations. *Health Care Management Review.* 2004;29(4):298–308.

Scheslinger M and Gray BH. How nonprofits matter in American medicine, and what to do about it. Health Affairs, Web exclusive, June 20, 2006. http://www.healthaffairs.org/WebExclusives.php

Smeltzer LR, Fann GL, and Nikolaisen VL. Environmental scanning practices in small business. *Journal of Small Business Management.* 1988;26(3):55–63.

Teece DJ. Profiting from technological innovations: Implications for integration, collaboration, licensing, and public policy. In: *The Competitive Challenge: Strategies for Industrial Innovations and Renewal.* New York, NY: Ballenger; 1987.

INDEX

H

I

N

Q

R

S

T

U

V

W